INSTRUCTOR RESOURCES FOR SUCCESS

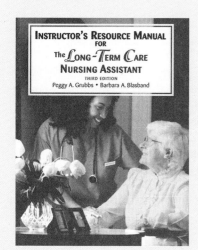

INSTRUCTOR'S RESOURCE MANUAL
FOR
The LONG-TERM CARE
NURSING ASSISTANT
THIRD EDITION
Peggy A. Grubbs • Barbara A. Blasband

Instructor's Resource Manual
ISBN: 0-13-118023-1

This manual contains a wealth of material to help faculty plan and manage the long-term care nursing assisting course. It includes learning objectives, detailed lecture suggestions, quizzes, a final exam, suggestions for classroom experiences, and more for each chapter.

Instructor's Resource CD-ROM
ISBN: 0-13-118026-6

This cross-platform CD-ROM includes an electronic version of the Instructor's Resource Manual, an electronic test bank with Competency Exam-style Multiple Choice Questions, PowerPoint slides with images and lecture suggestions, and a transition guide for a smooth changeover to the new edition. This supplement is available to faculty *free* upon adoption of the textbook.

Companion Website Syllabus Manager
www.prenhall.com/grubbs

Faculty adopting this textbook have *free* access to the online **Syllabus Manager** feature of the Companion Website, www.prenhall.com/grubbs. Syllabus Manager offers a whole host of features that facilitate the students' use of the Companion Website, and allow faculty to post syllabi and course information online for their students. For more information or a demonstration of Syllabus Manager, please contact a Prentice Hall Sales Representative.

BRIEF CONTENTS

The Long-Term Care Nursing Assistant

THIRD EDITION

Peggy A. Grubbs, RN, BSN

Nurse Consultant, Venice, Florida

Barbara A. Blasband, RN, BA

Health Occupations Instructor
Health Science Department
Hillsborough County Schools
Tampa, Florida

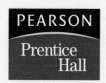

PEARSON

Prentice
Hall

Upper Saddle River, New Jersey 07458

Library of Congress Cataloging-in-Publication Data
Grubbs, Peggy A.
    The long-term care nursing assistant / Peggy A.
Grubbs, Barbara A. Blasband.—3rd ed.
      p. ; cm.
Includes bibliographical references and index.
ISBN 0-13-118022-3
    1.   Long-term care of the sick. 2.   Nurses' aides.
    3. Nursing home care.
      [DNLM: 1.   Long-Term Care—methods. 2.   Nurses' Aides.
    3. Nursing Care—methods.
      WY 152 G855L 2005] I. Blasband, Barbara A. II. Title.

RT120.L64G78 2005
610.73′6—dc22
                                                    2004011159

Publisher: *Julie Levin Alexander*
Assistant to the Publisher: *Regina Bruno*
Editor-in-Chief: *Maura Connor*
Executive Editor: *Barbara Krawiec*
Managing Development Editor: *Marilyn Meserve*
Development Editor: *Maureen Muncaster*
Editorial Assistant: *Jennifer Dwyer*
Director of Production & Manufacturing: *Bruce Johnson*
Managing Production Editor: *Patrick Walsh*
Production Liaison: *Mary C. Treacy*
Production Editor: *Karen Ettinger, The GTS Companies/ York, PA Campus*
Manufacturing Manager: *Ilene Sanford*
Manufacturing Buyer: *Pat Brown*
Design Director: *Cheryl Asherman*
Senior Design Coordinator: *Maria Guglielmo Walsh*
Manager of Media Production: *Amy Peltier*
Senior Media Editor: *John J. Jordan*
New Media Product Manager: *Stephen Hartner*
Media Development Editor: *Sheba Jalaluddin*
Senior Marketing Manager: *Nicole Benson*
Marketing Assistant: *Janet Ryerson*
Channel Marketing Manager: *Rachele Strober*
Composition: *The GTS Companies/York, PA Campus*
Cover Printer: *Lehigh Press*
Printer/Binder: *Von Hoffmann Press*

Pearson Education LTD.
Pearson Education Singapore, Pte. Ltd
Pearson Education, Canada, Ltd
Pearson Education—Japan

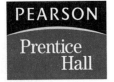

Pearson Education Australia PTY, Limited
Pearson Education North Asia Ltd
Pearson Educación de Mexico, S.A. de C.V.
Pearson Education Malaysia, Pte. Ltd
Pearson Education, Upper Saddle River, New Jersey

10 9 8 7 6 5 4 3 2 1
ISBN 0-13-118022-3

---

*D*edication

We would like to dedicate this edition to
Barbara Krawiec, Acquisitions Editor,
Prentice Hall/Pearson Education. We have
always been able to rely on her expertise and
guidance throughout the years.

NOTICE

The procedures described in this textbook are based on
consultation with nursing authorities. The author and
publisher have taken care to make certain that these
procedures reflect currently accepted clinical practice;
however, they cannot be considered absolute recommendations.

The material in this textbook contains the most current
information available at the time of publication. However,
federal, state and local guidelines concerning clinical
practices, including without limitation, those governing
infection control and standard precautions, change
rapidly. The reader should note, therefore, that new
regulations may require changes in some procedures.

It is the responsibility of the reader to familiarize himself or herself with the policies and procedures set by
federal, state and local agencies as well as the institution
or agency where the reader is employed. The authors
and the publishers of this textbook, and the supplements written to accompany it, disclaim any liability,
loss or risk resulting directly or indirectly from the suggested procedures and theory, from any undetected errors, or from the reader's misunderstanding of the text.
It is the reader's responsibility to stay informed of any
new changes or recommendations made by any federal,
state and local agency as well as by his or her employing
health care institution or agency.

In Memoriam

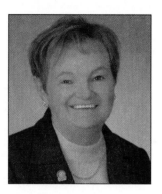

With gratitude for her many contributions as a distinguished Prentice Hall author, and with a profound sense of sorrow for her untimely passing, the Prentice Hall Health publishing team humbly share some reflections of Peggy A. Grubbs. Peggy has been part of our publishing family for the past ten years and her sudden death during the final production stages of this edition has saddended us greatly.

All who worked with Peggy remember her as a highly competent professional who worked tirelessly to meet the high standards of excellence she set for herself and for everyone associated with her projects. A no-nonsense woman of measured words and determined action, who held firmly to her convictions, Peggy was a model author. Her thoroughly meticulous work was always delivered with her distinctively no-fuss flair, on time or ahead of schedule.

It always seemed to us that what drove Peggy's unparalelled conscientiousness was that she wrote every word in her books as if to one nursing assistant at a time, mentoring each one, sharing the very best of what she had done and learned as a nurse and an educator, across a wide range of clinical and academic experiences. Anyone who reads *The Long-Term Care Nursing Assistant* or *Essentials for Today's Nursing Assistant* will recognize what a labor of love they were for Peggy, who still enjoyed pressing pencil to paper before composing on the computer. A true champion of the nursing assistants she taught and an advocate for the holistic care of their patients, Peggy was actively engaged in work on this book, even up to a few hours before she died.

Totally down-to-earth and unpretentious, Peggy A. Grubbs and co-author Barbara A. Blasband have been true pioneers in nursing assisting education. Grubbs and Blasband was the first author team to provide nursing assisting students with a textbook—*this same textbook that you hold in hand*—that focuses on a humanistic, restorative approach to caring for their patients.

Grubbs and Blasband's humanistic, restorative approach empowers and invites nursing assistants to give the best of themselves to caring for their patients in a way that is individually affirming, practical, and caring, without being sentimental. Peggy was like that herself: affirming, practical, and caring, without being sentimental. A wonderful nurse, educator, mother, grandmother, author, and friend, she will be missed by all who were influenced by the gift of herself that she shared generously in a style that was uniquely Peggy.

Peggy's graced wish for each nursing assistant student is an interesting, enjoyable nursing journey. For the next generation of nurses that begin their careers where Peggy left off, that is our wish as well.

We reserve the final sharing of thoughts to Peggy's dear long-time confidante, colleague, and collaborator: co-author Barbara Blasband.

The pages of this text are filled with Peggy's influence and the team spirit that existed between us as co-author. The book is an ongoing testimony to the excellence with which Peggy Grubbs lived her life. She was, although tiny in stature, an assertive woman who maintained a high level of motivation as she lived stoically through difficult and pain-filled days. Writing with her, although labor intensive, was fun and I will miss the satisfaction, balance, and teamwork that permeated the many years of our friendship.
Barbara Blasband

Guidelines

Important principles of care are highlighted throughout the text to guide your care for residents.

Procedures

When performing procedures, it's important to do every step correctly. That's why you'll find brightly colored procedure boxes throughout that clearly outline each procedure, from beginning to end, step by step, so you are sure to get it right every time.

Beginning Steps and Ending Steps

Directions for how to start and to conclude a procedure are included within each procedure box, so you have everything you need to know explained in one place.

Illustrations

Photographs and art show you key steps of the procedures.

---

120   Unit 3:   Basic Skills

Decreased activity may slow digestion. When this happens, the large intestine absorbs too much water from the stool, which becomes dry and hard. **Constipation** is the passage of hard, dry stool. One complication of constipation is a **fecal impaction** (a large amount of hard, dry stool). When constipation is not relieved, an impaction can fill the rectum. The impaction must be removed before the person can have a normal bowel movement. Nursing assistants do not remove impactions.

Inactivity causes circulation to slow down and become sluggish. When blood flow to the **extremities** (the arms and legs) slows, fluid collects in the tissues. This accumulation of fluid causes swelling and is called **edema**. Poor circulation is the major factor contributing to blood clots. It also plays a role in the development of pneumonia, urinary tract infections, and kidney stones.

Hypostatic pneumonia is a type of pneumonia that occurs when a person remains too long in one position. Gravity causes blood and other fluids to pool in one part of the lung, where infection can easily occur.

Limited activity can affect the resident's mental and emotional status. The lack of stimulation, combined with slowed circulation, may cause the resident to become **disoriented** (confused as to person, place, or time). Inactive people easily can become depressed. They may feel helpless and without hope. An active life is a healthy life. Inactivity damages the body and dulls the spirit.

RESTORATIVE TECHNIQUES

Restorative nursing care can prevent most of the complications of limited activity. Assisting the resident to move and exercise will give you many opportunities to use restorative techniques. Always encourage the resident to do as much as possible. This promotes the resident's mobility and increases body strength. It also helps to build his or her independence and self-esteem.

Remember the principles of restorative care that were described in Chapter 4 of this text:

* Treat the whole person.
* Start rehabilitation early.
* Stress ability—not disability.
* Encourage activity.
* Maintain a restorative attitude.

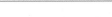

GUIDELINES

RESTORATIVE ACTIVITY TECHNIQUES

* Follow the principles of restorative care.
* Determine the resident's abilities and disabilities.
* Be aware of the resident's sense of balance.
* Know what special equipment will be needed.
* Be aware of the resident's motivation and ability to follow directions.
* Keep directions simple and consistent.
* Allow time for independent self-care.
* Watch for signs of fatigue or frustration.
* Use praise and encouragement frequently (see Figure 11-2 ■).
* Emphasize the positive and focus on success.

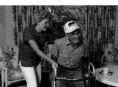

FIGURE 11-2 ■ Praise and encouragement are great motivators.

Chapter 11:   Moving and Exercising Residents   **125**

■ Ending Steps
To complete the procedure, perform the following steps:

Make the resident comfortable, positioning in good body alignment. Make the resident safe, placing the call signal within reach, lowering the bed, and raising the side rails, if appropriate. Wash your hands. Record and report the procedure as required.

PROCEDURE

Moving the Resident Up in Bed with a Lift Sheet

■ Beginning Steps
Before any procedure, you always must follow the five basic steps: wash your hands, collect the equipment, identify the resident, explain the procedure, and protect privacy.

Follow Standard Precautions

1. Arrange for a coworker to help you.
2. Raise the bed to a comfortable working height and lock the wheels.
3. Adjust the bed to as flat a position as possible.
4. Lower the side rail on your working side. Your assistant on the other side will do the same.
5. Place the pillow against the headboard.
6. Facing the head of the bed, stand with your feet apart (one in front of the other), bend your knees, and keep your back straight.
7. Roll the lift sheet close to the side of the resident's body (see Figure 11-8 ■) and straighten the linens.
8. Grasp the lift sheet with one hand at the resident's shoulder and the other hand at hip level.
9. On the count of "3" shift your weight from one foot to the other as you and your assistant move the resident up in bed.
10. Replace the pillow, unroll the lift sheet.

FIGURE 11-8 ■ Roll the lift sheet close to the sides of the resident's body when moving her up in bed.

■ Ending Steps
To complete the procedure, perform the following steps:

Make the resident comfortable, positioning in good body alignment. Make the resident safe, placing the call signal within reach, lowering the bed, and raising the side rails, if appropriate. Wash your hands. Record and report the procedure as required.

Moving a Resident Up in Bed With a Lift Sheet

Some residents, such as those who are helpless, critically ill, or comatose, will not be able to help move themselves up in bed. The easiest way to assist them is with a lift sheet (draw sheet). This procedure requires two people, one on either side of the bed (see Figure 11-8). A lift sheet supports body alignment and protects the resident's skin from friction. Lower the bed as flat as possible to make the procedure easier.

Moving the Resident to the Side of the Bed

It may be necessary to move the resident to one side of the bed when turning. The resident also will need to be moved to the side of the bed when being assisted to get up. Move the

Competency Exam Preparation

A variety of exercises are designed to expand your understanding of chapter material and help you prepare for the state certification exam. These exercises include vocabulary review, as well as multiple choice questions.

Communication Central

Tips and activities related to the content of each chapter help you develop the communication skills essential to delivering quality care.

www.prenhall.com/grubbs, a free website, provides chapter-specific on-line resources for students and educators!

Objectives—present the learning outcomes

Chapter Outline—provides the chapter-specific content outline for student reference

Audio Glossary—provides key terms, definitions, and correct pronunciations

Certification Exam-style Review Questions—provide practice and immediate feedback for exam-style questions

Case Study—provides a brief client scenario followed by critical thinking questions

Study Tip—provides helpful suggestions for learning challenging skills and concepts

Toolbox—provides additional handy reference material

Web Links—present hyperlinks

Faculty Office—provides lecture notes for your convenience

Syllabus Manager—allows faculty and students the convenience of creating and easily updating an electronic syllabus

---

CHAPTER 2   COMPETENCY EXAM PREPARATION

VOCABULARY REVIEW

Fill in the blank with the vocabulary term that best completes the sentence.

1. Understanding how another person feels is _____.

2. _____ is the opinion one has of oneself.

3. _____ are activities of personal care and hygiene performed daily.

4. Mental and physical tension or strain is _____.

5. _____ means rating each task in its order of importance.

6. A/an _____ lists the steps to be taken in performing a task.

7. Activities performed for health and cleanliness are _____.

8. _____ is the ability to accept change.

9. Temperature, pulse, respiration, and blood pressure are _____.

10. Nursing care that assists each resident to function at the highest possible level of indendence is _____.

CHECK YOUR UNDERSTANDING

The following questions cover the highlights of this chapter. Choose the best answer for each question.

1. Who supervises the work of a nursing assistant?
   A. the resident's family
   B. the doctor
   C. the nurse
   D. another nursing assistant

2. ADLs include which of the following?
   A. shopping
   B. personal hygiene
   C. driving
   D. getting a job

3. Providing restorative care is best accomplished by
   A. encouraging independence
   B. discouraging independence
   C. doing everything for the resident
   D. making the resident do everything

4. Which of the following is *not* a desirable quality for a nursing assistant?
   A. dependability
   B. flexibility
   C. empathy
   D. impatience

5. Which of the following is the most important reason for working together?
   A. to protect resident safety
   B. to finish as early as possible
   C. to have time for fun
   D. to please the charge nurse

6. Which of the following is a nursing assistant's responsibility?
   A. Give medications
   B. Measure vital signs
   C. Discontinue an IV
   D. Suction a resident

COMMUNICATION CENTRAL

AGE-SPECIFIC TIP

Long-term care facilities care for residents of all age groups. Consider the resident's age when communicating.

CULTURALLY SENSITIVE TIP

Cultural diversity challenges the staff of the long-term care facility to provide for a variety of resident choices. Always encourage residents to make choices by asking them what they prefer in every possible situation.

EFFECTIVE PROBLEM SOLVING

The nursing assistant notices that the bathroom in Room 202 is still dirty after the housekeeper finished cleaning. The nursing assistant says to the head of the housekeeping department, "The housekeeper who cleaned Room 202 doesn't know what she's doing."

Was the nursing assistant's communication appropriate? If not, what would have been more appropriate?

INTERPERSONAL COMMUNICATION

Fill in the answers.

You are angry with one of your coworkers because he refuses to help you move a heavy resident. You should take the problem to _____.

OBSERVING, REPORTING, AND RECORDING

You want to become a nursing assistant. List the requirements that you must fulfill in order to become employable.

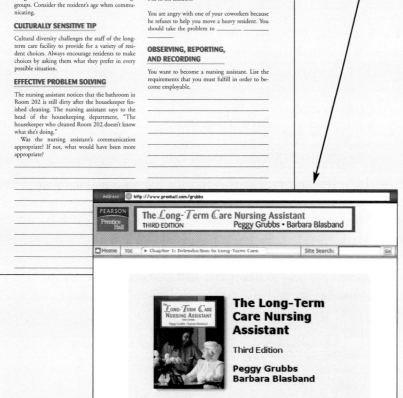

Address: http://www.prenhall.com/grubbs

PEARSON Prentice Hall

The Long-Term Care Nursing Assistant
THIRD EDITION   Peggy Grubbs • Barbara Blasband

Home | TOC | ▶ Chapter 1: Introduction to Long-Term Care | Site Search: | Go!

The Long-Term Care Nursing Assistant

Third Edition

Peggy Grubbs
Barbara Blasband

ABOUT THE AUTHORS

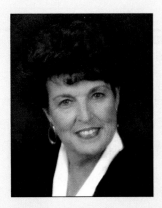

Barbara Blasband, RN, BA has 38 years of nursing experience, ranging from ICU and CCU to office nursing. She began her career in geriatrics and long-term care in 1976, when she became the staff development coordinator of a 120-bed long-term care facility. She was responsible for curriculum development, preservice training, and continuing education of the facility's health care team. In 1982, Barbara played a key role in the development of original curriculum used in Florida for preparing nursing assistants for state certification. She has been employed since 1983 as an instructor in the Health Science Department of Learey Technical Center, Hillsborough County School District in Tampa, Florida. Currently in her instructional position at Learey, Barbara teaches nursing assistant courses and provides in-service and continuing education for long-term care employees throughout Hillsborough County, Florida. In addition to coauthoring *The Long-Term Care Nursing Assistant,* Barbara authored the workbook that is a supplement to the Prentice Hall Health textbook *Essentials for Today's Nursing Assistant.*

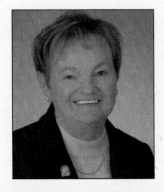

Peggy Grubbs, RN, BSN had nursing experience that included emergency room, pediatrics, medical-surgical, and supervisory roles in the hospital setting. She worked for 10 years in home health and was an administrator of a home health agency during that time. She served for several years on the board of directors of the Nurses Professional Registry in Tampa, Florida. She worked in hospice for 4 years, serving as a field nurse and as a patient care coordinator. She also did bereavement counseling, public relations, and teaching for hospice. Peggy worked as an instructor for Hillsborough County School District in Tampa, Florida, for 12 years. During her tenure with the school system she developed curriculum at the district level for the nursing assistant, the home health aide, and patient care assistant programs. She also participated in the development of the Florida Core Curriculum for Health Care and the Florida State Test Bank for CNA, HHA, and PCA. Peggy was a member of the ANA and the FNA. She served on the Board of Directors for FNA. District 4. In addition to coauthoring *The Long-Term Care Nursing Assistant,* Peggy published articles in nursing journals and had authored the Prentice Hall Health textbook *Essentials for Today's Nursing Assistant.* She had also written policy-and-procedure manuals for an assisted-living facility.

PREFACE

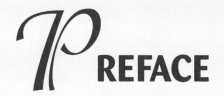

The third edition of *The Long-Term Care Nursing Assistant* is a modern, true-to-life textbook for today's nursing assistant students. It is designed to reflect changes in both the health care delivery system and the role of nursing assistants. It addresses new health care issues such as bioterrorism, anthrax, and workplace violence. Health care problems of recent emphasis such as end-of-life issues and reduction of medical errors are included, as well as the most current information available on infection control, safety, and emergency measures.

The third edition continues to focus on the restorative approach that has improved the quality of life for health care patients across the country. It places increased emphasis on cultural awareness and age-specific nursing to meet the individual needs of an increasingly diverse population. Communication will continue to be woven throughout the text. The Communication Central feature at the end of each chapter will be repeated in this edition. In response to recent trends and legislation, a separate chapter has been created on Alzheimer's disease and related disorders.

The third edition of *The Long-Term Care Nursing Assistant* follows the same format as the first two editions with a clean, colorful look that is refreshing and enjoyable. A simple, down-to-earth writing style makes it easy to read and understand. Each chapter opens with a list of specific, measurable objectives and vocabulary terms. End-of-chapter components include interactive communication exercises and activities to help students review and prepare for state competency exams.

The content of *The Long-Term Care Nursing Assistant* has been reorganized to meet the requests of nursing assistant training programs, educators, and students. Basic skills chapters have been moved closer to the front of the text. Additional guidelines have been included in an effort to decrease the amount of text while enhancing student understanding. These changes are reflected in the Contents.

Special Features

Easy Reading
A writing style that encourages the student to relate personally to the material. Detailed information is presented in a manner that makes reading enjoyable for students at various reading levels.

Objectives
Specific measurable objectives that are easily referenced in headings and subheadings.

Vocabulary Terms
A word list of key terms that are highlighted, defined in the text, and reviewed at the end of each chapter.

OBRA
Meets OBRA guidelines and accommodates state curricula.

Guidelines
Guidelines that contain the basic principles of care are presented in a concise, simple manner.

Procedures
Easy-to-follow procedures are well illustrated with line drawings.

Chapter Highlights
Chapter highlight contains a list of the most important information in each chapter.

Competency Exam Preparation
All end-of-chapter components provide questions and activities that will help students prepare for the state competency exam through the use of

vocabulary review, questions to stimulate critical thinking, and multiple-choice questions.

Vocabulary review
Questions encourage students to learn key medical terms.

Multiple-choice questions
Check the students' understanding of the chapter and improve test-taking skills.

Age-specific tips
Emphasize age-specific care and point out factors that need to be taken into account when performing a task or skill.

Culturally sensitive tips
Provide a tip that is culturally specific to the content of the chapter.

Effective problem solving
Helps students expand their understading by applying critical-thinking skills to real-world scenarios.

Interpersonal communication
Uses multiple types of questions to test the students' understanding of the chapter material.

Observing, reporting, and recording exercises
Ask the student to list specific items that should be reported and/or stimulate critical thinking by presenting a situation and asking "What would you do?"

Survey Process Reference Section
This section provides practical information to help nursing assistants understand the importance of the survey process in assuring quality care. It includes guidelines for performing confidently and competently in all types of resident care.

Glossary
The glossary contains key terms and their meanings.

Anatomy and Physiology Reference Section
This section stresses the interrelationship of the systems.

Index
Referenced and cross-referenced for easy location of topics.

Highlights of the Third Edition

- A separate chapter on the care of residents with Alzheimer's disease and related disorders.
- Continued emphasis on the importance of communication throughout the text.
- Addition of pertinent information on bioterrorism and anthrax.
- Addition of the prevention of medical errors in response to public and industry concerns.
- Addition of workplace violence.
- Increased emphasis on end-of-life issues.
- Current, updated information on infection control, safety, emergency procedures, HIV infection, hepatitis, tuberculosis, and Alzheimer's disease.
- Continued focus on restorative nursing and improving the patient's quality of life.
- Reorganization of content to move basic skills closer to the front of the book.
- A clear, simple writing style that meets the needs of students at various reading levels.
- Clear, step-by-step, simple procedures.
- Colorful photographs and clear line drawings to illustrate and clarify content and procedures.
- Guidelines and procedures boxed for easy identification. Guidelines present a simple, clear approach and are easy to read and understand.
- Addition of new guidelines and procedures.
- Continued emphasis on Competency Exam Preparation.
- Vocabulary reviews replace case studies in the end-of-chapter exercises.

Chapters New to This Edition

Chapter 24: Alzheimer's Disease and Related Disorders
Material has been reorganized so that techniques for caring for residents who are confused, aggressive, or depressed are grouped together. Many states have laws requiring that health care workers have specific training in caring for patients with Alzheimer's disease. This chapter will provide the information that is required for that training.

*P*rocedures New to This Edition

Admitting a Resident

Transferring a Resident

Discharging a Resident

Applying Elastic Support Hose

*G*uidelines New to This Edition

Staying Healthy

Personal Hygiene and Appearance

Prevent Medical Errors

Aid Victims of Domestic Violence

Protection against Workplace Violence

Protect Residents from Abuse

Handling Sharps

Transmission-Based Precautions

A Restorative Approach to Isolation

Terrorism Preparedness

Handling Emergencies

Recognizing Life-Threatening Conditions

Recognizing and Preventing Shock

Caring for the Resident with an Airway Obstruction

Caring for the Resident Who is Hemorrhaging

Emergency Care of a Resident Who is Suspected of Having a Stroke

Caring for the Resident Who is Experiencing a Seizure

Maintaining a Restorative Environment

The Care and Use of Equipment

A Restorative Approach to Bedmaking

Restorative Activity Techniques

Using a Mechanical Lift

Using a Wheelchair

Using a Stretcher

Assisting a Resident to Ambulate

Assisting the Resident with a Walker

Range-of-Motion Exercises

Providing Foot Care

Assisting and Providing Oral Hygiene

Providing Denture Care

Assisting with a Shower or Tub Bath

Assisting the Resident to Dress

Care and Use of Electronic Thermometers

Care and Use of a Glass Thermometer

Assisting the Resident in the Dining Room

Assisting Residents to Eat in Their Rooms

Care of the Resident with Edema

Preventing Dehydration

Measuring Fluid Intake

Measuring Urinary Output

Assisting with Elimination

Assisting the Resident to Use a Bedside Commode

Assisting the Resident to Use a Bedpan

Assisting the Resident to Use a Urinal

Assisting with Restorative Bladder Retraining

Assisting with Restorative Bowel Retraining

Measuring the Resident's Height on a Standing Balance Scale

Measuring the Height of a Resident Who Cannot Stand

Collecting a Fresh-Fractional Urine Specimen

Collecting a 24-Hour Urine Specimen

Verbal Communication

Observing

Reporting

Correcting a Charting Error

Working with Culturally Diverse Residents

Caring for Residents with Musculoskeletal Problems

Caring for Residents with Respiratory Problems

Caring for Residents with Circulatory Problems

Caring for a Resident Who has had a Stroke

Caring for Residents with Diabetes

Caring for Residents with Cancer

Improving Memory

Communicating with Residents with ADRD

Managing Problem Behavior

Managing Sexually Aggressive Behavior

Managing Aggressive Behavior in ADRD

Caring for the Depressed Resident

Assisting with Personal Care and Hygiene

Assisting with Nutrition

Assisting with Bowel and Bladder Problems

Assisting Family and Friends

Meeting the Dying Resident's Physical Needs

Meeting the Dying Resident's Psychosocial Needs

Helping the Dying Resident's Family

Assisting Other Residents to Cope with Grief

Coping with Staff Stress

Supplementary Materials

Student Workbook—Each chapter includes a Vocabulary Activity, a Case Study Activity, Test Taking Tips, Competency Review Questions, and Practice Exercises.

Instructor's Resource Manual—Includes Lesson Plans, Quizzes, Quiz Answer Keys, Workbook Answer Key, and Answer Key to End of Chapter Activities.

Companion Website—**www.prenhall.com/grubbs**—features chapter-specific modules for students and Syllabus Manager for instructors.

Instructor's Resource CD-ROM—This cross-platform CD-ROM includes an electronic version of the Instructor's Guide, an electronic test bank, PowerPoint slides, and a transition guide for a smooth changeover to the new edition.

Special Message to the Student

This textbook has been written to help you, the student, learn as easily and comfortably as possible. Through many years of teaching experience, we have gained an awareness of the students' needs and problems. We've learned how to meet those student needs and resolve your problems effectively.

In this edition, we have reorganized the content to allow you to begin learning skills and procedures early in your education. A chapter on Alzheimer's disease and related disorders has been designed to thoroughly meet the curriculum that is mandated in many states for preparation to work in long-term care. Each chapter ends with activities and questions designed to help you prepare mentally and emotionally for certification. We hope that your use of *The Long-Term Care Nursing Assistant,* third edition, will not only be educational, but also interesting and enjoyable.

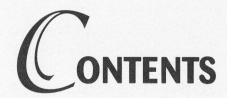

CONTENTS

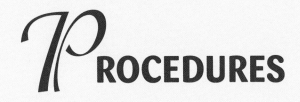

PROCEDURES

GUIDELINES

$\mathcal{A}$CKNOWLEDGMENTS

We would like to thank the many individuals who have lent their time, attention, and effort to the third edition of *The Long-Term Care Nursing Assistant.* Special thanks to our family and friends who are always supportive and understanding of the time and energy that writing demands of us. The students and instructors of the Health Science Department at Learey Technical Center of Tampa, Florida have been helpful in many ways. Their feedback and shared experiences provide a wealth of information and we are grateful for their contributions.

Special thanks to:

Cosette Whitmore, RN, MA for her leadership and inspiration as the Supervisor of Health Occupations, Cosmetology and Public Service, Hillsborough County School District.

Judy Thom, RN, MA for her guidance and continuing interest in the accuracy and usefulness of our publication.

Ann Marie Cupoli, RN for reviewing and critiquing the chapter on Alzheimer's Disease.

Patti Henderson, RN for her unwavering support and friendship.

We are appreciative of the professionally competent staff at Prentice Hall, who always produce a superior publication. Last but not least, we want to thank our acquisitions editor, **Barbara Krawiec,** who has been our beacon of hope through uncharted waters for many years.

Reviewers

We wish to thank the following professionals who have reviewed manuscript for this third edition of *The Long-Term Care Nursing Assistant.* Their careful reading helped to make this program a successful teaching tool.

For the Third Edition

Gloria Bizjak, MEd, EMT
Maryland Fire and Rescue Institute
University of Maryland
College Park, MD

Connie Davis, RN, MSN
Program Developer
Southwest Virginia Community College
Richlands, VA

Sally Flesch, PhD, RN
Professor
Black Hawk College
Moline, IL

Joanne Moats, RN, RMA
Program Manager
Seminole Community College
Sanford, FL

Rita Solander, MSN, RN
Nursing Assistant Instructor
Regional Occupational Program
Riverside County Office of Education
Riverside, CA

Carla Symons, RN, BSN
Instructor, Health Careers and Adult Education
Langdon Area High School
Langdon, ND

Sue Treitz, MA, BSN
Director, Health Careers Development
Arapahoe Community College
Littleton, CO

Sheri Weidman
Director of Nurse Aide Training
Harrisburg Area Community College
Harrisburg, PA

For the Second Edition

Neva Apsey Babcock
St. Thomas More Nursing & Rehabilitation
Center
A Future Care Managed Facility
Bowie, MD

Judith Benvenutti, PhD, RN
Coordinator for Health Occupations MGCCC
Perkinston, MS

Marie L. Boucher
Helping Hands Trade School
Waterville, ME

Shelly Burke
Inservice Instructor/Freelance Writer
Genoa, NE

Tammie Clark-Heller, RN, BSN
Regional Lead Coordinator/Instructor-Nurse
Aide Training Program
Harrisburg Area Community College
Harrisburg, PA

Connie L. Davis
Southwest VA Community College
Richlands, VA

Shahidah Doris Euchiti-Small
Academy for Career Excellence
Ridgeland, SC

Joncee Guido, RN, BSN
CNA Program Coordinator
Vegas Valley Convalescent Hospital
Las Vegas, NV

Cathy A. Learn, RN, BSN, MA
Director Mideast Ohio Vocational School
Nursing Program
Zanesville, OH

Susan Lewsen, RN, BSN, MA, Certification
Coordinator Utah Nurse Aide Registry
Kaysville, UT

Judith R. Mabrey, RN
Inservice Coordinator
NHC Health
Cookeville, TN

David R. Rank, RN, Med, President
TLC Institute, Inc.
Harrisburg, PA

Sarah P. Rogers, CPM
Stone County Hospital
Wiggins, MI

Frosini Rubertino
Health Corp, Inc.
Parma, OH

Racille Smith, RN-C, BSN, MSEd
Psychiatric Nursing & NATP Train the Trainer
Instructor
Clark State Community College
Springfield, OH

Gaye Studenic, RN, BSN
Staff Development Coordinator
Arbors at Marietta
Marrietta, OH

Martha Whited, RN
People Development Coordinator
Cloverlodge Care Center
St. Edward, NE

Joy Wolgamott, RN
Labette Community College
Parsons, KS

For the First Edition

Barbara Acello, RN
Director of Education
H.E.A. Management Group
Denton, TX

Sheila Chesanow, RN, BS
Care Enterprises
Education Department
Chico, CA

Margaret J. Denault, RNC, Med.
Staff Development
Heritage Hall Nursing and Rehabilitation Centers
Agawam, MA

Clair Dickey
Staff Development Coordinator
Living Centers of America (Windsor Health Care Center)
Windsor, CO

Cheryl L. Hoffman, BSN, RNC
Education Department
St. Luke's Extended Care Center
Spokane, WA

Ida A. Horvitz, Director
Continuing Education
University of Cincinnati
College of Nursing and Health
Cincinnati, OH

Beverly Long, RN
Staff Development
Yuma Life Care Center
323 West Ninth Avenue
Yuma, CO

Judith Pawloski
Child and Family Service of Washtenaw
Lifework Department
Ypsilanti, MI

Dr. Rosanne Pruit
College of Nursing
Clemson University
Clemson, SC

Gail Shoulders, PhD, RN
Gail Shoulders & Company
Toledo, OH

Lana B. Simonds, RN, MSN
Nursing Quality Advisor
Living Centers of America
Greeley, CO

Cynthia D. Voorhees
Medishare Health Education Learning Programs
Edison, NJ

Julia Walters, RN
Staff Development
Annaburg Manor
Manassas, VA

Credits

ACE is the registered trademark of Peg Bandage, Inc.

Acetest is the registered trademark of Miles, Inc., Diagnostics Div.

Band-Aid is the registered trademark of Johnson & Johnson Medical, Inc. and Johnson & Johnson Consumer Products, Inc.

Betadine is the registered trademark of Purdue Frederick

Clinitest is the registered trademark of Miles, Inc., Diagnostic Div.

Keto-Diastix is the registered trademark of Miles, Inc., Diagnostics Div.

K-Pad is the registered trademark of Katecho, Inc.

Lysol is the trademark of National Laboratories

T.E.D. is the registered trademark of The Kendall Co.

Tes-Tape is the registered trademark of Eli Lilly and Company

Toothette is the registered trademark of Halbrand Inc.

Velcro is the registered trademark of Velcro USA, Inc.

$\mathcal{I}$NTRODUCTION TO LONG-TERM CARE

$\mathcal{O}$BJECTIVES

1. List two reasons for the growth of long-term care.
2. Identify the purpose of federal and state regulations.
3. Explain the meaning and importance of the chain of command.
4. Identify four members of the health care team.
5. Identify the members of the nursing department and define their roles.
6. Explain the concept of the career ladder in health care.
7. Describe cross-training and multiskilling.

$\mathcal{V}$OCABULARY

The following words or terms will help you to understand this chapter:

Long-term care facility (LTCF)
Convalescence
Resident
Geriatrics
Rehabilitation
Restorative care
OBRA (Omnibus Budget Reconciliation Act)

Administrator
Chain of command
Health care team
Director of nurses (D.O.N.)
Assistant director of nurses (A.D.O.N.)

Registered nurse (R.N.)
Licensed practical nurse (L.P.N.)
Nursing assistant (N.A.)
Cross-training

In a world with rapidly advancing medical technology and spiraling costs of health care, long-term care is a growing segment of the medical industry. The average life span is increasing rapidly. People are living longer, healthier lives, and many are living well into their eighties. It is predicted that as the baby boomers pass their sixty-fifth birthday, the population will reach a statistic never before realized. Approximately one of every five citizens will be over sixty-five years of age.

Longevity and the accomplishments of medical science will create the ever-growing need for knowledgeable, caring nursing personnel with long-term care training and experience. The elderly population will continue to grow and will demand the special care they need and deserve as aging individuals.

$\mathcal{A}$ DESCRIPTION OF LONG-TERM CARE

With the shortened length of stays in hospitals and the current trend toward early posthospital care, tremendous growth in the number of the long-term care facilities is anticipated. A **long-term care facility (LTCF)** provides many levels of health care and activities for people who are not able to care for themselves at home but are not sick enough to be in a hospital. An LTCF may be known by many names, such as nursing home, convalescent center, or adult living facility (ALF).

For many elderly individuals, long-term care may be necessary until death occurs. The long-term care staff is responsible for maintaining the quality of life for the facility's residents. Staff members support residents' emotional, mental, and social well-being, as well as providing physical care. Through the use of a restorative approach, independence is encouraged and the focus is upon each resident's potential to live the best and most fulfilling life possible (see Figure 1-1 ■). You will find it rewarding to know that you are supporting each resident's health, success, and quality of life.

Due to the use of managed care and other attemps to control medical costs, many hospital patients are discharged before they are well enough to return home. They may be admitted to long-term care facilities for **convalescence** (the period of

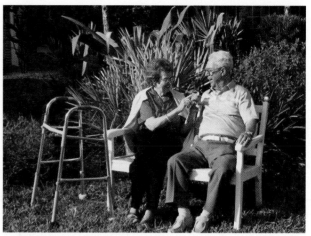

FIGURE 1-1 ■ Long term care encourages the residents to live the best and most fulfilling life possible.

recovery after an illness or injury). This trend has led to the development of subacute care units that provide care for individuals with specific needs such as rehabilitation or respiratory care. Subacute care units are discussed in detail in Chapter 25.

Although some people stay briefly in a long-term care facility, many live there until they die. A person who lives in a long-term care facility is called a **resident.** Although all adult age groups may reside there, the majority of the residents are elderly geriatric residents. **Geriatrics** is the branch of medical care that is concerned with the problems and disease of the elderly. Geriatrics is a specialized branch of health care.

$\mathcal{T}$ HE PURPOSE OF A LONG-TERM CARE FACILITY

Three important purposes of a long-term care facility are as follows:

Provision of Care

The main purpose of any health care facility is to provide care based on the resident's needs. A resident's needs change with improvement or decline of his or her condition. As changes occur, the plan of care is changed in order to support each resident as needed throughout the stay in the facility.

Prevention of Injury and Disease

The resident's safety and well-being are the most important concerns of the staff. Safety includes the prevention of infection and disease and protects the employees as well as the residents. Nursing assistants play a significant role as protectors of residents while they provide basic care on a daily basis.

Rehabilitation and Restorative Care

Rehabilitation is a method used to assist a person to achieve and maintain function at the highest possible level of independence. In the resident's daily life, rehabilitation is supported by the provision of restorative care. **Restorative care** is nursing care that assists each resident to function at the highest possible level of independence. Rehabilitation and restorative care focus on the mental, emotional, and social as well as physical functions and are the foundation of long-term care. Restorative care is addressed in Chapter 4 and throughout this textbook. It is applied to all areas of nursing care (see Figure 1-2 ■).

FEDERAL AND STATE REGULATIONS: OBRA

Long-term care facilities are regulated by state and federal rules. States must enforce federal regulations and may establish additional state regulations. These governmental regulations protect residents and ensure that they receive quality care. Annual state surveys are conducted for all facilities. Nursing assistants contribute significantly to the

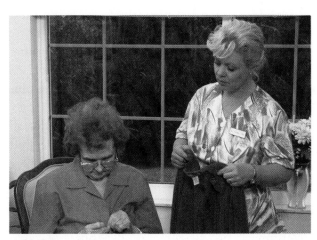

FIGURE 1-2 ■ One of the purposes of a long-term care facility is to promote independence and provide restorative care.

quality of care that is provided and they play an important role during surveys.

OBRA (Omnibus Budget Reconciliation Act) is a federal law that protects all long-term care residents by ensuring their quality of care and their safety, and well-being. OBRA was enacted in 1987 and went into effect three years later. This law addresses resident's rights and requires the education of nursing assistants. In addition, states require nursing assistants to pass a state test and obtain a state certificate. Their names are submitted to the Department of Law Enforcement for a background check to ensure that they have no criminal record.

ORGANIZATION OF THE LONG-TERM CARE FACILITY

Long-term care facilities may be owned either by a large corporation with facilities in widespread areas or by private individual owners. Facilities owned by corporations often have regional managers who are responsible for a number of facilities.

An **administrator** is responsible for the operation of the entire facility. All department heads report to the administrator, who then reports to the regional manager or owner. There are many departments in a facility, and in smaller facilities some departments may be combined. These departments may include nursing, social services, activities, dietary, business, housekeeping, and maintenance. All departments play an important role in the residents' lives.

THE CHAIN OF COMMAND

The **chain of command** is the order of authority and problem solving within a facility. To follow the chain of command, employees of all departments communicate with the person directly above them on the chain. If a problem is not resolved, it continues to move upward one level at a time. Each level is a link in the chain. Skipping links causes confusion and misunderstanding. The chain of command for a nursing department is depicted in Figure 1-3 ■. The nursing assistant reports all problems and requests to the nurse in charge of his or her assignment. As with all other departments, communication should

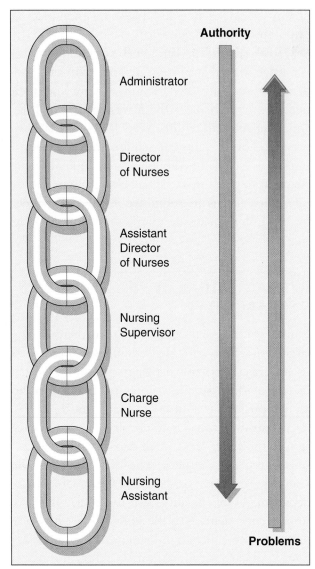

FIGURE 1-3 ■ An example of a nursing department chart. Always follow the chain of command.

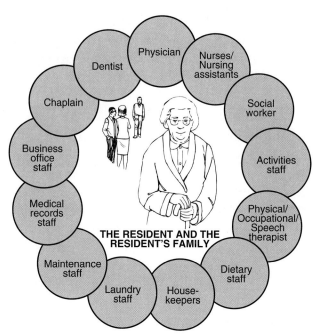

FIGURE 1-4 ■ All members of the health care team work with the resident and with each other.

flow smoothly in both directions when the chain of command is properly used.

𝒯HE HEALTH CARE TEAM

The **health care team** includes all the people who provide care and services for the residents. The team works together to care for the residents. Each person on the team has a role to carry out in caring for the residents, and it takes all team members working together to deliver quality care (see Figure 1-4 ■). The nursing assistant is the member of the health care team who provides basic care for the residents on a daily basis.

𝒯HE NURSING DEPARTMENT

Nursing is the largest department in any health care facility because it provides most of the direct patient care.

Responsibilities of Nurses

Nurses plan, provide, and oversee the care of residents, as well as teaching, giving medication, and providing treatments. The **director of nurses (D.O.N.)** is responsible for the nursing department and is assisted by the **assistant director of nurses (A.D.O.N.).** Other supervisory positions in the nursing department may include the nurse manager, case manager, or patient care coordinator. Nurse practitioners may work with physicians and may write orders and do assessments for residents.

A nursing supervisor may be responsible for all nursing units and nursing personnel on one shift and reports to the D.O.N. or A.D.O.N. Nurses are each responsible for one group of residents or one nursing unit, and they report to the nursing supervisor. The nursing assistant reports to the nurse, who determines work assignments. Regardless of variations in nursing titles that may be used in a facility, the chain of command is used for problem solving and communication. Nursing assistants first take problems or requests to the nurse in charge of their assignment. If problems are not resolved, they may continue up the chain of command.

Members of the Nursing Department

The nursing department members include registered nurses (R.N.s), licensed practical nurses (L.P.N.s), and nursing assistants (N.A.s). In some states, the L.P.N. is called a licensed vocational nurse (L.V.N.). Individual responsibilities depend upon education and training.

Registered Nurse The **registered nurse (R.N.)** is a person who is educated and licensed to plan, provide, and evaluate nursing care. Upon graduation from a two-, three-, or four-year program the student must take a state board examination to become an R.N.

Licensed Practical Nurse/Licensed Vocational Nurse The **licensed practical nurse (L.P.N.)** is a person who is educated and licensed to assist the registered nurse in planning, providing, and evaluating nursing care. This training is focused on technical nursing skills. Upon completion of a twelve- to eighteen-month training program, the graduate must pass a state board examination for licensure.

Nursing Assistant The **nursing assistant (N.A.)** assists the nurses in providing care for the residents (see Figure 1-5 ■). A nursing assistant may be called an aide, a nurse's aide, or a patient care assistant. In the past male nursing assistants have been called orderlies.

Nursing Assistant Training Prior to OBRA, there were no federal requirements concerning the training and competency of nursing assistants. Education varied from on-the-job training to state-approved certification. According to OBRA, every state must provide nursing assistant programs that contain at least 75 hours of instruction. States are permitted to increase the number of hours. Today, state minimum requirements for nursing assistant training vary between 75 and 150 hours. Some programs are much longer.

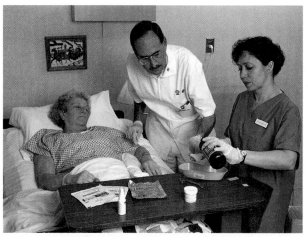

FIGURE 1-5 ■ The nursing assistant helps the nurse care for the resident.

OBRA also requires that nursing assistants demonstrate competency by passing a written test and a skills test. A state certificate and a registration number are issued after successful proof of competency. Your instructor will explain the requirements in your area. States maintain nursing assistant registries listing the nursing assistant's pertinent information. Any record of abuse, neglect, theft, or dishonesty will be added to the registry. A law enforcement background check may be done prior to certification. Employers are required to check the certification and legal records before hiring any nursing assistant. This portion of the law was designed to protect the safety of the residents.

The training of nursing assistants is very important because they provide most of the hands-on care to the residents. Helping the residents to eat, bathe, and dress are examples of activities in which a person's hands touch the resident's body. This is called hands-on care.

In many facilities, nursing assistants may function in expanded roles for which there are various titles, training, and responsibilities. The role of the nursing assistant will be discussed in detail in Chapter 2.

THE CAREER LADDER

The nursing assistant position is the first rung of the health care career ladder. Many job opportunities are available in the health care field. With additional training and education, you can move into higher levels of employment. If you decide that you would like to enter some other branch of health care, your training will be a valuable asset.

CROSS-TRAINING AND MULTISKILLING

Cross-training is accomplished by learning to perform additional specific skills that usually are performed by other members of the health care team. By learning additional skills that are outside the role of nurse assisting, you may serve a facility in a combined role. For instance, a nursing assistant may be trained to draw blood (phlebotomy) or to perform basic physical therapy or occupational therapy tasks. Learning multiple skills is called multiskilling.

Cross-training improves your employability and broadens your experience. It is more common in hospitals than in long-term care facilities. By receiving cross-training you will be able to experience a different job without leaving the one you have.

CHAPTER HIGHLIGHTS

1. Patients in long-term care facilities are called residents.
2. Geriatrics concerns the problems and diseases of the elderly.
3. Restorative care is the nursing care that encourages normal function and independence.
4. The purpose of federal and state regulations is to protect the residents and ensure quality care.
5. Members of the health care team always should follow the chain of command.
6. The health care team includes all the people who provide care and services to the residents.
7. Members of the nursing department include registered nurses, licensed practical nurses, and nursing assistants.
8. OBRA requires that nursing assistants demonstrate competency by passing a written test and a skills test.
9. Cross-training is accomplished by learning to perform additional specific skills that usually are performed by other members of the health care team.

VOCABULARY REVIEW

Fill in the blanks with the vocabulary term that best completes the sentence.

1. Individuals who live in long-term care facilities are called _____.

2. _____ is the nursing care that assists each resident to function at the highest possible level of independence.

3. _____ is the period of recovery after an injury or illness.

4. If you learn additional specific skills that are usually performed by another member of the health care team, you are _____.

5. The _____ is responsible for the operation of the entire facility.

6. All people who provide care and services for the residents are members of the _____ _____.

7. The _____ is the order of authority and problem solving within a facility.

8. The licensed nurse who assists the registered nurse is a/an _____.

9. A/an _____ cares for people who are not able to care for themselves at home but are not sick enough to be in a hospital.

10. A nurse who graduates from a two-, three-, or four-year program is called a/an _____.

CHECK YOUR UNDERSTANDING

The following questions cover the highlights of this chapter. Choose the best answer for each question.

1. The branch of medicine that is concerned with the problems and diseases of the elderly is
   A. pediatrics
   B. obstetrics.
   C. geriatrics
   D. orthopedics

2. The law that provides for the safety, and well-being of the residents is called
   A. OSHA
   B. OBRA
   C. cross-training
   D. chain of command

3. What is the purpose of using the chain of command?
   A. to keep communication about problem solving flowing smoothly
   B. to provide for more administrative positions
   C. to be sure that residents follow the facility rules
   D. to prevent residents from entering the nurses' station

4. Which member of the health care team provides basic care for the residents on a daily basis?
   A. the director of nurses
   B. the administrator
   C. the dietary aide
   D. the nursing assistant

5. Which person is responsible for the entire nursing department?
   A. the L.P.N.
   B. the D.O.N.
   C. the nursing assistant
   D. the charge nurse

6. What is the minimum number of hours required by OBRA for a nursing assistant program?
   A. 50
   B. 75
   C. 100
   D. 125

7. OBRA requires nursing assistants to demonstrate competence by which of the following?
   A. proving three years of work experience
   B. attending a nursing assistant training program
   C. passing a written test and a skills test
   D. providing letters of recommendation

AGE-SPECIFIC TIP

Long-term care facilities care for residents of all age groups. Consider the resident's age when communicating.

CULTURALLY SENSITIVE TIP

Cultural diversity challenges the staff of the long-term care facility to provide for a variety of resident choices. Always encourage residents to make choices by asking them what they prefer in every possible situation.

EFFECTIVE PROBLEM SOLVING

The nursing assistant notices that the bathroom in Room 202 is still dirty after the housekeeper finished cleaning. The nursing assistant says to the head of the housekeeping department, "The housekeeper who cleaned Room 202 doesn't know what she's doing."

Was the nursing assistant's communication appropriate? If not, what would have been more appropriate?

_____

_____

_____

_____

_____

_____

_____

_____

_____

_____

_____

INTERPERSONAL COMMUNICATION

Fill in the answers.

You are angry with one of your coworkers because he refuses to help you move a heavy resident. You should take the problem to _____ _____ _____.

OBSERVING, REPORTING, AND RECORDING

You want to become a nursing assistant. List the requirements that you must fulfill in order to become employable.

_____

_____

_____

_____

_____

_____

_____

_____

_____

_____

_____

_____

_____

_____

_____

_____

EXPLORE MEDIALINK

Check out www.prenhall.com/grubbs for additional chapter-specific interactive study and review activities.

THE NURSING ASSISTANT IN THE LONG-TERM CARE FACILITY

OBJECTIVES

1. Describe the role and responsibilities of the nursing assistant in the long-term care facility.
2. Explain the nursing assistant's responsibilities in providing restorative care.
3. List eleven desirable qualities and characteristics of the nursing assistant.
4. List four areas of importance in caring for yourself.
5. Identify eight measures to cope with stress.
6. Describe the procedure for conducting a job search, completing an application, and participating in an interview.
7. Identify four skills that will improve job performance.
8. Identify the five basic steps that are used with all procedures.

VOCABULARY

The following words or terms will help you to understand this chapter:

Activities of daily living (ADLs)	**Self-esteem**	**Procedure**
Vital Signs	**Stress**	**Prioritizing**
Empathy	**Hygiene**	

This chapter addresses the role and responsibilities of the nursing assistant in long-term care, as well as discussing desirable characteristics, employability skills, and guidelines for personal care, health, and hygiene of the nursing assistant.

THE ROLE OF THE NURSING ASSISTANT

It takes a very special kind of person to be a nursing assistant. Nursing assistants work very closely with residents and often develop special trusting relationships with them. Residents who have been separated from their families or who have no families depend on those closest to them for emotional support. If you choose to be a nursing assistant, you may be the one person who makes a difference in their lives. Nursing assistants help nurses provide care for residents. Working under the supervision of nurses, nursing assistants provide basic care, maintain health and hygiene, and promote physical comfort. They help to meet the residents' social, spiritual, and emotional needs as well as caring for their physical needs (see Figure 2-1 ■).

Today there are many jobs available for nursing assistants in clinics, adult care centers, assisted living facilities, home health, and long-term care facilities, as well as in hospitals. The majority of nursing assistants work in home health or long-term care facilities, providing most of the hands-on care for residents while supporting their emotional needs.

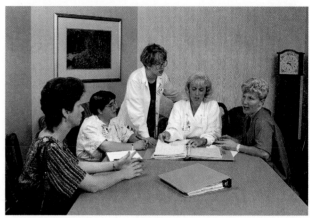

FIGURE 2-2 ■ The nursing assistant may participate in care plan meetings.

The emphasis on restorative nursing has created another role for the nursing assistant. This role may require the nursing assistant to participate in planning the residents' care (see Figure 2-2 ■). Although all nursing assistants are expected to provide restorative care, additional training may be obtained to specialize in rehabilitation.

There are other roles for the nursing assistant in long-term care such as area aide and hospitality aide. The titles, responsibilities, and qualifications for these roles vary from one facility to another.

RESPONSIBILITIES OF THE NURSING ASSISTANT

One of the most important responsibilities of a nursing assistant is performing correctly certain tasks, skills, or procedures. Instructions for performing these tasks are included in this textbook. Many of them involve assisting the resident with activities of daily living.

The nursing assistant provides basic care and assists residents with **Activities of daily living (ADLs)** under the supervision of nurses. ADLs are activities of personal care and hygiene performed daily. ADLs include personal care such as mouth care, bathing, hair care, skin care, foot and nail care, and shaving. Eating, drinking, getting dressed, and going to the bathroom are ADLs. Exercise, positioning, and moving are also ADLs that may require the nursing assistant's help (see Figure 2-3 ■).

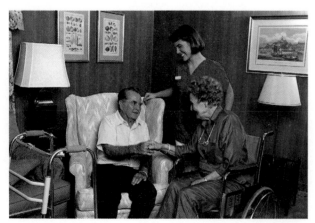

FIGURE 2-1 ■ The nursing assistant helps residents to meet their social needs.

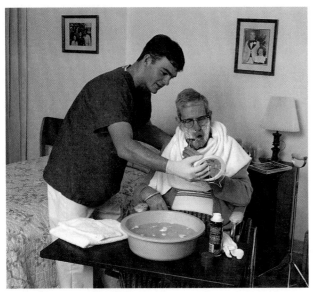

FIGURE 2-3 ■ The nursing assistant assists the residents with ADLs.

Other nursing assistant responsibilities include:

- Making beds
- Straightening the resident's room or area
- Caring for equipment
- Measuring the resident's temperature, pulse, respirations and blood pressure (**vital signs**)
- Measuring fluid intake and output
- Collecting specimens
- Performing urine tests
- Applying support hose
- Measuring height and weight
- Assisting in admitting, transferring, or discharging a resident
- Observing, reporting, and recording information

A job description lists the responsibilities of a nursing assistant. The tasks may not be the same in every facility. There are some tasks that a nursing assistant is not allowed to do. Education, training, and governmental guidelines determine the appropriate responsibilities.

The nursing assistant may not be allowed to:

- Give medications
- Perform sterile procedures
- Suction a resident
- Start, adjust, or discontinue an IV
- Supervise the work of another nursing assistant
- Change or replace urinary catheters

PROVIDING RESTORATIVE CARE

The objective of restorative care is to help the resident to achieve and maintain independence and to function at the highest possible level. All care that is given should include restorative care. Providing restorative care is one of the major responsibilities of the nursing assistant in long-term care. It is accomplished by encouraging the resident to function independently with as little assistance as possible. Residents will benefit most if they are encouraged to do as much as possible for themselves each day. The restorative approach should be used in all the nursing tasks that you perform. That is the best way to assist the resident with rehabilitation. Chapter 4 offers more detailed information about rehabilitation and restorative care.

PERSONAL QUALITIES AND CHARACTERISTICS OF THE NURSING ASSISTANT

Qualities and characteristics contribute to a person's attitude and can be learned at any point in life. The following qualities and characteristics are necessary for effective nursing care.

- Dependability
- Caring
- Patience and self-control
- Sensitivity and consideration
- Cultural awareness
- Courtesy and respect
- **Empathy** (understanding how another person feels)
- Cooperation and willingness to learn
- Flexibility
- Honesty and trustworthiness
- Positive **self-esteem** (one's opinion of oneself)
- Cheerful, positive attitude
- Coping skills for handling **stress** (mental and physical tension or strain)

TAKING CARE OF YOURSELF

In order to provide care for others, you must first be able to care for yourself. Taking care of yourself involves protecting your health, handling stress, developing proper hygiene practices, and presenting a good appearance. Stress, lack of rest, and poor nutrition can lead to illness.

Health

Good health and hygiene will allow you to move and think fast during your care of residents.

You have a responsibility to protect your own health. You cannot function safely as a nursing assistant unless you are physically and emotionally healthy. The following guidelines will help you to stay healthy.

GUIDELINES

STAYING HEALTHY

- Eat three well-balanced meals daily, beginning with a good breakfast.
- Diet only with a doctor's supervision.
- Avoid crash diets that may not provide adequate nutrition.
- Avoid eating junk food, and snack on fruit and vegetables.
- Get enough sleep. Most adults require eight hours of sleep. Be sure to meet your needs.
- Exercise regularly and choose a form of exercise that you enjoy.
- Exercise can help you relax and feel less tense. Thirty minutes of relaxation may also refresh you.
- Have regular checkups and follow your doctor's recommendations.
- Begin treatment promptly if you develop a cold or other health problem.
- Learn to recognize stress, and use coping skills and stress reduction tools.
- Avoid using alcohol and drugs.
- Practice proper hygiene on a daily basis.

Personal Hygiene and Appearance

Activities performed for health and cleanliness are called **hygiene**. Cleanliness helps prevent disease. You look better and feel better when you are clean. Residents and visitors often judge the

quality of care in a facility by the appearance of the employees (see Figure 2-4 ■). Lack of personal hygiene and grooming among employees may create a lack of confidence that proper care will be provided for residents. Consider the following guidelines:

GUIDELINES

PERSONAL HYGIENE AND APPEARANCE

- Bathe or shower every day.
- Use deodorant to prevent underarm odor.
- Brush your teeth at least twice a day.
- Wash your hair at least once a week.
- Clean your fingernails daily or as often as needed.
- Wash your hands frequently to remove germs.
- Practice correct posture.
- Wear a clean uniform every day.
- Change your underclothes daily.
- Keep your shoes polished and your shoelaces clean. Wear shoes that fit well and are in good repair.
- Make sure that your stockings have no holes or runs.
- Wear your hair in a neat style, off your collar and out of your face. Pin up long hair.
- You may wear a watch and wedding band. Jewelry collects germs and can scratch the resident.
- Apply cosmetics and cologne lightly.
- Do not wear nail polish. Germs collect in chipped polish.
- Male nursing assistants should shave daily. Beards should be kept neatly trimmed.
- Avoid smoking while in uniform.

Stress

Mental and physical tension or strain is stress. Your job as a nursing assistant in a long-term care facility can be stressful. Your responsibilities include the health and well-being of the residents, and you must perform with a high degree of accuracy at all times. Working with sickness and death is difficult. Your job is physically and emotionally

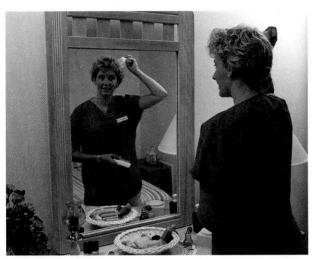

FIGURE 2-4 ■ A nursing assistant should always have a neat, well-groomed appearance.

demanding, and stress is unavoidable as you help others with their problems. You may have problems of your own. All these demands on your time can leave you overwhelmed and feeling out of control.

Stress may be relieved by playing a favorite sport and exercising. Your body will respond to stress more positively if you eat a well-balanced diet, get enough rest, and avoid drugs and alcohol. You may be able to eliminate some of the stress in your life, although a certain amount of stress is motivating. The following tools are useful in managing stress:

STRESS REDUCTION TOOLS	
Tool	Explanation
Laughter	Take time for humor each day because laughter relieves tension.
Talk	Talking to a friend relieves frustration and makes you feel less alone.
Reason	Think the problem through before you start worrying.
Assertiveness	Stand up for what you believe is right.
Flexibility	Be willing to accept change.
Relaxation	Do something you like. Have fun!
Self-care	Be nice to yourself. Be aware of your own needs.
Self-esteem	Give yourself credit for the good things you do.

Substance Abuse

Avoid using alcohol and drugs. These substances affect vision, balance, coordination, and judgment. A person under the influence of drugs or alcohol often makes mistakes. Alcohol or drugs should not be brought to the workplace. Do not come to work if you are under the influence of alcohol or drugs. Residents in your care will be endangered, and so will you. You can be fired for being under the influence of drugs or alcohol while you are at work.

EMPLOYABILITY SKILLS

Employability skills are necessary to get a job and keep it. A discussion of some employability skills follows.

Job Search

Friends and relatives may know of jobs that are available. You may check the Internet and newspaper employment listings, as well as facility listings in the telephone book. List employers that are of interest to you, including the contact person if available. Using your list of possible employers, decide the order in which you will apply for work. In making this decision, consider location and distance, transportation, salary, benefits, and working conditions. Some of this information may not be available until you interview.

Job Application

Call and inquire about a job before going to the facility. Be neat and well groomed, and go alone when you apply for a job because you may be interviewed at that time and without advance notice. Fill out the application honestly. The impression you make initially often will influence the decision to interview and hire you.

Information that will be needed for completing your job application includes:

• Educational background—List your graduation or GED date and location, as well as additional training or education that you have completed.

• Work experience—List the last three or four places where you have worked, including the addresses, phone numbers, and supervisors' names, as well as your position and responsibilities.

- References—Include the names, addresses, and phone numbers of people who will speak well of you. Choose professional people if possible and do not list relatives. Get permission from all persons before listing them as references.
- Documents—You will need to take your Social Security card, drivers' license, or other photo ID. Include pertinent documents such as a CPR card, HIV certificate, and NA certificate, as well as proof of other continuing education.

Job Interview

An interview is a meeting between an employer and an applicant at which both individuals obtain information related to employment. The decision to hire is often made during the interview. Questions that you might ask include available employee benefits such as insurance, retirement, and tuition reimbursement.

GUIDELINES

JOB INTERVIEW

- Be on time for the interview.
- Be prepared with the necessary information and documents.
- Present a neat, clean appearance.
- Communicate clearly.
- Show interest and enthusiasm.
- Be courteous and polite.
- Demonstrate self-confidence.
- Bring a pencil and notepaper.

Job Performance

When you begin a new job, you may spend a few days in orientation, during which you will learn about the employer's policies and procedures. A **procedure** is a list of the steps to be taken in performing a task. Procedures are contained in a procedure book, which may be located at the nurses' station in a long-term care facility.

A probationary period for new employees provides the employer an opportunity to evaluate your job performance. Evaluations will be done by your supervisor at least annually after the initial one that occurs at the end of your probationary period. If satisfactory, an evaluation can lead to a promotion or raise. Learning and using job performance skills such as teamwork, organization, planning, and prioritizing will help you improve your job performance and will have a positive effect upon your evaluation results. A discussion of these skills follows.

Teamwork

Care is delivered best when staff members work together. Cooperation makes the job easier and more pleasant for everyone concerned, while it protects the safety of both staff members and residents. After ensuring the safety of your own residents, assist your coworkers whenever possible. Working together often makes procedures more comfortable and safer for the residents. Staff members are responsible for individual assignments and should not expect others to complete the assignment for them.

Assignments may change daily. The nurse determines the assignments at the beginning of each shift. The ease or difficulty of your assignment may also change. All staff members are responsible for all residents even though each nursing assistant has a particular group of residents for whom to provide care.

Be sure to listen carefully to orders from the nurse and ask questions when you don't understand. Tell the nurse if you cannot do something, and report any time that you leave the unit. Develop and use communication skills, and avoid criticizing and arguing. Learn empathy, follow the chain of command, and leave personal problems at home.

Organization

Being a nursing assistant in a long-term care facility is not easy, and organization is necessary in order to complete your responsibilities in a timely, efficient manner. Organization is a skill that can be learned and improved. To be organized plan, prioritize, and manage your time well.

Planning and Prioritizing

Planning is the key to organization. The shift should begin with a brief visit with each resident included in your assignment. This will allow you to identify residents' needs, attend to immediate needs, ensure residents' safety, and reassure residents that you will be available if needed. An early visit made as soon as you have received your assignment will decrease residents' anxiety, and you will be less likely to be interrupted while you complete care for others.

List procedures that occur at specific times and intervals. Include planned events, appointments, visits, resident activities, and employee meetings and classes. Then determine what the priorities are. **Prioritizing** consists of rating each task in its order of importance. Anything that must be done at a specific time must be high on the priority list. Flexibility is important because needs change and therefore priorities must change. A sudden illness or a resident's need to go to the toilet must become priorities when they arise. A priority list will help you complete the most important tasks on time, and you will feel more finished and satisfied with your work (see Figure 2-5 ■).

Organization requires time management. Estimate how much time you will need for each task. Know facility routines and time frames for activities such as meals, and identify tasks that can be grouped together. For example, you may be able to make a resident's bed while the resident is in the bathroom. Plan ahead if you will need assistance or special equipment that must be shared. Determine what supplies and equipment you will

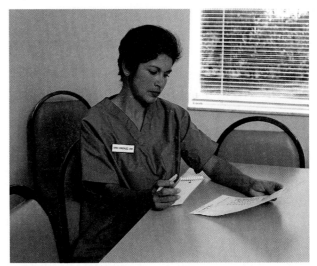

FIGURE 2-5 ■ Making a priority list will help you complete the most important tasks on time.

need for a task before you begin doing it. Take the equipment or supplies with you so that you will be prepared.

Prior to beginning any procedure, there are five basic steps that must be taken. If you learn and follow these steps, you will be safe, organized, and efficient. All procedures in this text will begin with a reminder to follow the basic beginning steps.

REMINDERS

FIVE BASIC STEPS BEFORE BEGINNING A PROCEDURE

- Wash your hands.
- Collect the equipment.
- Identify the resident.
- Explain the procedure.
- Provide privacy.

CHAPTER HIGHLIGHTS

1. The nursing assistant always works under the supervision of a nurse.

2. Tasks and responsibilities are not the same at every facility. You will be taught what is expected of you.

3. Dependability is an important quality for a nursing assistant.

4. A nursing assistant must be physically and emotionally healthy.

5. Never come to work under the influence of drugs or alcohol.

6. Having high self-esteem helps you to cope with stress.

7. You look and feel better when you are clean and well groomed.

8. Residents and visitors often judge the care of the residents by the appearance of the employees.

9. Cooperation makes everybody's job easier.

10. Being organized helps you to avoid stress and get your work done on time.

11. Planning, prioritizing, managing time, and organization are important employability skills.

12. The five basic steps before beginning any procedure are to wash your hands, collect the equipment, identify the resident, explain the procedure, and provide privacy.

VOCABULARY REVIEW

Fill in the blank with the vocabulary term that best completes the sentence.

1. Understanding how another person feels is _____.

2. _____ is the opinion one has of oneself.

3. _____ are activities of personal care and hygiene performed daily.

4. Mental and physical tension or strain is _____.

5. _____ means rating each task in its order of importance.

6. A/an _____ lists the steps to be taken in performing a task.

7. Activities performed for health and cleanliness are _____.

8. _____ is the ability to accept change.

9. Temperature, pulse, respiration, and blood pressure are _____.

10. Nursing care that assists each resident to function at the highest possible level of indendence is _____.

CHECK YOUR UNDERSTANDING

The following questions cover the highlights of this chapter. Choose the best answer for each question.

1. Who supervises the work of a nursing assistant?
   A. the resident's family
   B. the doctor
   C. the nurse
   D. another nursing assistant

2. ADLs include which of the following?
   A. shopping
   B. personal hygiene
   C. driving
   D. getting a job

3. Providing restorative care is best accomplished by
   A. encouraging independence
   B. discouraging independence
   C. doing everything for the resident
   D. making the resident do everything

4. Which of the following is *not* a desirable quality for a nursing assistant?
   A. dependability
   B. flexibility
   C. empathy
   D. impatience

5. Which of the following is the most important reason for working together?
   A. to protect resident safety
   B. to finish as early as possible
   C. to have time for fun
   D. to please the charge nurse

6. Which of the following is a nursing assistant's responsibility?
   A. Give medications
   B. Measure vital signs
   C. Discontinue an IV
   D. Suction a resident

AGE-SPECIFIC TIP

Use empathy when communicating with disabled elderly residents. Imagine yourself in the elderly resident's place.

CULTURALLY SENSITIVE TIP

It may be difficult to understand coworkers whose primary languages are different from your own. Ask for explanations if language barriers interfere with your ability to communicate with your coworkers.

EFFECTIVE PROBLEM SOLVING

The nursing assistant complains to his coworkers that his assignment is heavier than theirs. He says that he has more work to do than anyone else and asks another nursing assistant to trade assignments.

Was the nursing assistant's communication appropriate? If not, what would have been more appropriate?

_____

_____

_____

_____

_____

_____

_____

_____

_____

_____

_____

_____

INTERPERSONAL COMMUNICATION

Write a T or F in the space provided to indicate if a statement is true or false.

_____ It is not appropriate to ask questions about employee benefits during the job interview.

_____ It is proper to ask permission before giving a person's name as a reference to a prospective employer.

_____ Empathy is communicated by showing that you understand how another person feels.

OBSERVING, REPORTING, AND RECORDING

List ADLs that must be performed and recorded daily.

_____

_____

_____

_____

_____

_____

_____

_____

_____

_____

_____

EXPLORE MEDIALINK

ETHICAL AND LEGAL CONCERNS

OBJECTIVES

1. Identify seven rules of ethics to be followed by the nursing assistant.
2. Describe six examples of legal problems that may affect nursing assistant responsibilities.
3. Identify four guidelines to prevent medical errors.
4. Explain how advance directives can affect end-of-life issues.
5. Indentify 24 rights of the resident in a long-term care facility.
6. List four guidelines to help victims of domestic violence.
7. Identify six guidelines for protection against workplace violence.
8. Explain how and why the nursing assistant can prevent elderly abuse.
9. Describe the function of an Ombudsmen Committee.

VOCABULARY

The following words or terms will help you to understand this chapter:

Ethics
Assault
Battery
False imprisonment
Restraint
Invasion of privacy

Confidentiality
Negligence
Slander
Libel
Advance directive

Residents' bill of rights
Occupational Safety and
  Health Administration
  (OSHA)
Ombudsmen Committee

Legal and ethical issues have reached a high level of importance in health care today. The public is more aware of legal rights and is more likely to take action to protect them. New rules and regulations have been put in place to protect the individual rights of patients. This chapter contains information that will help you provide patient care in an ethical and legal manner. Prevention of medical errors is also included.

ᴇTHICS

Ethics are guidelines for defining right or wrong behavior. Ethics are formed by the moral code of our society and are influenced by our inner feelings. Professional ethics are rules of behavior that apply to members of a profession. Doctors, nurses, and teachers, for example, have developed ethical standards for their professions.

Nursing assistants can develop their own set of ethics, which might include the following:

- Treat each other with respect.
- Respect each resident as an individual.
- Protect the privacy of each resident.
- Protect each resident from harm.
- Avoid the use of illegal drugs or alcohol.
- Be honest and trustworthy.
- Be loyal to your employer and your coworkers.
- Do not steal. Stealing is unethical and illegal.
- Do the best job you can.
- Do not accept money or gifts.

Suggesting or accepting tips of money or gifts from residents or family members is unethical and may be against company policy. If you are offered a tip, politely refuse, and explain that caring for the resident is part of your job.

ʟEGAL RESPONSIBILITIES

There are certain legal responsibilities or laws that all health care workers must uphold. Laws are rules of conduct that are decided by the government and are enforced by the courts. The purpose of a law is to protect both the individual and society. It is a crime to break a law, and the person who commits

a crime may have to pay a fine, go to jail, or both. Legal terms that a nursing assistant should be aware of will now be discussed.

Assault

A threat to do bodily harm is **assault**. A threat to force a person to do something against his or her will is assault, as is any threat of punishment. Using hand gestures, such as shaking a fist at someone, could be considered assault.

Battery

Touching another person's body without permission is **battery**. Although battery may include hitting, pinching, or biting someone, it is not always that violent. Handling a resident roughly, hurrying, or forcing a resident is also considered battery. Performing a treatment or procedure without the resident's permission is also an example of battery.

False Imprisonment

Restraining or restricting a person's movements unnecessarily is **false imprisonment**. A **restraint** is a device that restricts a person's freedom of movement and may only be used for the safety of the resident. A resident may not be forced to stay or be locked in his or her room as punishment. Restraints may not be used to prevent wandering. Residents are never restrained for the convenience of the staff.

Invasion of Privacy

It is an **invasion of privacy** when the privacy of the resident's body or of personal information is not protected. Avoid unnecessary exposure of the resident's body during personal care. Protect the resident's privacy during personal care by closing the door and pulling the curtain. Always knock before entering the resident's room (see Figure 3-1 ■). Ask permission to look through the resident's belongings.

Personal information and medical care details must be kept confidential. **Confidentiality** means privacy of resident information. All questions from

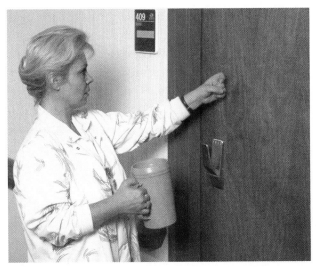

FIGURE 3-1 ■ Always knock before entering the resident's room.

family or friends concerning medical treatment should be referred to the nurse. Do not repeat personal information that the resident has chosen to share with you.

Negligence

The failure to give proper care, which results in physical or emotional harm to the resident, is **negligence**. Failure to perform a task may be considered negligence. It also is negligent to perform a task incorrectly. Examples of negligence include the following:

- A resident's signal light was on for 20 minutes. The resident got up alone to go to the bathroom, fell, and broke a hip.
- The nursing assistant dropped the resident's dentures (false teeth) and they broke.

Slander

A false statement that damages another person's reputation is **slander**. If the false statement is written, it is called **libel**. You can cause trouble by repeating gossip about a resident or coworker. Avoid this problem by refusing to repeat anything that you are not sure is true.

Legally, you are responsible for your own actions. This means that you can be sued if the resident is harmed because of something you did or some-thing you failed to do. If you are guilty of assault, battery, false imprisonment, invasion of privacy, negligence, slander, or anything else that harms someone, a lawsuit can be brought against you.

Working with Nurses

The nursing assistant always works under the supervision of a nurse. However, there may be times when you may not be able to follow the nurse's orders. For example, if the nurse asks you to do something that a nursing assistant is not allowed to do or that would harm the resident, you should politely refuse. If you perform a task or procedure that is only to be performed by a nurse, you may be guilty of practicing nursing without a license. Never ignore a nurse's order. Be sure the nurse knows that you are not going to carry out the order.

There are special situations in which you will need more information. For example if the nurse's order is not clear and you are not sure what to do or you're asked to do something that you haven't been taught, you will need more information. Talk to the nurse. Ask for a better explanation or tell the nurse that you do not know how to perform the task and would like to learn. Do not take any action until you know what you are doing, and do not attempt to do anything until you can do it safely.

PREVENTING MEDICAL ERRORS

Medical errors are a major concern for all health care workers. These errors contribute to the rising cost of health care and are one of the leading causes of death in the United States. A medical error occurs when a mistake is made during the delivery of health care.

Public attention is often focused on dramatic errors such as a surgeon amputating the wrong body part or a nurse giving the wrong medication. However, the majority of medical errors involve carelessness or negligence while providing routine patient care. Examples of medical errors by nursing assistants include failure to provide proper resident care, performing a procedure incorrectly, performing a procedure on the wrong resident, or recording information on the wrong chart.

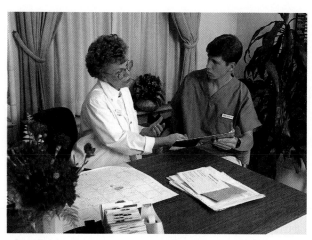

FIGURE 3-2 ■ Report medical errors to the nurse immediately.

GUIDELINES

To Prevent Medical Errors

- Follow each resident's plan of care.
- Identify residents by checking their identification bracelets.
- Perform procedures correctly.
- Follow safety and infection control guidelines.
- Record resident information promptly and accurately.
- Respect residents' rights.
- Behave in a legal and ethical manner.
- Report medical errors to the nurse immediately. (See Figure 3-2 ■).

---

*E*ND-OF-LIFE ISSUES

End-of-life issues have gained importance in recent years. Advances and changes in medical technology have affected the dying process. In earlier times, most people died suddenly of an acute illness or injury. Today, a person may live for years with a chronic illness that requires extensive treatment and medication. Individuals may be kept alive by machines long after body organs fail. Dying may progress slowly and painfully.

This modern technology has caused people to seriously consider what they want during the last days of their lives. End-of-life issues center on three themes—choice, control, and comfort.

Residents often want to be able to make informed choices about their health care. They may want to choose how much or how little treatment is given, who will deliver this treatment, and where they will spend their last days. Residents may want to be in control by making decisions and directing the course of their treatment. Loss of control can lead to depression and hopelessness. Most of all, residents want to be as comfortable and pain-free as possible at the end of life.

Avoid giving legal advice to a resident. Your role as a nursing assistant is to support the resident's decisions, whether you agree with them or not. Provide care in a way that allows the resident to maintain control. Do all that you can to make the resident as comfortable as possible and report complaints of pain to the nurse immediately.

The use of advance directives gives legal support to residents and caregivers regarding end-of-life issues.

Advance Directives

A document that provides instruction regarding a person's desires about health care is an **advance directive**. This document allows individuals to continue to have the right to make choices about treatment and care after becoming unable to express themselves. A law passed in 1990 established this right to make advance decisions. An advance directive is a legally binding document and becomes effective only when the individual is unable to state his or her wishes.

Living Wills and Powers of Attorney

A living will is a document in which a person may determine whether or not he or she wishes to have life prolonged when terminally ill. The living will should indicate whether food or fluids are to be given or withheld. A living will goes into effect when a person no longer can make decisions. The appointment of a power of attorney for health care also provides persons control of medical care after becoming unable to decide for themselves. The power of attorney becomes a part of the advance directive.

Wills

A will is a written document that states how a person wants property divided after his or her death.

You might be asked to witness the signing of a will. Although there is no legal reason why you cannot, it is better that you do not act as a witness. Your best response is to report the request to the nurse.

RESIDENTS' BILL OF RIGHTS

The **residents' bill of rights** is a list of the rights and freedoms of residents. Each right is guaranteed to all residents. Just as the Bill of Rights of the Constitution of the United States guarantees certain rights to the American people, all health care agencies must guarantee certain rights to all patients.

To meet federal regulations, long-term care facilities must have written policies to protect the rights of the residents. Violation of residents' rights is illegal and unethical. A more complete list of the residents' rights can be found in Figure 3-3 ■. Some of these rights are described in the paragraphs that follow.

The Right to Civil and Religious Liberties

The resident may take part in social, religious, or civic activities and is allowed to vote. This includes the right to contact government representatives as desired.

The Right to Complain Without Fear

A resident has the right to make complaints and suggest changes without fear of harm. A residents' committee may be formed to express complaints, concerns, and suggestions for change. Individuals may express grievances and concerns directly to the administration at any time.

The Right to Refuse

A resident has the right to refuse medication and treatment. Staff members should explain the importance of following the doctor's orders. However, the resident who continues to refuse has a right to do so.

The Right to Be Free from Unnecessary Physical Restraints

Restraints require a doctor's order and can be used only to protect the resident from harm. A violation of this right is considered false imprisonment.

RESIDENTS' RIGHTS

A long-term care facility must protect and promote the rights of each resident, including the following:

1. The right to civil and religious liberties.
2. The right to file complaints without fear.
3. The right to be informed of his/her rights, and the rules of the facility, upon admission.
4. The right to inspect his/her records.
5. The right to be informed of his/her medical condition and treatment, and to take part in planning the care.
6. The right to refuse medical treatment.
7. The right to information from agencies of inspection.
8. The right to be informed of responsibility for charges and services.
9. The right to manage his/her own financial affairs.
10. The right to receive adequate and appropriate health care.
11. The right to be free from unnecessary physical restraints and drugs.
12. The right to be free from verbal, mental, sexual, or physical abuse.
13. The right to personal privacy and confidentiality of information.
14. The right to be treated courteously, fairly, and with dignity.
15. The right to send and promptly receive mail that is unopened.
16. The right to have private communication with any person of choice.
17. The right to receive visitors at any reasonable hour.
18. The right to immediate access to family and friends.
19. The right to the right to choose a personal physician.
20. The right to have access to private use of a telephone.
21. The right to participate in social, religious, and group activities of choice.
22. The right to retain and use personal possessions and clothing as space permits.
23. The right to equal policies and practices regardless of source of payment.
24. The right to privacy during visits with a spouse, and to share a room when a married couple resides in the same facility.

FIGURE 3-3 ■ The residents' bill of rights.

The Right to Be Free from Mental or Physical Abuse

No resident has to endure abuse in any form. Physical abuse is the same as battery, and mental abuse may be assault.

The Right to Personal Privacy and Confidentiality

The resident has the right to personal privacy. This involves providing care in a way that does not expose the body unnecessarily. Pulling the privacy curtain, exposing only the part of the body involved in the care being given, and asking visitors to leave during personal care protect bodily privacy. Information about the resident must be kept confidential. It should not be discussed with anyone except those who participate in the resident's care. All records should be handled carefully and not left where they can be seen by people who are not involved in caregiving. A violation of this right is invasion of privacy.

The Right to Inspect Personal Medical Records

Residents should be encouraged to participate in planning their own care. This includes the right to see personal medical records. If the resident asks to see his or her medical record, communicate the request to the nurse.

The Right to Be Treated with Courtesy and Dignity

The resident must be treated with dignity as an individual. This means that all people are different and should be accepted as such. The resident is to be called by her proper name or the name she chooses.

The Right to Make Personal Choices

Each resident has the right to make personal choices. Examples include food, medication, and treatment choices; participation in social and religious activities; choice of physician; and planning health care.

The Right to Receive Proper Health Care

The resident has the right to receive adequate and appropriate health care. However, all citizens do not have the right to free medical care. The resident's care plan must be followed by all those who provide resident care. Failure to provide proper health care to residents may be considered negligence.

The Right to Personal Belongings

The resident may keep and use personal clothing and other belongings as space permits. The things residents bring are usually the most important and meaningful possessions they own. Their belongings are to be treated with care and respect.

The Right to Privacy for Married Couples

This right ensures a husband and wife privacy when a resident's spouse is visiting. It also permits them to share a room when both are residents.

A violation of any one of the resident's rights may be illegal, and it could be considered abuse. It is your responsibility to help protect each resident's rights.

PROTECTING RESIDENTS WHO HAVE ALZHEIMER'S DISEASE

Although health care workers are legally obligated to protect the safety and individual rights of all residents, those with Alzheimer's disease are at special risk because they are unable to protect themselves. They are not always able to make informed choices or behave in a logical manner. State and federal agencies have issued rules and regulations to ensure that residents suffering from Alzheimer's disease receive proper care. For example, legislation requires training for all nursing home employees who have contact with residents with Alzheimer's disease. This training is very specific in terms of structure and content. The information about the care of residents with Alzheimer's disease presented in this book follows the curriculum guidelines of that rule.

DOMESTIC VIOLENCE

Domestic violence is defined as violence or controlling behavior by one member of a household toward another member. It is a violation of basic human rights within a household. Women and children are the most common victims, although domestic violence may be directed at anyone in the home, including elder members such as parents or grandparents.

Forms of domestic violence include any assault, battery, or criminal offense causing injury or death. Domestic violence also includes name calling or verbal abuse, isolation from family and friends, withholding money, actual or threatened physical harm, and sexual assault.

Children who grow up in abusive households are significantly more likely to have abusive relationships in adulthood. Children who are raised with domestic violence are at higher risk for substance abuse as well as for juvenile delinquency. Many are injured while attempting to protect family members from abuse.

Characteristics of Abusers and Victims

Abusers generally experience low self-esteem, insecurity, jealousy, and substance abuse. They cope poorly with stress and have poor communication skills. Their victims usually have low self-esteem, are very dependent on the abuser, and earn less income than the abuser. Pregnant victims usually experience increased abuse. Usually both victims and abusers have grown up in abusive homes.

Signs of Domestic Abuse

Health care workers should be aware of injuries that don't match the stated causes. Injuries from abuse usually are under clothing, and victims may wear long sleeves or sunglasses to hide their injuries. Emergency room visits may be frequent, although victims will attempt to minimize their injuries. Victims often delay treatment and deny the abuse. The abuser usually attempts to stay near the victim to prevent communication with health care workers. There may be evidence of old and new injuries and bruises. Injuries caused by violence must be reported to law enforcement authorities by health care workers who are providing care for the victim.

Helping the Victim

Remember that violence is a control issue. Nothing the victim can do or say will stop the abuser. Trying to please the abuser is useless. It is important to emphasize that violence occurs not only to women, but to other household members as well. Domestic violence is always unacceptable.

GUIDELINES

TO AID VICTIMS OF DOMESTIC VIOLENCE

- Believe the victim. Listen and encourage the victim to talk.
- Respect the victim's need for confidentiality.

GUIDELINES (Continued)

- Don't tell the abuser.
- Don't encourage the victim to try harder to get along with the abuser.
- Avoid being judgmental. Offer emotional support.
- Allow the victim to make decisions.
- Provide information about legal protection, as well as about community shelters and other resources for assaulted individuals.
- Share warning signs and other information with the victim.
- Refer the victim to the appropriate person for help.

WORKPLACE VIOLENCE

Workplace violence has increased dramatically in the past few years. Almost daily we hear or see news reports of people being threatened, injured, or even killed at work. Health care is no exception. Violence can occur in a resident's room, in a common area, or in the parking lot. The person creating the violence can be a resident, a visitor, an employee, or a stranger. International terrorism has resulted in multiple injuries and deaths in the workplace on a worldwide scale.

There are many possible reasons for increased violence in health care settings. Frustration with health care delivery, inability to cope with sickness or death, dementia (confusion), and fear of contagious disease all contribute to the problem. Sometimes domestic violence spills over into the workplace.

OSHA Regulations

The **Occupational Safety and Health Administration (OSHA)** is a federal government agency that is concerned with the health and safety of workers. OSHA requires that all health care workers have training in recognizing, preventing, and responding to violence in the workplace. They require written policies addressing these issues. In response, many facilities have developed violence response teams that may include health care professionals, security guards, and law enforcement officers.

Preventing Workplace Violence

The best protection against violence is to prevent it from occurring when possible. Be aware of your environment at all times, and be alert to any problems. Notify your supervisor or the security guard immediately if you sense a dangerous situation.

GUIDELINES

PROTECTION AGAINST WORKPLACE VIOLENCE

- Be alert for danger.
- Do not take unnecessary risks.
- Be observant of people and report any unusual behavior or suspicious activities.
- Do not argue or become defensive with hostile people.
- Listen respectfully and try to stay calm when talking to an angry person.
- Watch for unspoken hostility such as facial grimaces or muscle tension.
- Trust your instinct if something seems to be wrong.
- Notify the nurse if you leave your work area.
- Do not go alone to isolated areas.
- Try to leave the building with other people and be especially alert in the parking lot.
- Report any threats, attempts, or actual violence immediately.
- If violence occurs, report it to the nurse and follow his or her instructions.

ABUSE OF THE RESIDENT

Abuse of the elderly can occur at home or in a health care facility. Most of the time, the abused person has physical or mental problems and requires a lot of care. The abuser often is the one who provides most of the care and may be a family member or a health care worker.

Abuse can be physical, verbal, sexual, material, and financial. Verbal abuse also may be called emotional abuse. Hitting, rough handling, shoving, or hurrying the resident are examples of physical abuse. Neglect is a form of physical abuse. Threats, curses, or anything said that makes the resident feel bad or that lowers his or her self-esteem is verbal abuse. Sexual abuse can involve physical contact,

gestures, or remarks. Material or financial abuse involves misuse of the resident's money or personal possessions. This can include anything from eating the resident's candy to stealing his or her money.

As a nursing assistant, you may be the first person to discover that a resident is being abused.

Signs and symptoms of abuse include the following:

- Physical injuries such as bruises, burns, or scratches
- Fear and anxiety
- Mood swings or changes in personality
- Frequent crying spells
- Avoidance of touch
- Withdrawal or depression
- Hostile, aggressive behavior

What kind of person would hurt a resident? Abusers often are people who are tired and overworked. They lose patience easily and do not handle stress well. They try to hold back their emotions and have difficulty saying what they feel. Many abusers have personal problems. Others have been abused themselves. They take their anger and frustration out on other people.

Protecting the Resident from Abuse

What can you do about resident abuse? Begin with yourself, and stay in tune with your feelings. If you find that the complaints and demands of a certain resident annoy you, it is time to withdraw. There is *never* an excuse for abusing a resident.

It is your ethical and legal duty to report resident abuse. If you fail to report abuse, you can be held legally responsible.

GUIDELINES

TO PROTECT RESIDENTS FROM ABUSE

- Know the signs and symptoms of abuse.
- Be observant and report anything suspicious.
- Observe the residents' skin carefully for signs of rough handling.
- Encourage residents to talk about their fears and anxieties.

GUIDELINES (Continued)

- Be aware of your own stress level and use appropriate coping techniques.
- Report abuse immediately if you witness or suspect it.
- Remember that negligence in care is a form of abuse.

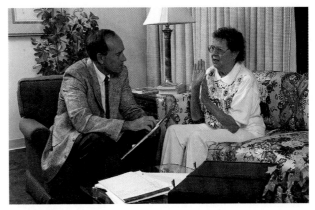

FIGURE   3-4 ■ A member of the Ombudsmen Committee will visit the long-term care facility to investigate a complaint of abuse.

Most areas have an abuse hotline that will be listed in the front of the telephone book. Your area also might have an Ombudsmen Committee to whom you may report abuse. The **Ombudsmen Committee** investigates complaints of resident abuse in health care facilities (see Figure 3-4 ■). This committee is composed of concerned citizens who usually are appointed by the governor of the state. The purpose of the Ombudsmen Committee is to protect the residents' rights. The resident, family, or facility may request the assistance of the Ombudsmen Committee.

CHAPTER HIGHLIGHTS

1. Ethics are guidelines for determining right or wrong behavior.
2. Privacy and confidentiality of resident information is important.
3. A nursing assistant who fails to give proper care is negligent.
4. Legally, you are responsible for your own actions.
5. Medical errors must be reported to the nurse immediately.
6. Advance directives allow residents to make choices and be in control at the end of life.
7. The purpose of the residents' bill of rights is to protect each resident's rights and freedoms.
8. Residents have the right to refuse medication and treatment.
9. Domestic violence is defined as violence or controlling behavior by one member of a household toward another member.
10. Government regulations have been issued to ensure that residents suffering from Alzheimer's disease receive proper care.
11. The best protection against workplace violence is to prevent it from occurring when possible.
12. The best way to protect residents from abuse is to be observant and report anything suspicious.

VOCABULARY REVIEW

Fill in the blanks with the vocabulary term that best completes the sentence.

1. _____ are guidelines for right or wrong behavior.

2. A threat to do bodily harm is a/an _____.

3. _____ is failure to give proper care that results in harm to the resident.

4. A document that provides instructions regarding a person's desires about health care is a/an _____.

5. The _____ is a group of concerned citizens who investigate complaints of resident abuse in health care facilities.

6. _____ means privacy of resident information.

7. Touching another person's body without permission is _____.

8. Restraining or restricting a person's movement unnecessarily is _____.

9. _____ is a federal government agency that is concerned with the health and safety of workers.

10. A/an _____ is a device that restricts a person's freedom of movement.

CHECK YOUR UNDERSTANDING

The following questions cover the highlights of this chapter. Choose the best answer for each question.

1. A resident's son offers you $20.00 for taking such good care of his mother. What is the best way to refuse the tip?
   A. "I'd get in trouble if I took the money."
   B. "Are you trying to bribe me?"
   C. "I appreciate the thought, but caring for your mother is part of my job."
   D. "That isn't enough money to pay for all the things I do for your mother."

2. Leaving the door open while you are bathing a resident is an example of

   A. assault   C. false imprisonment
   B. battery   D. invasion of privacy

3. The nursing assistant dropped the resident's dentures and broke them. This is an example of
   A. negligence   C. invasion of privacy
   B. assault   D. false imprisonment

4. Which of the following is *not* included in the residents' bill of rights?
   A. the right to free medical care
   B. the right to refuse treatment and medication
   C. the right to personal privacy
   D. the right to complain without fear

5. Mrs. Johnson refused to take a bath. The nursing assistant bathed her anyway. What right was violated?
   A. the right to privacy
   B. the right to complain
   C. the right to refuse
   D. the right to be free from unnecessary physical restraints

6. The nursing assistant tells the resident, "If you don't get ready for bed now, I'm going to leave you up all night." This is an example of
   A. battery and physical abuse
   B. false imprisonment
   C. invasion of privacy
   D. assault and verbal abuse

7. A resident has given her daughter power of attorney for her health care. What right does this give the daughter?
   A. The right to make decisions about her mother's health care
   B. The right to sign her mother's checkbook
   C. The right to sell her mother's home
   D. The right to divide up her mother's estate

8. Which of the following is *not* a guideline to prevent medical errors?
   A. Recording a procedure as soon as you complete it
   B. Identifying a resident by asking his or her name and room number
   C. Following infection control procedures
   D. Reporting a medical error to the nurse immediately

AGE-SPECIFIC TIP

Elderly residents often move slowly and may have difficulty following directions. Be patient, stay aware of your frustration level, and control the tone of your voice in order to avoid becoming verbally abusive.

CULTURALLY SENSITIVE TIP

Avoid expressing judgment toward victims of domestic violence who choose to remain in unsafe environments. Culturally established roles influence relationships.

EFFECTIVE PROBLEM SOLVING

Mrs. Frasier had prepared advance directives before being admitted to the long-term care facility. She is now in the last stage of terminal cancer. Her daughter tells the nursing assistant that she is going to support her mother's decision to not use a feeding tube. The nursing assistant replies, "If you don't let them put in a feeding tube, your mother will starve. Are you just going to let her die?"

Was the nursing assistant's communication appropriate? If not, what would have been more appropriate?

_____

_____

_____

_____

_____

_____

_____

INTERPERSONAL COMMUNICATION

Which incidents may lead to legal problems? Check the examples that may apply.

_____ Saying "If you don't take a bath, nobody will like you."
_____ Laughing at a resident who has trouble speaking.
_____ Referring visitors' questions to the nurse.
_____ Feeding a patient who is refusing to eat.
_____ Refusing to give a medication prepared by the nurse.

OBSERVING, REPORTING, AND RECORDING

You have orders to assist Jim Adams to walk in the hallway. When you return the resident to his bed, you say, "You did a good job, Mr. Adams." He responds, "I'm not Mr. Adams. I'm Mr. Brown." Is it necessary to report this to the nurse? Explain your answer.

_____

_____

_____

_____

_____

_____

_____

_____

EXPLORE MEDIALINK

Check out www.prenhall.com/grubbs for additional chapter-specific interactive study and review activities.

4

RESTORATIVE CARE: PROMOTING RESIDENT INDEPENDENCE

OBJECTIVES

1. Explain the meaning of rehabilitation and restorative care.
2. List the members of the rehabilitation team.
3. Describe six rehabilitation departments.
4. Explain the purpose of assistive equipment.
5. Identify the principles of restorative care.
6. List six guidelines for restorative care.
7. Identify ten restorative measures and six restorative programs.
8. List four guidelines to promote wellness.

VOCABULARY

The following words or terms will help you to understand this chapter:

Rehabilitation
Restorative care
Independence

Mobility
Prosthesis
Complication

Ambulate
Health

This chapter provides a brief overview of rehabilitation and restorative care. It identifies programs and techniques that are described in more detail in later chapters. Because restorative care is the central theme of this textbook, it is introduced early. This allows you to keep the principles of restorative care in mind throughout the text.

Rehabilitation is a method used to assist a person to achieve and maintain function at the highest possible level of independence. It also addresses the residents' emotions and the effects of problems and unmet needs. Rehabilitation is one of the best tools available to improve the quality of life.

INTRODUCTION TO REHABILITATION AND RESTORATIVE CARE

Restorative care brings rehabilitation into the total care of the resident. All daily activities are carried out with a focus on independence and the quality of the resident's life. Every staff member must be committed to meeting the challenge of assisting the resident, who may be struggling to cope with many problems. As a nursing assistant, you will be challenged to use enthusiasm, empathy, patience, and all your other emotional strengths. In return, your reward will be the joy and satisfaction of knowing you are making a significant difference in the resident's life.

Rehabilitation may be needed by any resident who has an impairment or a disability that causes a decrease in the ability to carry out daily activities. For example, a resident who has had a stroke might need rehabilitation in walking, talking, or self-care. Accidents, surgery, illness, or amputation might also create a need for rehabilitation.

Restorative care is the nursing care that assists each resident to function at the highest possible level of independence. All nursing care should be provided in a restorative manner that takes into consideration the culture and individual needs of each resident.

Promoting Independence

Independence means being able to care for yourself and being in control of your life. It means freedom and making your own decisions.

Of all life's gifts, independence is one of the most treasured. When the need for independence is not met, the resident may become angry, depressed, or demanding. How would you feel if someone else had to help you bathe, dress, and go to the bathroom?

You can help promote the residents' independence by allowing them to make their own choices. Encourage them to perform as much of their own personal care as possible.

OBRA Requirements

The Omnibus Budget Reconciliation Act (OBRA) requires that all health care facilities provide rehabilitation services. A rehabilitation plan must be prepared identifying the resident's needs and problems. The purpose of these requirements is to ensure that residents attain the highest possible quality of life with no decrease in the ability to perform ADLs.

THE REHABILITATION TEAM

The rehabilitation team is a group of people who work together to meet the resident's needs. The center of the rehabilitation team is the resident and the resident's family. The nursing assistant is an important member of the rehabilitation team. Other members of the team include doctors, nurses, physical therapists, occupational therapists, speech therapists, social workers, activity directors, and members of the clergy. All members of the health care team belong to the rehabilitation team.

REHABILITATION DEPARTMENTS

Every department in the long-term care facility might be called a rehabilitation department because all are concerned with keeping the resident in the best possible health. However, those that provide direct care to the resident have the greatest responsibility.

Nursing Department

The role of the nursing department in rehabilitation and restorative care is introduced in Chapter 1 and continues to be emphasized in every chapter of this textbook. Nurses and nursing assistants provide restorative nursing care whenever they are working with the residents. The members of the nursing department extend the efforts of other rehabilitation departments into the daily lives of the residents. The role of the nursing assistant is discussed later in this chapter.

Physical Therapy Department

The physical therapist and physical therapy assistant help the resident strengthen muscles and regain physical independence. Their responsibilities include evaluating and helping residents to regain muscle strength and **mobility** (ability to move). They also measure, fit, and help residents to use a **prosthesis** (an artificial body part). Physical therapists instruct residents in the use of canes, walkers, and crutches (see Figure 4-1 ■).

Occupational Therapy Department

The primary role of the occupational therapist is to help the resident perform ADLs. This might involve relearning previous skills or developing new ones. The therapist recommends equipment that can help the resident to function with a disability.

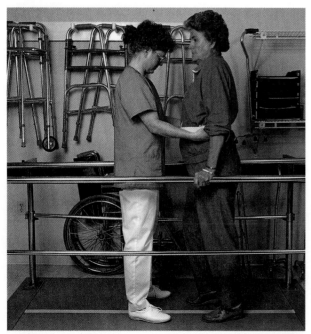

FIGURE 4-1 ■ The physical therapist helps the resident to learn to walk again.

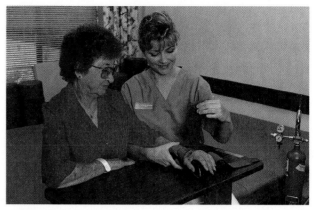

FIGURE 4-2 ■ The occupational therapist helps the resident to apply a hand splint.

For example, a resident who has a weak arm might need a splint to keep the hand in a normal position (see Figure 4-2 ■).

Speech Therapy Department

The speech therapist works with the resident who has a communication problem. Speech therapy involves planning and directing the treatment of residents whose ability to speak has been impaired. The speech therapist also works with residents who have hearing loss and residents with swallowing disorders.

Social Services Department

The social worker provides counseling to help the resident and the family adjust to the changes in their lives. Changes in health, independence, and living arrangements are upsetting, not only to the resident but to the family as well. The social worker helps them to work through their emotions and find ways to cope. Social services also helps the family to work out financial problems and provides information about community resources that are available.

Activities Department

The activity director and activity assistants provide programs that help the residents to socialize, keep busy, and feel worthwhile. They plan daily activities such as exercises, crafts, movies, shopping, and other outside trips. They meet with the residents to identify activities that will be of benefit and interest.

The activity department may post notices that indicate the date, weather, and special events that are planned. They help the residents celebrate birthdays and other holidays.

Other Departments

The responsibility of other departments in rehabilitation is discussed in later chapters. Although each department has specific responsibilities, their activities often overlap.

ASSISTIVE EQUIPMENT

Assistive equipment is the equipment that is used to help the resident adjust to a disability and function as independently as possible. A cane is an example of assistive equipment. A person with a weak leg uses a cane to assist in walking.

One type of assistive equipment is a prosthetic device that replaces or assists a body part to perform its function. Eyeglasses, false teeth, and artificial limbs are all examples of prosthetic devices.

There are many types of assistive equipment. Some are complicated and expensive; others are simple and easy to use. A straw is assistive equipment when you use it to drink milk out of a carton. It can provide independence for the resident who has difficulty holding a glass.

Wheelchairs, one of the most common pieces of assistive equipment, come in all shapes and sizes. Some are small, lightweight, and easily folded for transporting. Others recline and have headrests. There are electric wheelchairs for ease and convenience. There is also assistive equipment available for automobiles. These types of equipment increase the mobility of people who might be dependent on others for transportation (see Figure 4-3 ■).

These are only a few examples of assistive equipment and prosthetic devices. New equipment is being developed continually. It is the responsibility of the rehabilitation team to be aware of available equipment and to teach the resident how to use it. The nursing assistant must be familiar with the equipment and encourage the resident to use it (see Figure 4-4 ■). Be sure to report broken or defective equipment to the nurse promptly.

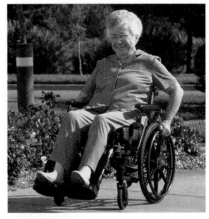

FIGURE 4-3 ■ Wheelchairs increase mobility and promote independence.

PRINCIPLES OF RESTORATIVE CARE

Restorative care requires commitment, thoughtful planning, and an understanding of the rehabilitation process. There are certain principles that will help you to practice restorative care.

* Treat the whole person.
* Start rehabilitation early.
* Stress ability, not disability.
* Encourage activity.
* Maintain a restorative attitude.

Treat the Whole Person

Rehabilitation is directed toward the needs of the whole person. It is not enough to treat only the physical needs; a person also has mental, emotional, social, sexual, and spiritual needs. When a person becomes ill, all those needs are affected and must be met in an individual manner.

Start Rehabilitation Early

Rehabilitation should begin at the first sign of illness or on admission to a health care facility. Early rehabilitation helps to prevent complications. A **complication** is an additional problem that results from a disease or another condition. Early rehabilitation also provides a positive approach that is encouraging to the resident. The fact that rehabilitation has begun increases the resident's self-esteem and lessens the chance of depression.

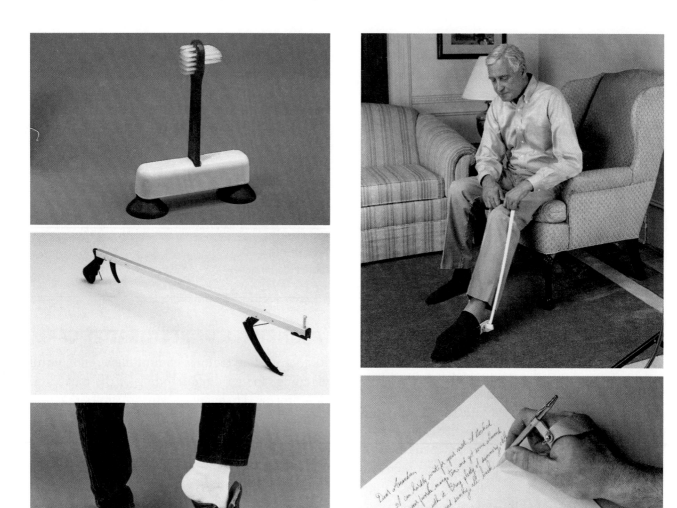

FIGURE 4-4 ■ There are many types of assistive equipment. *Sammons, Preston, Rolyan–U.S.A.*

Stress Ability, Not Disability

Restorative care emphasizes what the resident can do rather than what he or she cannot do. A person with a disability may be focused on the disability and give up many activities for fear of failure or embarrassment. A resident with a new disability may be depressed. Encourage the resident to perform ADLs to the best of his or her ability. The resident always should be encouraged to be as independent as possible.

Encourage Activity

It is important to encourage the resident to be active. Activity strengthens the mind and the body; inactivity weakens it. Activity improves circula-tion, digestion, elimination, and mobility. It helps prevent complications, increases mental alertness, and helps prevent depression (see Figure 4-5 ■). The active resident will be more independent and will have increased self-esteem. Independence motivates the resident to be active, and your praise and encouragement will help. Remember to watch for signs of fatigue and encourage rest periods between activities.

Maintain a Restorative Attitude

A restorative attitude includes positive feelings and beliefs. To be successful in providing restorative care, you must believe in its importance and in the resident's need for this care. You must believe that

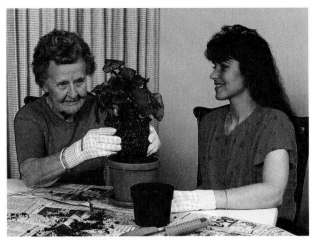

FIGURE 4-5 ■ Activity increases mental alertness and helps prevent depression.

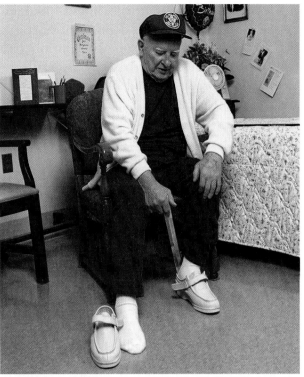

FIGURE 4-6 ■ Encourage the use of assistive equipment.

GUIDELINES

RESTORATIVE CARE

- Understand the resident's abilities and disabilities.
- Protect the resident's safety to make him or her feel more secure.
- Listen to the resident and be aware of his or her fears.
- Maintain a positive attitude.
- Encourage the use of assistive equipment (see Figure 4-6 ■) and check with the nurse to make sure that you know how to use the equipment correctly.
- Encourage the resident's involvement in restorative programs.
- Offer choices and encourage the resident to make decisions.
- Encourage family participation and support their efforts to help.
- Keep directions simple—one step at a time.
- Be consistent—do a task the same way every time, all the time.
- Arrange furniture and belongings for independence.
- Allow the resident to function independently with as little assistance as possible.
- Allow time—don't rush.
- Watch for signs of fatigue, exhaustion, or frustration and assist as necessary.
- Never scold or humiliate.
- Praise even the smallest effort.

restorative care will provide a better life for the resident. The resident can be influenced by your attitude, whatever it may be.

Positive feelings such as empathy, sensitivity, and patience contribute to a restorative attitude. Empathy, the ability to think how you would feel if you were the resident, helps you to understand the resident's feelings. Being in tune with the resident's feelings can mean the difference between success and failure. Relearning takes time, so patience is necessary to prevent frustration.

THE ROLE OF THE NURSING ASSISTANT IN RESTORATIVE CARE

Because nursing assistants provide most of the direct care of residents, they have many opportunities to use restorative measures. You can provide emotional support by following the principles of restorative care. Your support, praise, and encouragement contribute to the resident's sense of accomplishment. Learn to perform all your duties in a restorative manner. For example, while a resident is slowly dressing herself and buttoning her own blouse, you can be doing something else, like making the bed. That way, neither of you feels rushed or frustrated. Encourage family participation. You might ask the resident's daughter if she'd like to brush her mother's hair. This kind of activity benefits everyone. The guidelines for restorative care will help you provide nursing care in a restorative manner.

RESTORATIVE MEASURES AND PROGRAMS

Restorative measures are used to provide resident care and promote independence. These measures should be used seven days a week, 24 hours a day, whenever resident care is being provided.

Restorative programs are developed to meet the needs of residents who have difficulty performing ADLs. The purpose of each program is to promote independence and to enable the resident to perform the activities with as little assistance as possible. It is important to remember that a program must be adapted for each individual. The program then becomes a part of the resident's plan of care. All restorative care revolves around this plan.

Personal Hygiene and Grooming Program

This program helps the resident to meet hygiene and grooming needs independently. It includes such activities as bathing, mouth care, hair care, and dressing. Being unable to perform these simple, yet necessary, procedures causes distress. Personal hygiene and grooming are discussed in more detail in Chapter 13.

Restorative Dining Program

The restorative dining program is designed to help residents who are unable to feed themselves. The use of assistive equipment, learning new skills, and relearning old ones help the resident return to independent dining. Know which equipment to use. For example, the plate guard or scoop plate shown in Figure 4-7 ■ is helpful to a resident who can use only one arm. The restorative dining program is discussed in more detail in Chapter 15.

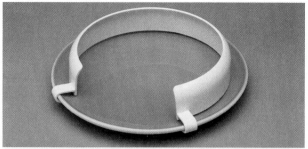
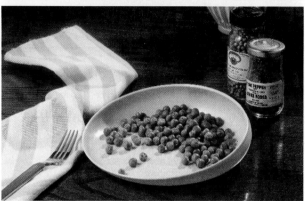
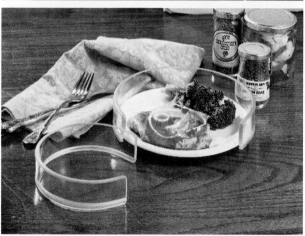

FIGURE 4-7 ■ Assistive equipment for independent dining. *Sammons, Preston, Rolyan–U.S.A.*

Bowel and Bladder Program

This program helps residents who are unable to control urine and bowel movements. The loss of the ability to control these body functions can be overwhelming to the resident and his or her family. It can cause physical, emotional, and social problems. The bowel and bladder program is discussed in more detail in Chapter 17.

Range-of-Motion Exercise Program

Restorative exercise programs help the resident who has limited mobility. Exercise benefits every

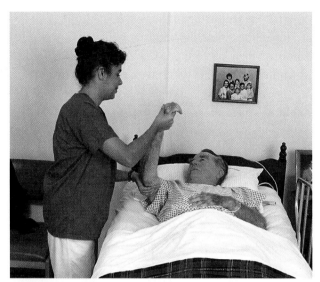

FIGURE 4-8 ■ Range-of-motion exercises help to prevent complications.

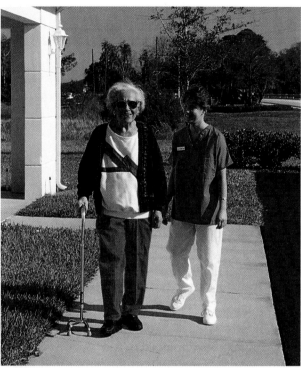

FIGURE 4-9 ■ Ambulation helps the resident to maintain independence.

system of the body. A resident who has had a stroke, broken bone, or paralysis will benefit from an exercise program.

Range-of-motion is a program in which the resident is encouraged to move and exercise. Exercise maintains muscle strength and prevents the joints from getting stiff. If the resident is not able to do the exercises without assistance, you must help (see Figure 4-8 ■). However, encouraging the resident's independent exercise will help to regain and maintain function. Range-of-motion and other exercise programs are discussed in more detail in Chapter 11.

Ambulation Program

The word **ambulate** means to walk. The purpose of this program is to increase or maintain the resident's ability to walk. It is hard to stay emotionally healthy and socially involved if you cannot walk. Ambulation helps keep the resident mobile and independent. The goal is to have the resident walk with as little assistance as possible (see Figure 4-9 ■). The ambulation program is addressed in more detail in Chapter 11.

Communication Program for the Sight-, Hearing-, and/or Speech-Impaired

Residents who have an impairment in sight, hearing, and/or speech may have difficulty communi-

cating. It can be frightening if you cannot see or hear what is happening. Being unable to put fears, needs, and concerns into words is very frustrating. There are special techniques to use when working with these individuals. Communicating with the sight-, hearing-, and/or speech-impaired resident is discussed in more detail in Chapter 19.

PROMOTION OF WELLNESS

The World Health Organization (WHO) defines health as follows: "**Health** is a state of complete physical, mental, and social well-being, not merely absence of disease and infirmity." Wellness means adapting to change in order to live life fully. Health and wellness are not the same. A person can have an illness and still have wellness. For example, the person with diabetes has a chronic illness that prevents good health. But wellness can be achieved by living the best life that is possible with the disease (see Figure 4-10 ■).

Wellness is physical, mental, emotional, social, and spiritual. It requires a positive attitude and a high degree of self-esteem and self-respect. The

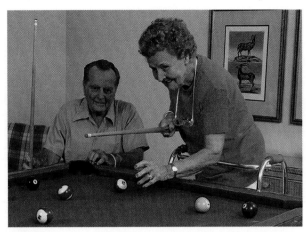

FIGURE 4-10 ■ Wellness is living life to the fullest.

It is very important that you help the resident to attain wellness, but do not forget your own wellness. You can apply to your life many of the guidelines to promote wellness. If you have a positive attitude and are moving toward wellness, you can better assist the residents to move in that direction.

ability to handle stress is important. Wellness is influenced by lifestyle and environment. Rehabilitation and restorative care help promote wellness. Restorative measures that increase self-esteem and independence also increase wellness. It is your responsibility as a nursing assistant to be concerned always with the wellness of the resident.

GUIDELINES

PROMOTE WELLNESS

- Remain aware of the resident's health.
- Encourage activity.
- Ensure personal hygiene.
- Use safety measures.
- Follow infection control policies.
- Assist with nutrition and fluids.
- Encourage rest, relaxation, and sleep.
- Provide continuity of care.

CHAPTER HIGHLIGHTS

1. Rehabilitation is a method used to assist a person to achieve and maintain function at the highest possible level of independence.
2. Restorative care assists the resident to maintain independence.
3. The center of the rehabilitation team is the resident and the resident's family.
4. Physical therapy helps the resident regain muscle strength and mobility.
5. Occupational therapy helps the resident perform the activities of daily living.
6. Rehabilitation is directed to the needs of the whole person.
7. Nursing assistants have many opportunities to use restorative measures as they care for residents.
8. The resident should be encouraged to function independently with as little assistance as possible.
9. Restorative measures that increase the resident's self-esteem increase wellness.
10. Work to achieve wellness in your own life.

VOCABULARY REVIEW

Fill in the blank with the vocabulary term that best completes the sentence.

1. _____ means being able to care for yourself and being in control of your life.

2. An artificial body part is called a/an _____.

3. A/An _____ is an additional problem that results from a disease or another condition.

4. "A state of complete physical, mental, and social well-being, not merely absence of disease and infirmity" is the World Health Organization's definition of _____.

5. To _____ means to walk.

6. The ability to move is _____.

7. _____ is nursing care that assists each resident to function at the highest possible level of independence.

8. A _____ are activities of personal care and hygiene performed daily.

9. Caring for the _____ includes meeting the physical, mental, emotional, social, sexual, and spiritual needs.

10. _____ is understanding how another person feels.

CHECK YOUR UNDERSTANDING

The following questions cover the highlights of this chapter. Choose the best answer for each question.

1. The method used to bring a resident back to as nearly normal function as possible is called
   A. mobility
   B. prosthesis
   C. complication
   D. rehabilitation

2. What department is responsible for evaluating and assisting with muscle strength and mobility?
   A. speech therapy
   B. physical therapy
   C. social services
   D. activities

3. The speech therapist is responsible for assisting residents who have
   A. speech problems
   B. hearing loss
   C. swallowing problems
   D. all of the above

4. A resident who is in an ambulation program seems to tire easily. What is your best response?
   A. encourage her to walk as far as possible.
   B. encourage her to spend a lot of time in bed.
   C. encourage her to rest when necessary.
   D. encourage her to ask for more help.

5. A resident who is relearning to dress himself is very slow, and you have a lot of work to do. What is the best way to handle the situation?
   A. dress him yourself and go on to some other chore.
   B. do some other task while he is dressing and help only if necessary.
   C. leave him alone to dress himself and check back in an hour.
   D. tell him to hurry because you have a lot of work to do.

AGE-SPECIFIC TIP

Changes of aging may interfere with the independence of elderly residents. Make positive comments about even the smallest accomplishments of the resident to encourage independence.

CULTURALLY SENSITIVE TIP

Cultural roles may determine the amount of family participation in the resident's care. Support the family's efforts to help, and accept their decisions.

EFFECTIVE PROBLEM SOLVING

A resident who is in a restorative personal hygiene program is trying to bathe herself. You observe that she did not wash under her arms or cleanse properly. You say to her, "Mrs. Jones, you're not cleaning yourself very well and you've skipped certain areas altogether. I'll finish bathing you now." Was your communication appropriate? If not, what would have been more appropriate?

_____

_____

_____

_____

_____

_____

_____

_____

_____

_____

_____

INTERPERSONAL COMMUNICATION

Which statements best reflect a restorative approach? Check the examples that are appropriate.

_____ "You've managed some of the buttons on your shirt, and that's the hardest part."

_____ "You've buttoned your shirt crooked, and I'll have to do it right."

_____ "You do what you can by yourself and I'll help if necessary."

_____ "You're not well enough to dress yourself."

OBSERVING, REPORTING, AND RECORDING

The nursing assistant observes that a resident is having difficulty feeding himself. He can use only one hand and accidentally is pushing most of the food off the plate. What piece of assistive equipment would be most helpful to the resident's independence?

_____

_____

_____

_____

_____

_____

_____

_____

_____

_____

_____

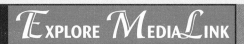

$\mathcal{I}$NFECTION CONTROL

$\mathcal{O}$BJECTIVES

1. Explain the purpose of infection control.
2. Explain the difference between pathogens and nonpathogens.
3. List five ways microorganisms are spread.
4. Identify five signs and symptoms of a localized infection.
5. List eight guidelines for aseptic practices.
6. Explain the importance of handwashing.
7. List nine guidelines for standard precautions.
8. Identify and describe three types of transmission-based precautions.
9. List four guidelines for using a restorative approach to isolation.

10. Identify the cause, methods of transmission, prevention practices, and legal issues related to HIV.
11. Briefly describe hepatitis A, B, and C.
12. Explain the purpose of the bloodborne pathogens standard.
13. Identify the symptoms and describe the treatment of tuberculosis.
14. Describe three ways that anthrax pathogens may enter the body.
15. Perform the procedures described in this chapter.

$\mathcal{V}$OCABULARY

The following words or terms will help you to understand this chapter:

Infection
Communicable disease
Microorganisms
Nonpathogens
Pathogens
Normal flora
Susceptible

Asepsis
Disinfection
Sterile
Contaminate
Standard precautions
Transmission-based
  precautions

Bloodborne pathogen
HIV (human immunodeficiency virus) infection
AIDS (acquired immune deficiency syndrome)
Biohazardous medical waste
Bioterrorism

This chapter describes the dynamics of infection and immune function and provides guidelines and procedures for maintaining infection control. Bioterrorism is also addressed.

𝒯HE PURPOSE OF INFECTION CONTROL

The purpose of infection control is to prevent the spread of infection and disease in a health care facility. **Infection** is a disease caused by harmful microorganisms (germs). A disease or infection that spreads easily from one person to another is a **communicable disease.** Preventing the spread of infection is the responsibility of all members of the health care team. It is a primary responsibility of nursing assistants because they provide most of the hands-on care of residents. Infection control reduces the risk to residents, visitors, employees, and their families. Each facility has developed policies and procedures to reduce the spread of infection. It is your responsibility to know the policies and procedures of the facility in which you work. In this chapter, you will learn general infection control practices and procedures.

𝒯HE BODY'S RESPONSE TO MICROORGANISMS

Microorganisms

Microorganisms (microbes) are small living things that cannot be seen without the aid of a microscope. Microorganisms commonly are called "germs." They can cause infection and disease by entering the body and changing cells. We are surrounded by microorganisms. Remember that while microorganisms are too small to be seen without a microscope, they are always present on our skin, and in food, air, and water (see Figure 5-1 ■). Some microorganisms are harmful, and some are helpful.

Microorganisms that do not cause an infection are called **nonpathogens.** Some are useful, as in the creation of cheese, yogurt, and alcohol for example. Even penicillin (a medication) is created by the use of nonpathogens.

Microorganisms that are harmful and cause infection are called **pathogens.** Because the signs of

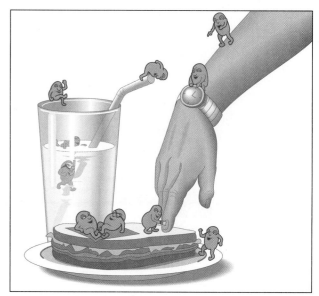

FIGURE 5-1 ■ We are surrounded by microorganisms.

infection do not occur immediately upon contact with pathogens, it is easy to forget how harmful they can be. The danger of pathogens would be much more real to us if they were visible.

Normal flora are microorganisms that are necessary for good health and are harmless when found in certain locations. Normal flora exist on the skin to help protect it from infection. The intestine also contains normal flora that help to break down food particles. Normal flora can become harmful and cause infection if they enter another part of the body. For example, the normal flora of the intestine can cause infection if they enter the urinary system or an open wound. Figure 5-2 ■ illustrates the differences between pathogens, nonpathogens, and normal flora.

Conditions That Promote the Growth of Microorganisms

Microorganisms live in humans, animals, plants, water, food, and dirt. All microorganisms need water and food, and most of them need oxygen. They thrive in a dark, warm (50° to 110° Fahrenheit), moist area. It is no surprise that humans are infected so easily because there are many areas of the body that provide excellent conditions for the growth of microorganisms. Germs grow best in the body's dark, warm, moist areas.

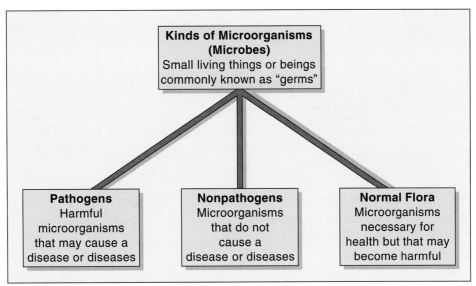

FIGURE 5-2 ■ The differences between pathogens, nonpathogens, and normal flora.

Spread of Microorganisms

Microorganisms enter and leave the human body through the eyes, nose, mouth, rectum, vagina, and urethra. They also enter and exit by way of the bloodstream and through mucous membranes, and broken skin. When a microorganism leaves the body, it can be transmitted to another person. Microorganisms spread in the following ways:

- Direct contact: touching the infected person
- Indirect contact: touching an object that has been in contact with pathogens
- Droplet: inhaling fine drops of moisture caused by talking, sneezing, or coughing
- Airborne: inhaling pathogens that are floating in the air
- Vehicle: entering the body in food, water, blood or medication that contains pathogens.

Infection can be spread by a carrier. A carrier is a person who has the pathogen but has no signs or symptoms of infection. The carrier can give the pathogen to others who may become infected.

The Immune System

The body's immune system attacks invading microorganisms and helps protect against infection. We are always in contact with pathogens. However, because the immune system is working, an infection does not always develop. Poor nutrition, lack of rest, stress, chronic illness, and chemotherapy (a treatment for cancer) can weaken the immune system and make the resident less able to fight infection. A weakened immune system makes a person susceptible to disease. **Susceptible** means having an increased risk of developing an infection.

SIGNS AND SYMPTOMS OF INFECTION

An infection may be localized (located in one part of the body), or generalized (affecting the entire body). Signs and symptoms of localized infection are redness, swelling, heat, drainage, and pain. Signs and symptoms of generalized infection are fever, headache, fatigue, increased pulse and respirations, nausea, and vomiting.

It is important to observe for and recognize signs and symptoms of infection and to report them immediately to the nurse. The resident's verbal complaints are as important as the signs that you can see.

PREVENTING THE SPREAD OF INFECTION

Asepsis

Asepsis is the absence of pathogens. When asepsis is practiced, clean procedures prevent the spread of pathogens and lower the risk of infection. When something is clean, it is free of pathogens.

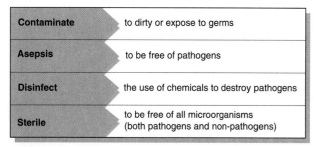

Contaminate	to dirty or expose to germs
Asepsis	to be free of pathogens
Disinfect	the use of chemicals to destroy pathogens
Sterile	to be free of all microorganisms (both pathogens and non-pathogens)

FIGURE 5-3 ■ Infection-control terms.

Disinfection is the use of chemicals to destroy many or all pathogens on objects. Disinfectants include Lysol™, bleach, hydrogen peroxide, and alcohol, among others.

An object is **sterile** when it is free of *all* microorganisms. Sterile items always will be in a package that is sealed. If the seal is broken, the items inside no longer are sterile. The difference between "clean" and "sterile" may be demonstrated by using gloves as an example. Sterile gloves are individually wrapped in sealed packages. The gloves in an open box are clean, but they are not sterile.

A sterile procedure requires sterile gloves. Because the hands cannot be sterilized, they must be covered to prevent contaminating a sterile area. To **contaminate** means to dirty or to expose to microbes. Although you may not perform sterile procedures, you may assist the nurse. Figure 5-3 ■ illustrates the differences between asepsis, disinfection, sterility, and contamination.

Aseptic Practices

Aseptic practices reduce the spread of infection by keeping everything as clean as possible. Any cleaning task you perform is asepsis. Everyone should follow aseptic practices at all times. (See the guidelines for aseptic practices.)

Handling Sharps

Infection can be spread by contaminated sharp objects such as needles, razors, and surgical instruments. Needle sticks are a source of infection in health care. Although nursing assistants do not handle needles and syringes as frequently as nurses do, there is still a risk. Handle all sharps carefully and dispose of them promptly after use.

GUIDELINES

ASEPTIC PRACTICES

- Always clean from the cleanest area to the dirtiest area.
- Use gloves and other protective equipment when appropriate.
- Wash your hands before and after giving resident care.
- Wash your hands before handling food; after using the toilet, sneezing, coughing, or blowing your nose; and before and after eating.
- Do not handle contact lenses in patient care areas.
- Change your uniform immediately if it becomes wet or contaminated.
- Keep fingernails short and avoid wearing artificial nails.
- Cover your nose and mouth when coughing, sneezing, or blowing your nose
- Don't come to work if you have a fever, a cold, or diarrhea.
- Report all open sores on your body or on a resident's body to the nurse.
- Dispose of tissues properly.
- Place unused personal care items in the bedside table and do not share them with another resident or return them to supply storage.
- Carry linens and other items away from your uniform.
- Never put linen on the floor.
- If clean linen touches the floor, it must be placed in the soiled linen hamper.
- Don't take supplies or equipment from one resident's room to another's.
- Don't place bedpans, urinals, soiled linen, or other soiled items on the overbed table. The overbed table is a clean area.
- Wipe stethoscope earpieces and diaphragm with alcohol before and after use.
- Take dirty or contaminated items to the dirty utility room.
- Wash and dry soiled mattresses when changing the bed.
- Do not store food in the refrigerator with lab specimens or blood.

GUIDELINES

HANDLING SHARPS

- Dispose of needles, syringes, and other sharp objects promptly.
- Do not bend, break, or recap needles.
- Wear gloves when handling sharp objects such as razors.
- Handle sharps carefully to avoid cutting or sticking yourself.
- Dispose of sharps in a labeled, puncture-proof container (see Figure 5-4 ■).
- Do not force objects into the sharps container.
- Notify the nurse when the sharps container is full.
- Keep the sharps container near the area of use.

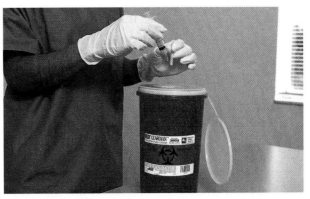

FIGURE 5-4 ■ Dispose of needles and syringes carefully.

A REMINDER

ALWAYS WASH YOUR HANDS

- Before and after eating
- After using the bathroom
- After combing your hair
- Before and after removing gloves, handling contact lenses, using lip balm, or applying makeup
- Before handling food
- After coughing, sneezing, or blowing your nose
- After smoking
- Before and after giving care to each resident
- After handling soiled items

*H*ANDWASHING

Handwashing is the most important procedure used to prevent the spread of infection. Proper handwashing protects the residents, visitors, yourself, other staff members, and your families. The Centers for Disease Control (CDC) recommends washing the hands for at least 15 seconds. Your instructor will teach you the accepted time frame in your area. (See the procedure for handwashing on page 46.)

Remember: Just because you can't see the pathogens doesn't mean they aren't there!

Use of Hand Sanitizers

In addition to regular handwashing the CDC recommends the use of alcohol-based handrubs (sanitizers). These products are easy to use and fast-acting. When using an alcohol-based handrub, apply the product to the palm of one hand and rub the hands together, covering all surfaces of the hands and fingers. Continue to rub all surfaces of your hands until they are completely dry. Hands should always be washed with soap and water if they are visibly soiled or have had contact with blood, body fluids, or body substances. They should also be washed periodically throughout the day in addition to the use of handrubs.

*I*SOLATION PRECAUTIONS

As a result of research, infection control practices are continually changing. It is important that you be aware of the most current information. A few years ago, the CDC established two levels of isolation precautions to be observed in health care. These levels include standard precautions and transmission-based precautions.

Standard Precautions

Standard precautions are procedures that are used in the care of *all* residents to protect the health care worker from exposure to blood, body fluids, and body substances. These precautions are used with all residents whether or not they have an infectious disease. Standard precautions should be used any time there is a possibility of contact with blood, body fluids, and or body substances. This includes

PROCEDURE

Handwashing

1. Remove your watch or push it out of the way.
2. Stand back so that your uniform doesn't touch the sink.
3. Turn the faucet on and adjust the water to a warm temperature.
4. Wet your hands and wrists thoroughly by holding them under running water. Hold your hands lower than your elbows, with the fingertips down (see Figure 5-5A ■), so that water runs off your fingertips.
5. Apply soap to your hands and work up a lather.
6. Wash your hands and wrists vigorously for at least 15 seconds. Apply friction to all surfaces of your hands as follows:
   a. Wash the palms and backs of your hands. Do not forget the outside surface of your thumbs.
   b. Interlace your fingers and thumbs (see Figure 5-5B ■). Move your hands back and forth to clear between your fingers.
   c. Wash your wrists (see Figure 5-5C ■) and lower arms 3 or 4 inches above the wrists using rotating movements.
7. Clean around the cuticles and under the fingernails.
8. Rinse well, starting above your wrists and ending with your fingertips, keeping your hands lower than your elbows, with your fingertips down.
9. Dry your hands thoroughly, using a separate paper towel for each hand. Discard the towels.
10. Use a paper towel to turn the water off (see Figure 5-5D ■) and open the door. Discard the paper towel.

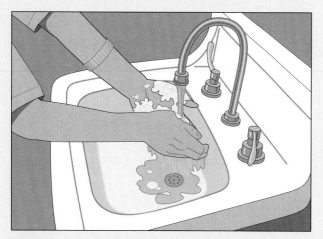

A Hold hands lower than elbows.

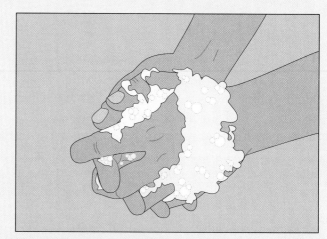

B Interlace fingers and thumbs.

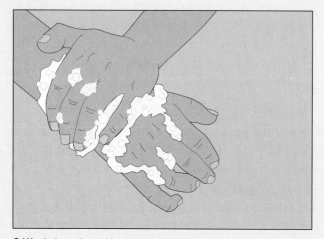

C Wash the wrists with a rotating motion.

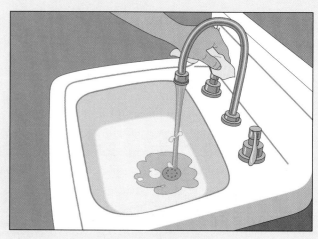

D Turn the water off with a dry paper towel.

FIGURE 5-5 ■ Handwashing procedure.

GUIDELINES

STANDARD PRECAUTIONS

- Use standard precautions when caring for all residents.
- Wash your hands after accidental contact with blood, body fluids, secretions, excretions (except sweat), nonintact skin, or mucous membranes.
- Wash your hands before applying gloves and after removing gloves.
- Wear gloves when you may be touching blood, body fluids, secretions, excretions (except sweat), nonintact skin, or mucous membranes.
- Wear gowns when your uniform might come into contact with blood, body fluids, secretions, excretions (except sweat), nonintact skin, or mucous membranes.
- Wear masks, face shields, and protective eye wear when contact with droplets or splashes of blood, body fluids, secretions, or excretions is possible.
- If a sprayer is used to rinse bedpans or urinals, wear gloves, gown, mask, and goggles to protect yourself from splashes.
- Handle soiled equipment and supplies in a manner that prevents contact with skin, mucous membranes, or clothing. Clean and disinfect soiled equipment according to facility policy.
- Treat all soiled linen as infectious.
- Carefully dispose of sharp objects in the proper container.

contact with broken skin or mucous membranes (thin sheets of tissue that line body openings). Follow the guidelines for standard precautions to protect yourself and others from infection.

Transmission-based Precautions

Transmission-based precautions include procedures that are used in the care of residents who are contagious or are suspected of being infected with communicable diseases. Three types of transmission-based precautions include contact, droplet, and airborne precautions. These precautions are used in addition to standard precautions.

Contact precautions reduce the risk of the transmission of infection by direct contact (between the infected person and another) or by indirect contact with surfaces or items that have been contaminated by the infected person. Some diseases that are transmitted by contact include skin or wound infections, scabies, enteric (intestinal) infections, impetigo, conjunctivitis (pink eye), shingles, and hepatitis A (see Figure 5-6 ■).

Droplet precautions reduce the risk of infections by pathogens that are carried in droplets of moisture. These droplets are exhaled when the infected person coughs, sneezes, sings, or talks. Diseases that are transmitted by droplets include pneumonia, influenza, meningitis, rubella (measles), mumps, streptococcal infections of the throat, and the common cold (see Figure 5-7 ■).

Airborne precautions reduce the risk of transmission of infection by pathogens that are carried in

CONTACT PRECAUTIONS

Visitors report to nursing station before entering room.

- *Patient Placement:* Private room (if not available, place patient with another patient with a similar microorganism but with no other infection).
- *Gloves:* Wear gloves when entering the room and for all contact with patient and patient items, equipment, and body fluids.
- *Gown:* Wear a gown when entering the room if it is anticipated that your clothing will have substantial contact with the patient, environmental surfaces, or items in the patient's room.

- *Masks and Eyewear:* Indicated if potential for exposure to infectious body material exists.
- *Handwashing:* After glove removal while ensuring that hands do not touch potentially contaminated environmental surfaces or items in the patient's room.
- *Transport:* Limit the movement and transport of the patient.
- *Patient-care Equipment:* When possible, dedicate the use of noncritical patient care equipment to a single patient.

Always Use Standard Precautions.

FIGURE 5-6 ■ Contact precautions.

DROPLET PRECAUTIONS

Visitors report to nursing station before entering room.

- *Patient Placement:* Private room (if not available, place patient in a room with a patient who has active infection with the same microorganism).
- *Gloves:* Must be worn when in contact with blood and body fluids.
- *Gowns:* Must be worn during procedures or situations where there will be exposure to body fluids, blood, draining wounds, or mucous membranes.
- *Masks and Eyewear:* In addition to *Standard Precautions,* **wear a mask when working within**

FIGURE 5-7 ■ Droplet precautions.

small droplets that remain suspended in the air after being exhaled and may be inhaled by others. Some diseases that may be transmitted by suspended droplets and that require airborne precautions are measles, chicken pox, shingles, and tuberculosis (see Figure 5-8 ■).

*P*ERSONAL PROTECTIVE EQUIPMENT AND SUPPLIES

Both standard precautions and transmission-based precautions require the appropriate use of gloves, gowns, masks, face shields, and protective eyewear, as indicated in each set of precautions, when there is a risk of exposure to blood, body fluids, secretions, excretions (except sweat), nonintact skin, or mucous

AIRBORNE PRECAUTIONS

Visitors report to nursing station before entering room.

- *Patient Placement:* Private room. Negative air pressure in relation to the surrounding areas. Keep doors closed at all times.
- *Gloves:* Same as for *Standard Precautions.*
- *Gown or Apron:* Same as for *Standard Precautions.*
- *Mask and Eyewear:* For known or suspected pulmonary tuberculosis: Mask N-95 (respirator) must be worn by all individuals prior to entering the room. For known or suspected airborne viral disease (for example, chicken pox or measles), a standard mask should be worn by any person entering the room unless the person is not suscepti-

FIGURE 5-8 ■ Airborne precautions.

3 feet of the patient (or when entering the patient's room).

- *Handwashing:* Hands must be washed before gloving and after gloves are removed.
- *Transport:* Limit the movement and transport of the patient from the room to essential purposes. If it is necessary to move the patient, minimize patient dispersal of droplets by masking the patient if possible.
- *Patient-care Equipment:* When using common equipment or items, they must be adequately cleaned and disinfected.

Always Use Standard Precautions.

GUIDELINES

TRANSMISSION-BASED PRECAUTIONS

- Always use standard precautions.
- Place the appropriate precaution sign on the door of the resident's room.
- Follow the instructions on the precautions sign.
- Wear gloves for all types of transmission-based precautions.
- Wear gowns, masks, and other personal protective equipment when appropriate.
- Wash your hands before gloving and after removing gloves.
- Discard protective equipment in the proper container.

---

ble to the disease. When possible, persons who are susceptible should not enter the room.

- *Handwashing:* Hands must be washed before gloving and after gloves are removed. Skin surfaces must be washed immediately and thoroughly when contaminated with body fluids or blood.
- *Patient Transport:* Limit the transport of the patient to essential purposes. If transport is necessary, place a mask on the patient if possible.
- *Patient-care Equipment:* When using equipment or items (stethoscope, thermometer), they must be adequately cleaned and disinfected before use by another patient.

Always Use Standard Precautions.

membranes. All personal protective equipment that is required in performing your job must be provided by your health care facility at no charge to the employee. Training for use of this equipment also must be provided by the facility. Guidelines and procedures follow that will help you learn how to use gloves, gowns, and masks. Facility policies and procedures may vary.

GUIDELINES

THE USE OF GLOVES

- Wear gloves any time there is a possibility of exposure to blood, body fluids, secretions, excretions (except sweat), nonintact skin, or mucous membranes.
- Always wash your hands before putting on new gloves and after removing gloves.
- Check for defects before putting on gloves.
- Avoid excessive stretching of gloves.
- Wear a clean pair of gloves for each resident and for each task.
- Do not wear gloves outside of the resident's room.
- Nonlatex gloves must be provided by the facility if you are allergic to latex.

GUIDELINES

THE REMOVAL OF GLOVES

- The outside surface of the glove is contaminated and should not touch your skin or any clean surface.
- The inside surface is considered clean.
- Remove the first glove with the gloved fingers of the other hand by grasping the glove 1 inch below the cuff on the outside and pulling it over your hand while turning it inside out (see Figure 5-9A ■).
- Place the ungloved middle and index fingers inside the cuff of the remaining glove (see Figure 5-9B ■).
- Carefully turn the cuff down, pulling the glove inside out and over the other glove as you remove it from your hand (see Figure 5-9B).
- Discard the gloves according to facility policy and wash your hands.

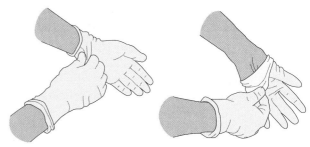

A Grasping the glove just below the cuff with the gloved fingers of the other hand, pull the glove over your hand while turning it inside out.

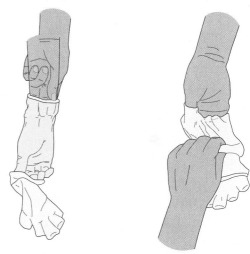

B Place the ungloved index and middle fingers inside the cuff of the glove, turning the cuff downward, pulling it inside out, as you remove it from your hand.

FIGURE 5-9 ■ Guidelines for removing gloves.

Use of Gloves

Although handwashing is very important for protection against infection, gloves provide additional protection. They must be checked for defects before they are used, and removal of gloves must be followed by thorough handwashing to ensure the most complete protection. (See the guidelines for the use of gloves and their removal.)

Use of Gowns and Masks

Disposable gowns and masks also may be necessary as indicated in the guidelines for standard precautions and guidelines for transmission-based precautions. The guidelines and procedures on pages 50 to 52 will instruct you in the use of gowns and masks.

GUIDELINES

THE USE OF DISPOSABLE GOWNS

- Gowns protect your clothing from pathogens.
- Wear a disposable gown any time there is a possibility that your uniform might come in contact with blood, body fluids, secretions, excretions (except sweat), nonintact skin, or mucous membranes.
- Gowns open at the back and have ties or adhesive strips at the waist and neck.
- The gown must cover your entire uniform.
- The gown must be changed immediately if it becomes damp.
- Ties at the neck of a gown are considered clean and are untied after glove removal and handwashing.
- The outside surface of the gown is contaminated.
- Do not wear gowns outside of the resident's room.

GUIDELINES

USE OF MASKS

- Masks prevent blood, body fluids, secretions, and excretions from getting into your mouth and nose. They also prevent microorganisms exhaled by the resident from entering your respiratory system.
- Protective eyewear or a face shield may be necessary with the mask.
- The mask must fit snugly over your mouth and nose without blocking your vision.
- The mask must be changed immediately if it becomes damp.
- The mask must be changed at least every 30 minutes.
- Do not touch the surface of the mask because microorganisms collect over the nose and mouth.
- Remove the mask by touching only the strings.
- Do not wear a mask outside of the resident's room.

PROCEDURE

Putting on a Gown

1. Wash your hands.
2. If you need to wear a mask, put it on first.
3. Let the clean gown unfold without touching any surface.
4. Slide your hands and arms through the sleeves.
5. Tie the neck ties.
6. Overlap the back of the gown.
7. Fasten the waist ties.
8. If gloves are required, put them on last. Pull them up over the cuffs of the gown (see Figure 5-10 ■).

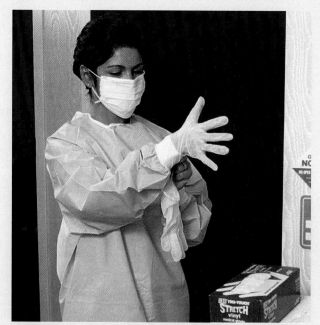

FIGURE 5-10 ■ Pull gloves up over the cuffs of the gown.

$\mathcal{P}$ROCEDURE

Removing a Gown

1. Untie the waist belt or ties.
2. If you are wearing gloves, remove them (see Figure 5-11A ■).
3. Wash your hands (see Figure 5-11B ■).
4. Untie the neck ties.
5. Pull the sleeve off by grasping each shoulder at the neck line (see Figure 5-11C ■).
   a. Do not contaminate your hands by touching the outside of the gown.
   b. Turn the sleeves inside out as you remove them from your arms (see Figure 5-11D ■).

6. Holding the gown away from your body by the inside of the shoulder seams, fold it inside out, bringing the shoulders together (see Figure 5-11E ■).
7. Roll the gown up with the inside out and discard (see Figure 5-11F ■).
8. Wash your hands (see Figure 5-11G ■).
9. If you are wearing a mask, remove it, touching only the strings, and wash your hands (see Figures 5-11H ■ and 5-11I ■).

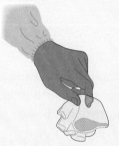

A Remove gloves.

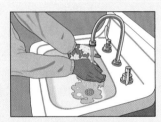

B Wash your hands.

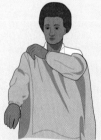

C Grasp each shoulder of gown near neck to remove sleeves.

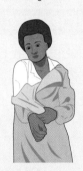

D As you remove sleeves, turn them inside out.

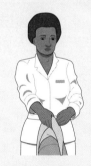

E Fold the gown inside out, holding it away from you.

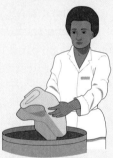

F Roll up the gown and discard it.

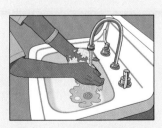

G Wash your hands.

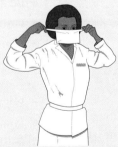

H If you are wearing a mask, remove it at this time.

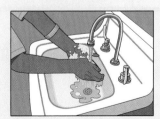

I Wash your hands.

FIGURE 5-11 ■ Preparing to leave an isolation room.

PROCEDURE

Putting on a Mask

Put on the mask before putting on the gown or gloves.

1. Wash your hands.
2. Holding the mask by the upper ties or ear loops, place it over your nose or mouth. Be sure the upper edge is under your glasses. Tie the upper strings at the back of your head or place the ear loops over your ears.
3. Be sure the lower edge of the mask covers your chin while you tie the bottom strings at the nape of your neck.
4. Form the top edge of the mask to your nose to prevent microorganisms from entering behind the mask.
5. Wash your hands.

Removing a Mask

1. Follow procedures to remove the gloves and gown before removing the mask.
2. Wash your hands. (Microorganisms can spread to your head and neck from your hands or from the gloves.)
3. Untie and discard the mask by touching only the strings. Untie the lower strings before untying the upper strings.
4. Bring the upper strings together as you remove the mask from your face.
5. Wash your hands after discarding the mask.

Changes in Isolation Procedures

Changes in infection control have led to the elimination of practices and procedures that are no longer necessary. The dishes, eating utensils, and trash of all residents are handled as if they are infectious; therefore, additional precautions are not needed for contagious residents. Melt-away bags and double-bagging of linen and trash are not necessary because all linen and trash are considered infectious.

Previously, reverse or protective isolation was used to protect residents who were at increased risk for infection. Because it was determined that these efforts were often ineffective, they were discontinued in most facilities. Always learn and follow the policies and procedures of the facility in which you work. If your facility requires the use of procedures that are not taught in this text, your employer will provide training for you.

USING A RESTORATIVE APPROACH TO ISOLATION

Isolation can affect the resident both physically and emotionally. It may cause him or her to become depressed and less motivated. Being isolated also can cause feelings of rejection and fear. The resident may feel "dirty," and his or her self-esteem may be affected. The resident may resent being confined and wish visitors and staff members could stay longer. A restorative approach to isolation can help to meet all the resident's needs. See the guidelines for a restorative approach to isolation.

GUIDELINES

A RESTORATIVE APPROACH TO ISOLATION

- Encourage self-care and independence.
- Listen attentively to the resident's fears and concerns.
- Use your communication skills to promote self-esteem and emotional well-being.
- Let the nurse know if the resident or family has questions you cannot answer.
- Be aware of your own feelings about isolation.
- Discuss your fears and concerns with the nurse.
- Learn to perform isolation procedures correctly.
- Maintain the resident's safety and answer call signals promptly.
- Help the family adjust to the insolation practices.
- Remind yourself and the resident that it is the pathogens that are being isolated, not the person.
- Spend as much time with the isolated resident as you would with any other resident (see Figure 5-12 ■).

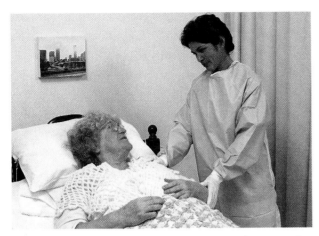

FIGURE 5-12 ■ Remind yourself and the resident that it is the pathogens that are being isolated and not the resident.

UNDERSTANDING INFECTIOUS DISEASES

A disease or infection that spreads easily from one person to another is called a "communicable disease." Of particular concern to health care workers are the diseases caused by **bloodborne pathogens** (disease-causing microorganisms found in blood, blood products, and body fluids that contain blood). HIV infection (AIDS), hepatitis B, and hepatitis C are examples of bloodborne pathogens. This chapter will also address tuberculosis and anthrax. While they are not bloodborne, they are infectious diseases of national concern.

HIV INFECTION (AIDS)

HIV (human immunodeficiency virus) infection is a disease that destroys the immune system and leaves the body unable to fight infection. **AIDS (acquired immune deficiency syndrome)** is the term used to describe the final stage of HIV infection AIDS.

The disease is caused by the HIV virus, which enters the bloodstream, where it continues to live and reproduce. The virus attacks and destroys cells in the immune system. The death of these cells leaves the body unable to fight other infections and diseases. Once a person is infected with HIV, even if there are no symptoms, he or she is contagious and can transmit the disease to someone else. Although the number of HIV infections and AIDS-related deaths appears to be leveling off in the United States, there is an epidemic of AIDS worldwide. In fact, it is the leading cause of death in some countries.

Risk Groups

A risk group includes people who are susceptible to a disease. The following is a list of risk groups for HIV:

- men who have sex with men
- injectable drug users
- sexual partners of persons infected with HIV
- babies of HIV-infected mothers
- people who receive blood transfusions
- hemophiliacs

Transmission

HIV usually is transmitted by

- sexual contact with an infected person
- HIV-contaminated needles and syringes
- an HIV-infected mother to the unborn baby
- transfusion of blood contaminated by HIV

Since 1985, all blood collected for transfusions is tested for evidence of the virus. If the blood tests positive for HIV, it is discarded. This practice has reduced the risk to those who receive blood transfusions or blood products.

How Contagious Is HIV?

It is not easy to get HIV. The virus is not airborne and cannot live long outside the human body. Every exposure does *not* result in infection. There is no evidence that HIV is spread by casual contact, toilet seats, mosquitoes, coughing, sneezing, or working or eating with HIV-infected persons.

Prevention

Because HIV is transmitted primarily by sexual contact, some changes in behavior must be made to stop its spread. People must remain aware of the danger of casual sex and of having multiple sex partners. The practice of "safe sex" with the use of condoms also helps to prevent the spread of HIV.

The safest behavior is to have a trusting relationship with only one sexual partner who is not HIV-infected.

The second most common way that HIV is spread is by using needles and syringes that are contaminated with the virus. Usually this type of transmission occurs in the illegal use of drugs that are injected into the body. Some states furnish clean needles and syringes to addicts to prevent sharing. Shared needles and syringes can cause HIV infection.

Occupational Prevention

Aseptic techniques currently required in health care facilities are sufficient to prevent the spread of HIV and other diseases on the job. Follow standard precautions and wash your hands frequently. Use protective barriers like gloves, gowns, and masks when necessary. Handle sharp objects such as needles and razors carefully and dispose of them promptly in labeled, puncture-proof containers. Dietary, laundry, housekeeping, and maintenance departments have policies and procedures in place that prevent the spread of HIV.

On surfaces HIV is killed easily by chemicals commonly found in the facility. These chemicals include alcohol, Lysol, peroxide, and any other approved germicide. Even in a diluted solution, bleach, the most commonly available disinfectant, will kill the virus. Mix one part bleach with 10 parts of water, and make a new solution every 24 hours.

Education

One means to stop the spread of HIV is education. Health care facilities are required to provide in-service education about HIV, so be sure to attend. Information changes continually. It is your responsibility, as a member of the health care team, to stay informed of current information about HIV.

Testing

There are tests to find out if a person has developed antibodies to the virus. An antibody is a substance that is produced by the immune system when a foreign body (a virus, for example) is present.

However, it takes several weeks after infection for the antibodies to develop. There is a period of time when a person who is infected might test negative. During that time, the infected person could infect someone else. If no antibodies develop within five or six months after an exposure to HIV, the exposed person probably has not been infected and will not develop AIDS. *Not every person who is exposed to HIV becomes HIV-positive.*

Signs and Symptoms

Persons who are infected with HIV may have no symptoms for a period of time. They may not be sick and may not realize that they are infected. When symptoms appear, they may include fatigue, diarrhea, weight loss, fever, night sweats, and loss of appetite. An opportunistic disease may develop because of the weakened immune system. Pneumonia, cancer, tuberculosis, fungal infections, and shingles are examples of opportunistic diseases that may occur in HIV-infected patients. Most AIDS patients die because of infection with the opportunistic diseases.

Care and Treatment of HIV

At the present time, there is no vaccine available to prevent HIV infection and there is no cure for AIDS. However, many drugs now are being used for treatment. AZT and DDI have been used for several years. Replication (production of more viruses) is reduced by protease inhibitors. Treatment usually includes a combination of drugs. With early, aggressive treatment, many persons infected with HIV can live longer and more comfortable lives.

As a nursing assistant, you may be caring for persons with HIV infection and AIDS. The person with HIV will need your help in dealing with many emotions, such as anger, fear, depression, anxiety, or guilt. All these feelings are normal responses to the problems associated with HIV infection.

Your attitude toward HIV will affect your response to the resident with HIV. It is important to develop a supportive, nonjudgmental attitude. Tact, sensitivity, and empathy are necessary. Show acceptance and compassion by touching and spending time with the HIV-infected resident. The resident

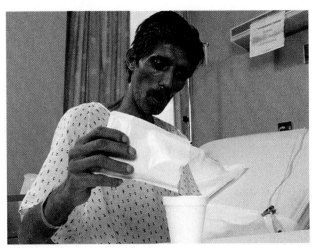

FIGURE 5-13 ■ You may be caring for residents with AIDS.© *Yoav Levy/Phototake*

with HIV is entitled to the same loving care you give to the other residents (see Figure 5-13 ■).

Legal Issues

Federal and state laws have been passed concerning HIV. They cover reporting, education, testing, confidentiality, and discrimination. Laws vary among states and constantly change. It is your responsibility to keep up with current legal issues in your area.

HEPATITIS

Hepatitis is a disease that affects the liver and causes the skin to look yellow. The three most common types of hepatitis are hepatitis A, hepatitis B, and hepatitis C. Although they have similar symptoms and are contagious, they are not transmitted in the same way. Hepatitis A is transmitted by the oral-fecal route. Hepatitis B and hepatitis C are caused by bloodborne pathogens, as is HIV. Hepatitis B is the bloodborne pathogen that is most easily transmitted to health care workers.

Hepatitis A

Hepatitis A is caused by a virus that may be found in contaminated food or wastes. The virus can enter the mouth and cause infection when the hands are not washed correctly after handling contaminated body wastes. An attack of hepatitis A provides lifelong immunity. The disease does not become chronic and has no carrier state. Although

modern sanitation practices have reduced the incidence of hepatitis A in the United States, the disease is still prevalent in some Third World countries. Prevention consists of using good hygiene and sanitation practices. The most important method of prevention is good handwashing.

Hepatitis B

Hepatitis B is caused by a virus called "hepatitis virus B (HBV)." It is spread in the same way that HIV is spread, through sexual contact and contaminated blood. HBV is able to live longer outside the human body than HIV and is more difficult to kill. HBV can infect people who do not get the disease but become carriers. A carrier can transmit the disease to someone else. Symptoms of hepatitis B include a yellow color of the skin, mucous membranes, and eyes. Other symptoms may include fever, fatigue, and nausea. The disease may become chronic with acute outbreaks. Complications include cirrhosis, liver cancer, and death.

Because HBV is transmitted in the same way as HIV, the same methods of prevention are necessary. Follow standard precautions with all residents and wash your hands frequently. There is a vaccine to prevent hepatitis B. The vaccine provides immunity to hepatitis B and has few side effects or reactions. It does not prevent any other type of hepatitis. The hepatitis B vaccine will be offered to you by your employer at no cost to you.

Hepatitis C

Hepatitis C is caused by a bloodborne virus. It is transmitted primarily by blood transfusions and contaminated needles. It also may be transmitted sexually. The disease usually becomes chronic and progresses slowly. The symptoms of hepatitis C are similar to those of hepatitis B. Unfortunately, by the time symptoms appear, the disease already may have caused severe liver damage. Hepatitis C is the leading reason for liver transplants in the United States.

As with HIV infection and hepatitis B, many people who have hepatitis C do not know they are infected. Persons who are infected with hepatitis C may become carriers and infect others. Prevention is best accomplished by following standard precautions and infection control practices.

BLOODBORNE PATHOGENS STANDARD

The bloodborne pathogens standard was developed by the Occupational Safety and Health Administration (OSHA) to help protect health care workers who come into contact with blood or other infectious materials. The bloodborne pathogens of most concern in health care today are HIV, hepatitis B, and hepatitis C. OSHA places responsibility on both employers and employees. Employers are required to establish an exposure control plan that includes:

- identification of workers at risk of exposure to blood and other infectious material
- methods to protect employees from bloodborne pathogens
- providing personal protective equipment such as gloves, gowns, and masks
- training of new employees and annual training of all employees
- proper disposal of needles and sharp objects
- proper environmental controls

The employer must offer hepatitis B vaccine, at no cost, to employees who are at risk of exposure to bloodborne pathogens.

Employees are responsible for protecting themselves by attending training sessions and by following standard precautions. All the infection control policies of the facility must be followed. Possible exposures to bloodborne pathogens must be reported immediately. Facilities are required to provide a post-exposure program of testing, counseling, and medications when necessary.

Biohazardous Medical Waste

There also are requirements in place for the proper handling of **biohazardous medical waste** (waste material that has been contaminated with blood, body fluids, or body substances that may cause infection). Examples of biohazardous medical waste include used gloves, needles and syringes, drainage bags, facial tissues, and wound dressings. Contaminated material must be placed in a separate container and must not be discarded in the regular trash. A biohazard label is placed on the bag, box, or container to indicate that the contents are infectious.

TUBERCULOSIS

Tuberculosis (TB) is caused by bacteria that enter through the respiratory system. The lungs are the most common site of infection. TB is transmitted primarily by airborne droplets from a person with active tuberculosis. The droplets are sent into the air when the infected person coughs, sneezes, talks, or sings.

Symptoms of TB include a chronic cough, fever, chills, night sweats, fatigue, weight loss, and loss of appetite. As the disease advances, the person may begin spitting blood. Treatment involves multiple drugs over an extended period of time. A person who has been treated successfully for active TB and has recovered is said to have inactive TB. Active TB is infectious, and inactive TB is *not* infectious. However, once a person is infected, he or she always will test positive for TB. Residents with active TB will be in isolation under airborne precautions. Follow the procedures and policies of your facility when caring for residents with TB.

Tuberculosis Testing

Routine screening and annual Mantoux testing is the major method used to control the spread of TB. Annual testing is required for all health care workers (see Figure 5-14 ■).

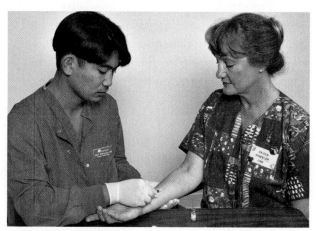

FIGURE 5-14 ■ Annual TB testing is required for health care workers.

Multidrug-Resistant Tuberculosis

Multidrug-resistant tuberculosis is a strain of TB that is resistant to current drugs and frequently is fatal. It develops when infected persons do not follow the drug program, so only some of the bacteria are destroyed. The pathogens that remain become resistant to treatment.

ANTHRAX

Anthrax is an infectious disease that is rarely passed from one person to another. Anthrax is a disease that infects animals such as cattle and sheep. People get the disease through contact with infected animals or animal products. The anthrax pathogens enter the body through skin contact, through inhalation (breathing in), or by eating contaminated meat. The majority of cases in the United States have been skin infections. Inhalation anthrax was rare until October 2001, when anthrax bioterrorism occurred. **Bioterrorism** is an act intended to destroy large numbers of people by the release of biologically harmful agents. The first incident involved anthrax material enclosed in a letter that came through the U.S. Postal Service.

Symptoms of skin anthrax infection include swelling, fever, and headache. Inhalation anthrax symptoms include fever, headache, cough, fatigue, joint pain, nausea, and vomiting. Inhalation anthrax can be fatal. Most anthrax is curable if treatment is started early. Antibiotic therapy should be started as quickly as possible after exposure, even before symptoms appear. Early treatment of anthrax may be delayed because the symptoms are similar to those of influenza and other infections. Although an anthrax vaccine is available, it is not commonly used. The vaccine injections must be repeatedly administered for an extended period of time and may produce a variety of side effects. Research is underway to produce a vaccine that is safer, more effective, and easier to administer.

Following the infection control practices outlined in this chapter will prevent exposure to anthrax at work. Remember that the disease is not communicable between humans. Prevention of anthrax would be extremely difficult if it was used in bioterrorism. Open your mail carefully, and be suspicious of any letter or package that has no return address or seems bulkier than usual. Persons coming into contact with a material suspected to be anthrax should remove their clothing as soon as possible and wash their bodies with soap and water. However, there is little reason to suspect exposure unless an incident occurs where you work or live.

CHAPTER HIGHLIGHTS

1. Preventing the spread of infection is the responsibility of all employees and will protect you as well as visitors, residents, and family members.

2. Pathogens are microorganisms that cause infection.

3. All microorganisms prefer darkness, warmth, moisture, and food. Most need oxygen.

4. It is important to observe for and recognize the signs of infection and report them immediately.

5. Aseptic practices reduce the spread of pathogens by keeping everything as clean as possible.

6. Dispose of sharps such as needles or razors in a labeled, puncture-proof container.

7. Handwashing is the most important procedure that is used to prevent the spread of infection.

8. Standard precautions are used with all residents whether or not they have an infectious disease.

9. Wear gloves when you may be touching blood, body fluids, secretions, excretions (except sweat), nonintact skin, or mucous membranes.

10. Transmission-based precautions are used when caring for residents who are infected or suspected of being infected with specific communicable diseases.

(*Continued*)

CHAPTER HIGHLIGHTS *(Continued)*

11. A gown or mask must be changed immediately if it becomes damp.

12. All used linen, dishes, eating utensils, and trash are considered infectious.

13. Encourage the isolated resident's independence by using restorative measures.

14. HIV infection destroys the immune system and leaves the body unable to fight infection.

15. With early, aggressive treatment, many persons infected with HIV can live longer and more comfortable lives.

16. The bloodborne pathogen standard was developed by OSHA to protect health care workers who come into contact with blood or other infectious materials.

17. The bloodborne pathogens of most concern in health care today are HIV, hepatitis B, and hepatitis C.

18. TB is transmitted primarily by airborne droplets from a person with active tuberculosis.

19. Biohazardous medical waste must be labeled and discarded according to facility policy.

20. Anthrax pathogens may enter the body through skin contact, through inhalation, or by eating contaminated meat. Anthrax is not communicable between humans.

VOCABULARY REVIEW

Fill in the blank with the vocabulary term that best completes the sentence.

1. A _____ is a disease that spreads easily from one person to another.

2. Microorganisms that are harmful and cause infection are called _____.

3. An object that is _____ is free of all microorganisms.

4. To _____ means to dirty or expose to microbes.

5. _____ is the use of chemicals to destroy pathogens.

6. _____(_____) are small living things that cannot be seen without the aid of a microscope. They are commonly called _____.

7. Procedures that are used for the care of all residents to protect the health care worker from infection through exposure to blood, body fluids, and body substances are _____.

8. Procedures that are used in the care of residents who are contagious or are suspected of being infected with communicable diseases are ____.

9. _____ are microorganisms that do not cause an infection.

10. _____ is the absence of pathogens. This is the use of clean procedures to prevent the spread of infection.

CHECK YOUR UNDERSTANDING

The following questions cover the highlights of this chapter. Choose the best answer for each question.

1. Which of the following environments promotes the growth of microorganisms?
   A. cool, dark, and moist
   B. warm, dark, and dry
   C. warm, sunny, and moist
   D. dark, warm, and moist

2. You used one swab, out of a package of three, to clean Mrs. Smith's mouth. What should you do with the remaining two swabs?

A. Use them for the resident in the next bed.
B. Throw them in the waste basket.
C. Close the package and place it in Mrs. Smith's bedside table.
D. Close the package and return it to the clean utility room.

3. Signs and symptoms of a localized infection include
   A. pale, clammy skin
   B. stiff, sore joints
   C. redness, swelling, and heat
   D. rapid, irregular, weak pulse

4. You have taken an extra sheet into the resident's room. What should you do with it?
   A. Store it in the closet.
   B. Place it in the dirty linen hamper.
   C. Return it to the clean linen storage.
   D. Use it on another resident's bed.

5. How should you hold your hands while washing them?
   A. fingertips pointed upward
   B. hands held above the elbows
   C. fingertips down, below the elbows
   D. hands level with the elbows

6. You used a disposable razor to shave the resident. What should you do with it?
   A. Clean the razor and place it in the appropriate storage.
   B. Throw the razor in the resident's waste basket.
   C. Put the razor in your pocket and discard it when you have more time.
   D. Place the razor immediately in a labeled sharps container.

7. Which of the following statements about standard precautions is true?
   A. Use standard precautions only with residents who are infected.
   B. Use standard precautions with all residents.
   C. Wear gloves throughout all care that is provided.
   D. Only wet linen is handled as infectious.

8. HIV infection is transmitted primarily by
   A. sexual contact   C. coughing or sneezing
   B. casual contact   D. toilet seats

AGE-SPECIFIC TIP

Elderly residents with chronic illnesses are more susceptible to disease. Protect them from infection by using aseptic techniques and standard precautions.

CULTURALLY SENSITIVE TIP

Avoid discussing the HIV-infected resident's lifestyle with individuals who are not directly participating in the resident's care.

EFFECTIVE PROBLEM SOLVING

A resident who has been placed on isolation precautions is upset because of all the restrictions. The nursing assistant, in an attempt to explain, says, "You have a bad infection, and we don't want to catch it. It is not pleasant for us to wear these protective garments. We wish you were not in isolation, either."

Was the nursing assistant's communication appropriate? If not, what would have been more appropriate?

_____

_____

_____

_____

_____

_____

_____

_____

INTERPERSONAL COMMUNICATION

Write a T or F to indicate if the statement is true or false.

_____ Cleaning the top of the resident's bedside table is a form of asepsis.

_____ Dirty linen may be placed on the floor until you finish making the resident's bed.

_____ Recap needles and syringes before you discard them.

_____ Wear gloves for all types of transmission-based precautions.

_____ Anthrax is not communicable between humans.

OBSERVING, REPORTING, AND RECORDING

List six signs and symptoms of infection that should be reported to the nurse.

_____

_____

_____

_____

_____

_____

_____

_____

_____

_____

_____

EXPLORE MEDIALINK

Check out www.prenhall.com/grubbs for additional chapter-specific interactive study and review activities.

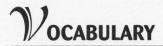

6

SAFETY IN THE LONG-TERM CARE FACILITY

OBJECTIVES

1. List five reasons why elderly residents have accidents.
2. Identify four accidents that are common to the elderly.
3. List ten safety measures to prevent accidents.
4. List six guidelines for using body mechanics.
5. Identify six substitutes for restraints.
6. List six guidelines to be followed when applying restraints.
7. List four rules of fire prevention.
8. Explain the purpose of a disaster plan.
9. List four guidelines for terrorism preparedness.

VOCABULARY

The following words or terms will help you to understand this chapter:

Toxic
Suffocation

Body mechanics
Restraint

Bioterrorism

The prevention of medical errors and safety concerns of the elderly are discussed, and safety measures and guidelines are provided in this chapter.

SAFETY CONCERNS OF THE ELDERLY

Elderly people have more accidents than persons in any other age group except children. Reasons for this include physical changes of aging, disease process, mental impairment, life changes and losses, and medications.

Physical Changes of Aging

Changes of aging that increase the elderly person's risk of accidents include slower blood circulation, weak muscles and stiff joints, brittle bones, vision and hearing loss, decreased sense of touch, and slowed reflexes. Slowed blood circulation has the most dramatic effect. Dizziness results from insufficient blood flow to the brain and often occurs when the elderly person sits up or stands suddenly.

Disease Process

There are many diseases that place the elderly resident at risk for accidents. For example, many geriatric residents suffer from arthritis, a joint disease that interferes with movement. This can lead to loss of balance and falls. The desire for independence may cause the resident to attempt to do things that are unsafe.

A stroke may result in paralysis, poor balance, and poor coordination. A stroke that affects the ability to speak or to think clearly also increases the risk of an accident. Paralyzed residents are also more at risk for accidents.

Mental Impairment

Diseases like Alzheimer's disease or chronic brain syndrome can cause the elderly resident to be confused or disoriented. Confused people accidentally can injure themselves or others. Unconscious residents are even more at risk because they are totally dependent on others for their safety. Any decrease in awareness creates a hazard.

Life Changes and Losses

Leaving home and being admitted to a long-term care facility requires a major adjustment. The environment has changed drastically, and everything is unfamiliar. The resident may wake up at night and be unable to find the bathroom. An accident may occur because furniture isn't arranged the way it was at home.

Although some people adjust quickly to the change, others do not. Many become depressed, which makes them less concerned for their safety. The elderly person may have lost a spouse, a home, and friends. Loss of health or even loss of life no longer seems important.

Medications

As people age, they react differently to medications. Medications may have a stronger effect, and the effects may last longer. The need for several medications increases the risk of drug interaction. Some medication causes confusion or drowsiness. A confused or drowsy resident is at great risk.

TYPES OF ACCIDENTS

An accident may be caused by carelessness or negligence. Some examples include

- Failure to identify the resident
- Delay in answering the call signal
- Incorrect moving and lifting
- Failure to lock brakes on equipment wheels
- Lack of knowledge about using equipment
- Failure to clean up spills
- Failure to place call signal in reach

Some types of accidents involving the elderly include

- Falls
- Burns
- Poisoning
- Suffocation

Falls

A fall is the most frequent accident in the long-term care facility. The most common cause of falls is wet, slippery floors. Water or any other

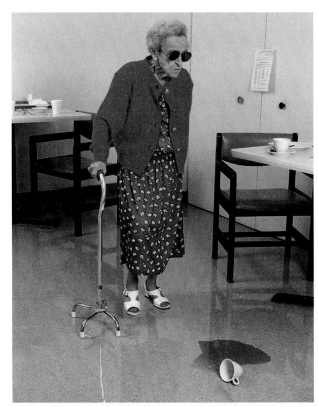

FIGURE 6-1 ■ The confused or vision-impaired resident may not be aware of spills.

liquid spilled on the floor creates a hazard for everyone. The resident with poor vision and unsteady gait is more likely to slip on wet floors. Picture the blind resident coming down the hall, totally unaware that directly ahead is a puddle (see Figure 6-1 ■). The result likely will be a fall. The following list includes other factors that can cause a fall:

- Improper footwear
- Poor lighting
- Clutter
- Staff carelessness or negligence

Burns

Burns sometimes are caused by careless smokers. Hot water and other liquids also may cause burns. Extra precautions are necessary when performing any procedure involving heat or cold. A decreased sensitivity to heat can result in a burn. Burns can be caused by negligence.

Poisoning

Residents who have poor vision or are confused may pick up a toxic substance and eat or drink it. **Toxic** means poisonous. Cleaning solutions and disinfectants are examples of toxic substances.

Suffocation

Suffocation means the interruption of respiration. Some causes of suffocation include choking, drowning, smoke inhalation, and electrical shock.

*S*AFETY MEASURES TO REDUCE MEDICAL ERRORS AND PREVENT ACCIDENTS

The purpose of safety measures in the long-term care facility is to reduce medical errors and prevent accidents. The following is a list of safety measures:

- Correctly identify the resident.
- Follow each resident's plan of care.
- Perform procedures correctly.
- Follow facility policies.
- Keep the call signal in reach.
- Clean up spills immediately.
- Use safety equipment.
- Encourage the resident to use safety bars and rails.
- Make sure the resident is wearing proper footwear.
- Raise side rails when appropriate.
- Follow aseptic practices to prevent the spread of infection.
- Lock wheels on beds, chairs, and other equipment.
- Provide adequate lighting.
- Report faulty equipment and other safety hazards.
- Return beds to the lowest position and fold bed cranks out of the way.
- Keep hallways and rooms free of clutter.
- Use correct procedures.
- Get help when necessary.
- Use proper body mechanics.
- Chart promptly and correctly.

Correct Identification

Correct identification of the resident is a very important safety measure. The safest way to identify

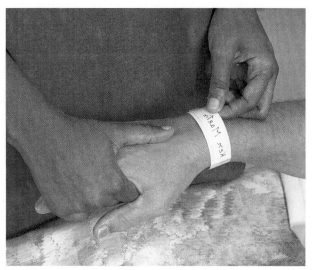

FIGURE 6-2 ■ Always check the identification bracelet before you perform resident care.

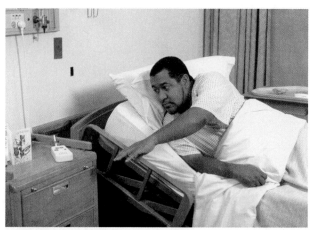

FIGURE 6-3 ■ Always place the call signal within the resident's reach.

the resident is by checking the identification bracelet. Never rely on calling the resident by name because the wrong person may answer.

You cannot depend on checking the room number or the name on the bed. Residents sometimes enter the wrong room and occasionally get into the wrong bed. Always check the I.D. bracelet (see Figure 6-2 ■).

Using the Call Signal and Intercom

The call signal should be placed where the resident can reach it. Even if a resident is confused or unconscious, the call signal must be in reach at all times. A fall may occur when a resident tries to use a call signal that is out of reach (see Figure 6-3 ■). Check to be sure the call signal is working and that the resident knows how to use it. Answer all call signals promptly. Delay in answering call signals is a frequent cause of accidents. A resident who needs to go to the bathroom may fall in an attempt to get up without assistance. A confused resident who is out of the room in a wheelchair and away from the call signal should be positioned within sight of staff members.

Some facilities have intercom systems for communication between the residents' rooms and the nurses' stations. Be sure to explain the use of the intercom when the resident is admitted. The intercom does not replace personal contact. Visit the resident at regular intervals. Intercoms that are used between departments can be noisy and disturbing to residents and should not be overused. Do not use the intercom to residents' rooms for paging employees. The intercom should be used sparingly at night.

Cleaning Up Wet Floors and Spills

Cleaning up spills is everyone's responsibility. The person who sees the spill first should take action to prevent an accident. If you are unable to clean it up yourself, tell someone else immediately. Observe "Wet Floor" signs, and remind residents and visitors to avoid those areas.

Wearing Proper Footwear

The resident should wear nonskid shoes when out of bed or walking. Check to be sure that shoes fit properly and are in good repair. Tie shoestrings and fasten buckles as needed. Bedroom slippers should not be worn unless they provide support and have nonskid soles. The resident should not attempt to walk in stocking feet. Any footwear with an open heel is unsafe. The safest shoe for the elderly person is one that has nonskid soles and a closed heel and toe. This is also the safest type of shoe for you to wear to work.

BODY MECHANICS

Body mechanics refers to the use of the body to move. Correct body mechanics (see Figure 6-4 ■) means using the body in a careful and efficient manner. The three most important reasons for using correct body mechanics are to protect the resident from injury, to protect you from injury, and to save energy and prevent fatigue.

Use correct body mechanics all the time, not just at work. Read the guidelines that follow and consider how you could use them while sitting, standing, walking, working, lifting, or moving objects. To prevent fatigue and back strain, change your position frequently, stretch and relax occasionally, and use correct body mechanics.

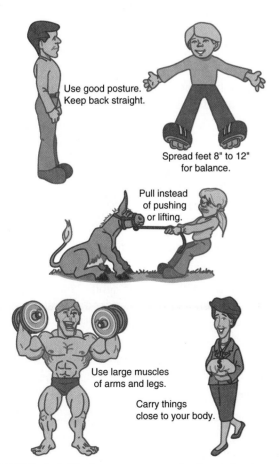

FIGURE 6-4 ■ Always use correct body mechanics.

GUIDELINES

USING CORRECT BODY MECHANICS

- Maintain a wide base of support by standing with your feet 8 to 12 inches apart for balance.
- Bend at your knees, not at your waist.
- Keep your back straight.
- Use the large muscles of your legs and arms. The strongest muscles are in your thighs and the weakest are in your back.
- Stand close to the object or the person you are working with. Hold the object or person you are lifting close to your body.
- Turn your whole body at once; don't twist.
- Use smooth, coordinated movements.
- Push or pull an object rather than lift it.
- Use correct posture.
- Keep beds and other surfaces at the proper working height when possible.
- Plan ahead and get help if needed.

OSHA (THE OCCUPATIONAL SAFETY AND HEALTH ADMINISTRATION)

OSHA is a government agency that is concerned with the health and safety of workers. These concerns include infection-control practices and other safety issues. Rules specify the types of protective supplies, equipment, and techniques to be used in the health care facility.

Hazard Communication Standard

OSHA's Hazard Communication Standard states that you have the right to know what hazards you may be exposed to at work. This standard also requires that you protect yourself against possible hazards. All hazardous material must be labeled. The employer must provide information and training to help you understand labels and safe procedures.

INCIDENT REPORTS

An incident is an event that occurs that is not a part of the routine of the facility. An accident is one type of incident. An error in performing resident care is another type. An incident report provides written documentation of an incident. It includes information such as the persons involved; the date, time, and location of the incident; witnesses; and injuries, if any.

An incident must be reported immediately any time you are involved in an accident or make an error that could result in an injury.

An incident should be reported even if there are no obvious injuries or if the persons involved think they are not hurt. If an injury develops later as a result of the incident, all the facts will be available.

RESTRAINTS

A **restraint** is a device that is used to restrict a person's freedom of movement. A restraint may be used only for the safety of the resident, *never* for the convenience of the staff.

Legal Issues

There are federal and state laws regarding the use of restraints. OBRA (the Omnibus Budget Reconciliation Act) specifically addresses the use of restraints in long-term care facilities. Restraining a resident unnecessarily is false imprisonment. It is also abuse and a violation of the resident's rights. A restraint requires a doctor's order.

Effects of Restraints

Being restrained affects the resident physically and emotionally. Physical effects can include

- Skin breakdown
- Constipation
- Pneumonia
- Blood clots
- Muscle weakness
- Loss of mobility

Emotional effects of being restrained can include

- Loss of dignity, independence, and control
- Decreased self-esteem
- Confusion and disorientation
- Anxiety and restlessness
- Frustration and anger
- Decreased communication and social activity

Most people don't like to have their movements restricted. It causes them to become upset and angry. If the resident is already angry or combative, a restraint will only increase his or her anger. Your goal should be to calm the resident down.

Residents who suffer from chronic wandering, such as those with Alzheimer's disease, should not be restrained except in extreme situations. Always try to encourage independence. It is important to protect the resident without damaging self-esteem.

GUIDELINES

APPLYING RESTRAINTS

- A restraint requires a doctor's order.
- Use a restraint only when necessary, never for convenience.
- Use restorative techniques first (activities or recreation).
- Use the least restrictive device when possible (a soft belt restraint instead of a safety vest, a mitt instead of a wrist restraint).
- Remember that a geri-chair (geriatric chair) is considered a restraint.
- Explain what you are doing and why you are doing it.
- Use the correct size and type of restraint.
- Apply the restraint properly.
- Tie a knot that can quickly be released (half-bow).
- Apply the restraint over clothing.
- Cross the vest restraint in the front.
- Provide padding for a wrist restraint.
- Do not tie the restraint too tightly. You should be able to insert four fingers under the waist of the vest restraint and two fingers under the wrist restraint.
- Tie the bed restraint to the bed frame, never to the side rail.
- Never use a sheet as a restraint.
- Do not restrain a resident to the toilet or a bedside commode.
- Allow as much movement as possible.
- Protect the resident's rights.

Substitutes for Restraints

A restraint should be the last resort, used only after other methods have failed to protect the resident. As a substitute for restraints, you may do the following:

- Interrupt behavior that might lead to the need for restraints.
- Use music to calm the resident.
- Use TV and radio for diversion.
- Encourage activities as an outlet for energy.
- Closely observe confused residents.
- Allow residents to walk in safe areas.
- Encourage family participation.
- Use pillows, padding, and other equipment for support.

The facility may use bed alarms, door alarms, and arm band alarms to signal the location of the confused resident. Always respond immediately to the sound of an alarm.

Types of Restraints

There are many types of restraints designed to protect the resident in different situations (see Figure 6-5 ■). The doctor decides which type of restraint,

---

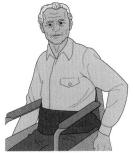

A A soft belt restraint

A soft belt restraint is used to prevent the resident from falling out of a bed or wheelchair.

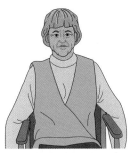

B A safety vest

A safety vest is used to prevent the resident from falling from a chair or bed. It provides more support than a belt.

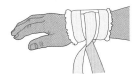

C A wrist restraint

A wrist restraint is used to prevent the resident from removing dressings or pulling out tubes that are a part of the treatment.

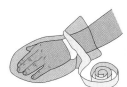

D A mitt restraint

A mitt restraint is used for the same purpose as a wrist restraint but is less restrictive. It looks like a big mitten without a thumb.

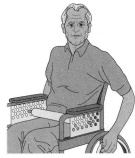

E A safety bar kit

A safety bar kit can be applied to a wheelchair to help prevent a resident from falling. It is less restrictive than a belt or vest.

FIGURE 6-5 ■ Types of restraints.

GUIDELINES

AFTER RESTRAINTS HAVE BEEN APPLIED

- Visually check the resident's safety every 30 minutes.
- Check wrist restraints every 15 minutes.
- Remove the restraint every 2 hours, provide exercise and skin care, and reposition the resident. Offer toileting and fluids at this time.
- Observe for complications such as skin irritation, injury, circulatory impairment, or increased anxiety.
- Observe for comfort and body alignment.
- Reassure the resident frequently.
- Keep the call signal within reach.
- Make sure the restraint is clean and undamaged.
- Keep the restraint free of wrinkles.
- Document the type of restraint and the times of application and removal.

for what length of time, and in what circumstance it may be used. Following the guidelines for applying restraints and the guidelines after restraints have been applied will help you to use restraints correctly and safely.

FIRE SAFETY

Fire safety focuses on the prevention of fires. It also includes information on how fires start and the correct response to a fire. Health care facilities are built with safety features to prevent fires and to reduce the need for evacuation. These safety features include fire exits, closed stairwells, smoke detectors, sprinkler systems, and automatic fire door closers.

Elements of a Fire

The three elements needed for a fire are fuel, oxygen, and a spark. Draperies, linens, clothing, wood, or any material that will burn provide fuel. Because there is fuel almost everywhere and oxygen is found naturally in the air, all that is needed for a fire is a spark.

Causes of Fires

Fire is often the result of improper disposal of matches or cigarette butts. Most health care facilities do not allow smoking in the building. Not only does this reduce pollution from tobacco smoke, but it also lessens the chance of a fire.

Defective electrical equipment can cause fires. Frayed wires, overloaded circuits, and ungrounded plugs are dangerous. Electrical appliances that are used improperly or are in need of repair are another hazard.

Other factors that contribute to fires include improper trash disposal, cooking materials, flammable liquids, and oxygen equipment.

Sometimes the resident will need more oxygen than is present in the air. This oxygen usually is provided by a tank, wall outlet, or concentrator. Because oxygen can explode and burn, special rules apply when it is used. The following guidelines will help you to practice fire safety when oxygen is being used.

GUIDELINES

FIRE SAFETY WHEN OXYGEN IS BEING USED

- Remove radios, televisions, and electric razors from the area.
- Use cotton blankets, not wool or synthetic fabrics.
- Remind residents and visitors not to smoke in the room.
- Dispose of waste material correctly.
- Store flammable liquids properly.
- Check electrical equipment and report any hazards.
- Observe all the rules for oxygen safety.

Fire Emergency Rules

If a fire occurs, it is important that you stay calm and do not panic, run, or scream. Reassure residents and visitors. The first step in the event of fire is to remove residents who are in immediate danger. The fire should be contained by closing doors. Halls should be cleared of people and equipment to allow easy access by the fire department. Each facility has a policy and procedure for fire, and it is your responsibility to know the correct procedure to follow. One system that is used in many public buildings is the RACE system (see Figure 6-6 ■).

A smoldering fire is very dangerous. In a fire, more people die from smoke inhalation than from the fire itself. Smoke can kill even if there is no flame. If you are in a room that is smoke-filled, drop to your knees on the floor, cover your mouth and nose, and crawl to an exit.

Fire Extinguishers

There are several kinds of fire extinguishers. Your facility will provide in-service classes to show you which type to use in any situation. These classes often are taught by the local fire department. When you are using a fire extinguisher, you should point the nozzle toward the base of the fire.

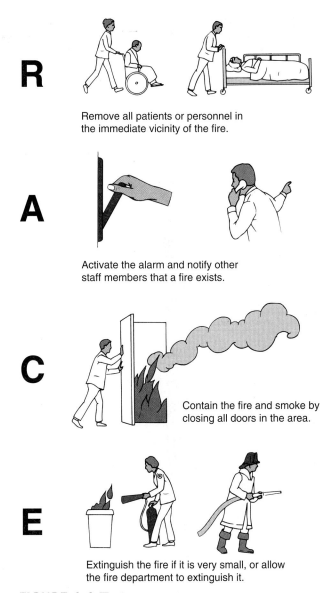

R Remove all patients or personnel in the immediate vicinity of the fire.

A Activate the alarm and notify other staff members that a fire exists.

C Contain the fire and smoke by closing all doors in the area.

E Extinguish the fire if it is very small, or allow the fire department to extinguish it.

FIGURE 6-6 ■ The RACE system.

Fire Drills

Your facility will have regular fire drills in which everyone participates. It is your responsibility to know the fire emergency plan for your facility. You must be able to respond quickly and correctly.

*D*ISASTER PLANNING

A disaster is an event that may cause injury or death to a large number of people. It also may cause great property damage. Some examples of disasters include explosions, bomb threats, fires, transportation accidents, earthquakes, floods, hurricanes, tornadoes, or other severe weather conditions.

Every health care facility must have a disaster plan that describes the role of all employees. The plan includes policies and procedures for the protection of the residents and the staff. There also are procedures for handling large numbers of people and providing medical care for the wounded.

Disaster safety drills are held on a regular basis in a health care facility. They may be combined with a community disaster drill. In this way, the authorities can evaluate the ability of the entire community to handle an emergency.

*T*ERRORISM

Worldwide terrorist threats and activities have increased in recent years. After September 11, 2001, the president of the United States declared a war on terrorism. That is a frightening concept. A conventional war is usually fought by trained military personnel, whereas a terrorist war consists of random acts of violence against civilians. Terrorist activities might include bombs, fires, or transportation disasters. There is also a possibility of bioterrorism with the release of toxic chemicals or disease germs such as anthrax or smallpox. **Bioterrorism** is an act intended to destroy large numbers of people by the release of biologically harmful agents.

Additional emphasis has been placed on disaster plans to cover these kinds of emergencies. Health care workers must be prepared to handle large numbers of victims, but they must also be concerned with the safety of themselves and their families. All this can cause worry and anxiety because we don't know when terrorist activities will occur. The best tools to use in dealing with terrorism are knowledge and preparedness. Health care facilities regularly update their policies and procedures and provide ongoing education and training. The following guidelines will help you be knowledgeable and prepared.

GUIDELINES

TERRORISM PREPAREDNESS

- Attend educational and training programs at your facility.
- Be aware of current safety levels and warnings.
- Follow facility policies and procedures.
- Carefully consider sources of information. Not everything you hear or read is reliable.
- Keep calm and don't panic.

GUIDELINES (Continued)

- Be alert for unusual and dangerous situations.
- Open your mail carefully and report anything suspicious.
- Make sure vaccinations are current for yourself and your family members.
- Report any suspicious activities to the proper authorities.

CHAPTER HIGHLIGHTS

1. Elderly people and children have the most accidents.
2. Any decrease in awareness creates a safety hazard.
3. The most common accident in a long-term health care facility is a fall.
4. Keep the call signal in reach at all times, even if the resident is confused or unconscious.
5. The safest way to identify the resident is by checking the identification bracelet.
6. Correct body mechanics include standing with your back straight and your feet apart.
7. OSHA regulations help protect the safety of workers.
8. An incident report protects you, the resident, visitors, and the facility.
9. A restraint may be used only to protect the resident.
10. Try restorative techniques before using a restraint.
11. Restraints must be removed every 2 hours.
12. Fire prevention is everybody's responsibility.
13. In case of fire, remove the residents who are in immediate danger first.
14. A disaster plan describes the role of the employees in an emergency.
15. The best tools to use in dealing with terrorism are knowledge and preparedness.

VOCABULARY REVIEW

Fill in the blank with the vocabulary term that best completes the sentence.

1. _____ refers to the use of the body to move.

2. The interruption of respirations caused by choking or drowning is called _____.

3. A/An _____ is a device used to restrict a person's freedom of movement.

4. The release of disease germs such as anthrax as a threat to the general population is called _____.

5. _____ means poisonous.

6. _____ is a joint disease that interferes with movement and may lead to falls.

7. _____ is a government agency that is concerned with the health and safety of workers.

8. Restraining or restricting a person's movements unnecessarily is _____.

9. The failure to give proper care that results in harm to the resident is _____.

10. _____ is the law that went into effect in 1990 and focused on the care of the elderly in long-term care facilities.

CHECK YOUR UNDERSTANDING

The following questions cover the highlights of this chapter. Choose the best answer for each question.

1. What is the *best* way to identify a resident?
   A. Call the resident's name.
   B. Check the room number.
   C. Ask the roommate.
   D. Check the ID bracelet.

2. You find water spilled on the floor. What should you do?
   A. Clean it up immediately.
   B. Determine who spilled it.
   C. Clean it up as soon as you have time.
   D. Wait for someone else to do it.

3. A confused resident is wearing a mitt restraint to prevent her from pulling out a feeding tube. How often must the restraint be removed?
   A. every 30 minutes
   B. every hour
   C. every 2 hours
   D. every 4 hours

4. Where should the call signal be placed if the resident is confused?
   A. on the wall over the bed
   B. fastened to the side rail
   C. within the nurse's reach
   D. within the resident's reach

5. How should you stand while lifting something?
   A. back straight and feet apart
   B. back straight and feet together
   C. knees locked and feet apart
   D. knees bent and feet together

6. What is the first thing you do in the event of a fire?
   A. Remove residents from immediate danger.
   B. Put out the fire.
   C. Sound the alarm.
   D. Close the doors.

AGE-SPECIFIC TIP

Be aware of elderly residents' need for independence while protecting their safety.

CULTURALLY SENSITIVE TIP

Invite the resident to talk about his or her culture. This may help the resident feel accepted, cope with life changes, and adapt more safely.

EFFECTIVE PROBLEM SOLVING

The nursing assistant has been assigned to give an enema to Mrs. Jones in Room 412B. Going to the first bed in Room 412, the nursing assistant asks the resident, "Are you Mrs. Jones?" The resident replies, "Yes, dear." The nursing assistant explains what she is going to do. The resident in the second bed says, "I am Mrs. Jones."

Was the nursing assistant's communication appropriate? If not, what would have been more appropriate?

_____
_____
_____
_____
_____
_____
_____
_____
_____
_____
_____
_____
_____

INTERPERSONAL COMMUNICATION

A resident becomes angry and strikes out at you. You are trying to calm the resident and protect her from harm. Check the examples that are appropriate.

_____ "If you don't calm down, I'll have to restrain you."

_____ "I can see you're upset. Would you like to talk about it?"

_____ "Maybe some milk and cookies will make you feel better."

_____ "I'll only leave the restraint on until you calm down."

OBSERVING, REPORTING, AND RECORDING

You observe a resident falling in the hallway. List the information you will need to report and record the fall.

_____
_____
_____
_____
_____
_____
_____
_____
_____
_____
_____
_____
_____

EXPLORE MEDIALINK

7

FIRST AID AND EMERGENCY CARE

OBJECTIVES

1. Identify ten guidelines for handling emergencies.
2. List seven guidelines for recognizing life-threatening conditions.
3. Explain how to recognize and prevent shock.
4. Describe the emergency care for airway obstructions, hemorrhage, strokes, and seizures.
5. Demonstrate the procedures described in this chapter.

VOCABULARY

The following words or terms will help you to understand this chapter:

First aid
Pulse
Respiration
Trauma
Assess

Hemorrhage
Cyanosis
Cardiopulmonary resuscitation (CPR)
Aspirate

Heimlich maneuver
Sternum
Cerebrovascular accident (CVA)
Seizure

This chapter discusses first aid and emergency care of the long-term care resident.

INTRODUCTION TO FIRST AID

First aid is immediate care for injuries or sudden illness. It is given to prevent further injuries and save lives. When an emergency occurs at work, it is your responsibility to stay with the resident who needs first aid, call for the nurse, and begin first aid. When the nurse arrives, you will continue emergency care as directed. Your facility will have written procedures that you should follow when handling emergencies.

You will be better prepared for handling emergencies after you complete a course of first aid offered by the American Red Cross or the National Safety Council. You also may prepare yourself for cardiac and respiratory emergencies by taking a CPR course offered by the American Heart Association, the National Safety Council, or the American Red Cross. This chapter will discuss emergency care for situations that might occur in a long-term care facility.

HANDLING EMERGENCIES

Some guidelines to be followed in every emergency situation follow.

GUIDELINES

HANDLING EMERGENCIES

- Call for help and stay with the resident.
- Check the environment to be sure that it is safe for you and the resident.
- Stay calm and reassure the resident frequently.
- Use standard precautions as needed.
- Move the resident only if necessary to prevent injury and to ensure your own safety. Avoid twisting the resident's back and neck if movement is necessary.
- If you must provide ventilations for the resident, use a protective device such as a face mask (familiarize yourself with the device provided by your facility and know how to use it in advance of an emergency).

GUIDELINES (Continued)

- Know your limitations and follow the facility's plan.
- Observe for life-threatening conditions.
- Monitor consciousness, **pulse** (heartbeat), and **respirations** (breathing).
- Keep bystanders away.
- Keep the resident as comfortable as possible.

Staying calm helps you to function well. The resident may develop shock as a result of **trauma** (physical injury or emotional upset). Staying calm will help reduce the resident's anxiety. Movement may cause additional injuries and can be especially dangerous if the resident has head, neck, or spinal injuries. Remember that when you are in the facility, you must call for the nurse and work under his or her direction.

Observing for Life-Threatening Conditions

Life-threatening emergencies must be treated first. When injury or sudden illness has occurred, you must first **assess** (check or evaluate) the resident's condition to determine whether it is life-threatening. Some situations that threaten life are cardiac arrest (the absence of heartbeats), respiratory arrest (absence of breathing), drowning, smoke inhalation, electric shock, **hemorrhage** (severe bleeding), and stroke.

GUIDELINES

RECOGNIZING LIFE-THREATENING CONDITIONS

- Observe for danger in the environment.
- Check for unresponsiveness.
- Observe for an open airway, breathing, and circulation.
- Observe for **cyanosis** (a blue color of the skin, lips, and nails due to lack of oxygen).
- Observe for blood or fluid in the mouth or nose.
- Observe for signs of shock and stroke.
- Examine the resident's entire body for life-threatening injuries.

The heart, lungs, and brain depend upon each other for survival. If any one fails, they all fail. Every cell of the body must have a constant flow of oxygenated blood to continue functioning. When breathing or heart action stops, the oxygenated blood will not be available to cells, and the cells will begin to die. Death of brain and heart cells could make recovery impossible and immediate steps must be taken. The procedure for emergency care to restore heart and lung function is called **cardiopulmonary resuscitation (CPR)**. This procedure is described later in this chapter. It is recommended that you take a CPR course.

Calling for Help (Activating the EMS System)

When beginning care for life threatening conditions, the emergency medical service (EMS) must be called. The nurse will either call EMS or designate someone else to do so. Information to be given should include your location (with the name of the nearest cross street), the nature of any injuries, number of residents needing emergency care, and emergency care that is being given. Always wait to hang up after the operator disconnects. To activate the EMS System, dial 911 or call the operator.

Recognizing and Preventing Shock

In any emergency situation, shock may result from a drop in blood pressure. This may happen because of loss of blood or physical injury. Emotionally upset bystanders and victims with minor injuries also may experience shock. If the blood pressure drops too low, the vital organs will not receive oxygenated blood and death will result. Attempt to prevent shock in all emergency situations.

GUIDELINES

RECOGNIZING AND PREVENTING SHOCK

- Notify the nurse and call for help.
- Use standard precautions as needed.
- Observe for signs of shock including rapid respirations and pulse, cyanosis, cool and damp skin, thirst, dilated pupils, and nausea and vomiting.
- Calm and reassure the resident.
- Maintain a normal body temperature and prevent chilling.
- Place the resident in a flat position (see Figure 7-1A ■). The feet may be elevated if there is no evidence of breathing difficulty, broken leg bones, or head injury.
- Turn the resident to the side if you observe vomiting or bleeding at the nose or mouth (see Figure 7-1B ■).
- Identify and control bleeding.
- Avoid offering food or fluids.
- Stay with the resident.

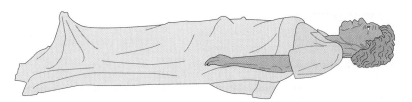

A To prevent shock, the resident must lie flat and be kept warm.

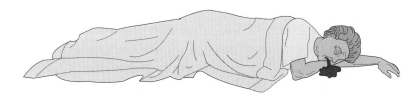

B If the injured resident is vomiting or hemorrhaging from the mouth or nose, she must be placed on her side to prevent aspiration.

FIGURE 7-1 ■ Positioning the shock victim.

*E*MERGENCY CARE FOR AIRWAY OBSTRUCTION

In the long-term care facility, you may encounter respiratory distress due to airway obstruction. Severe respiratory distress is a life-threatening condition and must be treated as a priority.

Causes of Airway Obstruction

The most common cause of airway obstruction for a conscious person is choking on food. Because elderly residents may have weakened swallowing muscles, they may **aspirate** (choke) on fluids or food. Laughing or talking during meals also can cause choking. An unconscious resident may develop respiratory distress because the tongue falls back into the throat and blocks the air passage. The resident may be turned to the side or a small pillow may be placed beneath the shoulders of the unconscious resident to maintain the proper airway position.

Signs of Airway Obstruction

Be aware of signs of respiratory distress and choking so that you can provide immediate assistance to correct this problem. A person who is choking on a foreign object may have a partial or complete airway obstruction. If the obstruction is partial, the resident may cough or make unusual noises while breathing. These noises include wheezing, gurgling, or crowing. As the obstruction becomes more severe, the cough will become weak. With a complete airway obstruction, there may be no cough or no movement of air. The resident may indicate choking by grabbing the throat with the hands. This is referred to as the "universal sign for choking" (see Figure 7-2 ■). A response is urgent and must begin immediately.

Caring for Airway Obstructions

The immediate first aid for an airway obstruction is the **Heimlich maneuver**. See the procedure on page 77.

In order to prevent the possible transmission of disease during ventilations, use a barrier to deliver mouth-to-barrier ventilations (see Figure 7-4 ■). Mask devices and face shields of many styles are available and should be positioned over the resident's

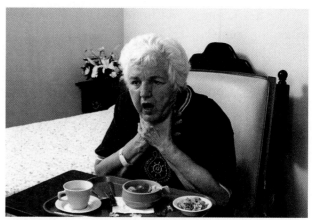

FIGURE 7-2 ■ The universal sign of choking.

GUIDELINES

CARING FOR THE RESIDENT WITH AN AIRWAY OBSTRUCTION

- Notify the nurse and call for help if you observe an airway problem.
- Stay with the resident and provide encouragement if the cough is effective.
- Observe for signs of poor or absent air exchange such as lack of chest movement, inability to speak, a weak cough (or no cough), and cyanosis.
- Observe for the universal sign of choking.
- Perform the Heimlich maneuver.
- If the resident is unresponsive, position him or her on the back and perform the procedure for care of the unconscious resident with an airway obstruction. (The procedure is included in this chapter.)

---

mouth and nose to ensure an adequate seal. Familiarize yourself with the device provided by your facility and learn how to use it properly. You may wish to purchase a personal device that may be carried with you for use in emergencies outside of your facility. Frequent recertification training is necessary to remain current with changing procedures in emergency care.

If the resident is unresponsive and the airway is opened, you must check for signs of circulation (breathing, coughing movement and pulse). When a pulse is present but the resident is not breathing, you must perform rescue breathing by giving one slow breath every 5 to 6 seconds. Monitor the pulse periodically to determine the need for CPR.

PROCEDURE
Heimlich Maneuver

Follow standard precautions.

1. Identify the universal sign for choking (see Figure 7-2 ■).
2. Check for complete or severe obstruction (no air movement, no chest movement, no speech, cyanosis, and/or weak cough).
3. Say, "Are you choking? I can help."
4. Stand behind the resident.
5. Wrap your arms around the waist with the resident's arms free.
6. With your hand held in a fist, place the thumb side of your hand against the resident's abdomen, in the midline, an inch or two above the naval (see Figure 7-3 ■).
7. Keep your fist away from the rib cage.
8. Wrap your other hand around your fist and sqeeze inward and upward with repeated thrusts toward the abdomen until the obstruction is cleared.

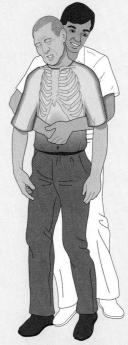

FIGURE 7-3 ■ The Heimlich maneuver is the immediate first aid procedure used to remove an airway obstruction.

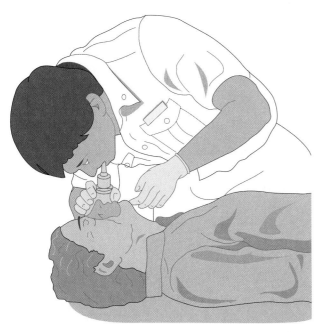

FIGURE 7-4 ■ Care of the unconscious resident who is not breathing.

CARDIOPULMONARY RESUSCITATION FOR CARDIAC ARREST

Cardiopulmonary resuscitation (CPR) is an emergency procedure that is used to replace lung and heart function when respiratory and cardiac arrest have occurred. Artificial ventilations are given by the rescuer, to provide oxygen for the body, when respiratory arrest has occurred. During emergency care for a cardiac arrest, chest compressions circulate blood and replace contractions of the heart. A person may experience respiratory arrest before cardiac arrest. However, cardiac arrest soon will follow respiratory arrest because the heart cannot continue to function without oxygen.

All body functions stop when cardiac arrest occurs. Cardiac arrest is clinical death. When cardiac

PROCEDURE

Care of the Unconscious Resident with an Airway Obstruction

Follow standard precautions.

1. Determine unresponsiveness by shaking gently and shouting, "Are you okay?"
2. If there is no response, call for help.
3. Kneel beside the unconscious resident and open the airway by using the head tilt/chin lift method. Tilt the head back with one hand while you lift the chin with the other.
4. Place your cheek close to the resident's face. Take 3 to 5 seconds to look at the resident's chest while you listen and feel for air movement against your cheek (see Figure 7-5A ■).

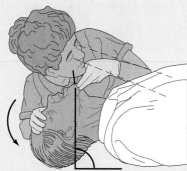

FIGURE 7-5A ■ Use the head tilt/chin lift method to open the airway. Look, listen, and feel.

5. If there is no air movement, give two ventilations. If the air will not enter the airway, reposition the head in order to open the airway and attempt two additional ventilations.
6. If air still does not enter the airway, kneel and straddle the resident's thighs.
7. Place the heel of one hand on the abdomen, slightly above the navel, at the midline. Place your other hand on top of the first hand. Your fingers should point toward the resident's chest (see Figure 7-5B ■).

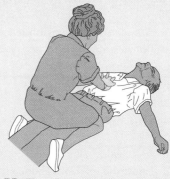

FIGURE 7-5B ■ Place the heel of one hand on the abdomen slightly above the navel at the midline. Place your other hand on the top of the first hand and give up to five abdominal thrusts.

8. Press inward and upward for up to five abdominal thrusts.
9. Open the resident's mouth using the tongue-jaw lift and perform a finger sweep. Insert the index finger of your other hand into the resident's mouth and sweep it along the inside surfaces to the base of the tongue (see Figure 7-5C ■). Hook your finger slightly to dislodge and remove any object you find.

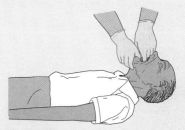

FIGURE 7-5C ■ Perform a finger sweep to dislodge and remove any objects.

10. Attempt ventilation again.
11. Repeat the series of five abdominal thrusts, finger sweep, and attempts to ventilate. ■

arrest occurs, the heart fails to circulate blood that carries oxygen to the cells. Cells and tissues will begin to die within 4 to 6 minutes of a cardiac arrest because of a lack of oxygen. This death of cells is called "biological death."

One-Rescuer CPR

The cardiac arrest victim must lie flat on a firm surface so that the heart can be compressed between the **sternum** (breastbone) and the spine. Chest compressions and ventilations replace the heartbeat and breathing.

$\mathscr{P}$ROCEDURE

One-Rescuer CPR

1. Determine unresponsiveness by gently shaking the resident and shouting, "Are you okay?"
2. Call for help and activate the EMS system.
3. Open the airway by using the head tilt/chin lift method (see Figure 7-6A ■).

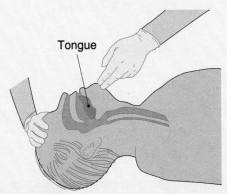

Tongue

FIGURE 7-6A ■ Use the head tilt/chin lift method to open the airway.

4. While holding the airway open, place your cheek near the resident's mouth and nose. Look at the resident's chest while you listen and feel for air movement against your cheek (see Figure 7-6B ■).

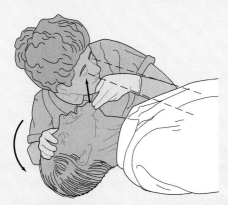

FIGURE 7-6B ■ Look, listen, and feel for breathing.

5. Provide two breaths (1½ to 2 seconds each) into the resident's airway. If the air will not enter the lungs, reposition the head and try again.

6. Check for circulation by feeling the carotid pulse (see Figure 7-6C ■), which is located in the groove between the Adam's apple and the large muscle of the neck. This should take 5 to 10 seconds.

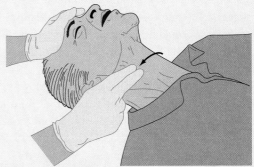

FIGURE 7-6C ■ Check for circulation by feeling the carotid pulse on either side of the neck.

7. If no pulse is present, use the index and middle fingers of your hand nearest the resident's feet to locate the compression site. Follow the edge of the rib cage to the notch where the ribs join the sternum (see Figure 7-6D ■).

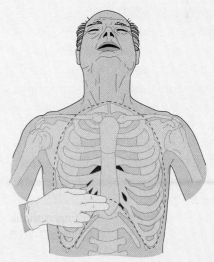

FIGURE 7-6D ■ Locate the compression site by following the edge of the rib cage to the notch where the ribs join the sternum.

(continued)

8. Place your fingers on the notch and place the heel of your other hand in the midline of the chest, just above and next to your fingers.

9. Place the heel of the hand used to locate the compression site on top of the positioned hand. Interlock the fingers of the top hand in order to lift all fingers off the chest. Keep your shoulders directly above your hands and lock your elbows. Begin compressions and compress the chest 1½ to 2 inches (see Figure 7-6E ■) at a rate of 100 compressions per minute.

10. Alternate 15 compressions with two ventilations, and repeat this sequence for four full cycles or 1 full minute. Do not lift your hands from the chest during compressions.

11. Finish the four cycles with two ventilations before rechecking the pulse. Do not interrupt CPR for more than 5 seconds. If the pulse is still absent, continue the cycles of chest compressions and ventilations. Correctly locate the hand position each time after

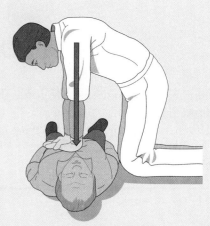

FIGURE 7-6E ■ Position your hands and begin chest compression.

you lift your hands from the chest. Check the pulse every few minutes thereafter. If the pulse is present, resume rescue breathing and continue to monitor the pulse. ■

To perform chest compressions and ventilations properly, remember these important points:

- Keep your shoulders directly above your hands and lock your elbows.
- Do not lift your hands from the chest during compressions.
- Correctly locate the hand position each time you lift your hands from the chest.
- Compress the chest 1½ to 2 inches.
- Lean toward the resident's head to give ventilations. Do not move your knees back and forth between ventilations and compressions.
- Continue cycles of 15 compressions and two ventilations for four cycles or 1 full minute. Check for recovery of the pulse. If the pulse is present, resume rescue breathing and continue to monitor the pulse. If the pulse is not present, resume CPR.

*E*MERGENCY CARE FOR HEMORRHAGE

Hemorrhage is a life-threatening condition because severe loss of blood can quickly result in shock and death. Immediate first aid to control bleeding is necessary.

GUIDELINES
CARING FOR THE RESIDENT WHO IS HEMORRHAGING

- Stay with the resident and reassure him or her.
- Call for help and notify the nurse.
- Observe for signs of shock and respond appropriately if observed.
- Use standard precautions as needed.
- Apply pressure directly over the hemorrhage site by holding an appropriate dressing with your gloved hand (see Figure 7-7 ■).
- If the dressing becomes saturated, do not remove it. Add additional dressings as needed while continuing to apply pressure.
- If hemorrhage continues while maintaining direct pressure over the wound, elevate the bleeding areas (if it is an extremity) above the heart and continue the direct pressure on the wound.
- If hemorrhage continues after elevation, apply pressure to the artery supplying blood to the area of the injury.

Pressure points are places where arteries supplying blood lie over a bone near the surface of the skin (see Figure 7-8 ■). If you observe evidence of a broken bone in the area of the injury or if it is painful to elevate a limb, do not elevate it. Do not

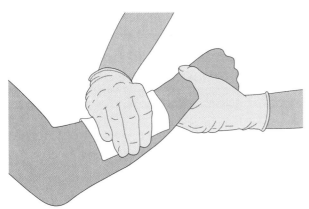

FIGURE 7-7 ■ Apply direct pressure to stop a hemorrhage.

discontinue one step in controlling hemorrhage to replace it with another. The steps must be done simultaneously as they are added.

*E*MERGENCY CARE FOR A STROKE

Blood vessels in the brain may rupture or a clot may lodge and block blood flow. In medical terminology the term for stroke is **cerebrovascular accident (CVA).** A stroke is the interruption of blood flow in the brain and can be life-threatening. See Chapter 23 for more information about strokes. The following guidelines will help you care for a resident who is experiencing a stroke until medical help arrives.

GUIDELINES
EMERGENCY CARE OF A RESIDENT WHO IS SUSPECTED OF HAVING A STROKE
• Notify the nurse and call for help.
• Stay with the resident and be reassuring.
• Maintain an open airway and provide CPR if it becomes necessary.
• Maintain normal body temperature and avoid chilling.
• Protect paralyzed limbs.
• Do not provide food or fluids.
• Slightly elevate the head and shoulders.
• If there is danger of aspiration, position the resident on the side.
• Monitor pulse, respirations, and blood pressure.
• Observe for signs and symptoms and report them to the nurse.

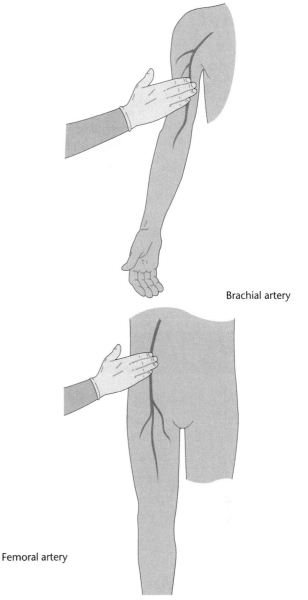

Brachial artery

Femoral artery

FIGURE 7-8 ■ Pressure points may be used, in addition to the use of direct pressure, to stop hemorrhage.

Signs and symptoms of a stroke include the following.

- Seizures
- Headache
- Drooling
- Unequal pupils
- Vision or speech problems
- Change in the level of consciousness
- Confusion
- Paralysis
- Difficulty breathing

EMERGENCY CARE FOR SEIZURES

A **seizure** (convulsion) is a sudden spasm of muscles that is caused by abnormal brain activity. The resident may have tremors, and loss of conciousness often occurs. The intensity, length, and extent of seizures vary. Observe and report the length and progression of the seizure and the involvement of parts of the body.

Learning first aid procedures will help you to protect your family and friends, as well as the residents in your care. If an injury or sudden illness occurs while you are at work, you should stay with the resident and call the nurse, who will direct further care.

GUIDELINES

FOR CARING FOR THE RESIDENT WHO IS EXPERIENCING A SEIZURE

- Call for help and notify the nurse.
- Stay with the resident and be reassuring.
- Prevent further injury.
- Loosen tight clothing at the neck.
- Observe the progression of the seizure.
- Do not attempt to place anything in the resident's mouth.
- Do not attempt to restrain the resident's movements.
- Maintain an open airway.
- Report your observations to the nurse.

CHAPTER HIGHLIGHTS

1. First aid is immediate care for injury or sudden illness that is given to prevent further injury and save lives.
2. The American Red Cross, the National Safety Council, and the American Heart Association offer courses on handling emergencies.
3. Check the environment for safety.
4. Move the resident only if necessary to prevent injury and ensure safety.
5. Staying calm helps you to function well.
6. Life-threatening emergencies must be treated first.
7. Dial 911 or the operator to summon the emergency medical service (EMS).
8. Keeping the resident flat and warm helps to prevent shock.
9. Severe respiratory distress is a life-threatening condition.
10. The Heimlich maneuver is the first aid for an airway obstruction.
11. CPR replaces lung and heart function when respiratory and cardiac arrest have occurred.
12. Pressure is used to stop hemorrhage.
13. A stroke is life-threatening.
14. The first aid for seizures is the prevention of injuries.
15. If an injury or sudden illness occurs, you should stay with the resident, call for the nurse, and follow instructions.

VOCABULARY REVIEW

Fill in the blanks with the vocabulary term that best completes the sentence.

1. A medical term that means severe bleeding is _____.

2. _____ (____) is the procedure for emergency care to replace heart and lung function.

3. The heartbeat is the _____.

4. Breathing is called _____.

5. _____ is physical injury or emotional upset.

6. Immediate care for injuries or sudden illness is called _____.

7. To inhale food or fluids or to choke is to _____.

8. A stroke is also called a _____ _____ and is abbreviated _____.

9. To _____ means to check or evaluate.

10. A blue color of the skin, lips, and nails due to lack of oxygen is _____.

CHECK YOUR UNDERSTANDING

The following questions cover the highlights of the chapter. Choose the best answer for each question.

1. You find a resident lying on the floor beside his bed and moaning. What should you do?
   A. Call for help and stay with the resident.
   B. Get the nurse immediately.
   C. Call 911 immediately.
   D. Get the resident up and into the bed.

2. Which of the following conditions is considered life-threatening?
   A. hemorrhage
   B. fainting
   C. diarrhea
   D. vomiting

3. How should the victim who is in shock be positioned?
   A. sitting up
   B. lying down
   C. with the head raised
   D. with the feet apart

4. Which of the following is a symptom of stroke?
   A. extreme hunger
   B. bruised skin
   C. paralysis
   D. equal pupils

5. The emergency procedure for an airway obstruction is called
   A. cardiopulmonary resuscitation
   B. seizure precautions
   C. the Heimlich maneuver
   D. the White maneuver

6. The resident you are ambulating begins to have a seizure. What should you do *first*?
   A. Place a padded tongue blade between the teeth.
   B. Loosen the resident's clothing.
   C. Lower the resident to the floor.
   D. Take the resident's blood pressure.

AGE-SPECIFIC TIP

Because of sensory changes that occur with aging, you may need to take special care to communicate and provide reassurance for the elderly resident in an emergency. For example, be sure that the hearing-impaired resident can see your lips when you are communicating.

CULTURALLY SENSITIVE TIP

Reassurance can be communicated nonverbally. In an emergency situation, be aware of the message you convey by your facial expression, movements, and voice tones.

EFFECTIVE PROBLEM SOLVING

A resident is choking at mealtime. She is unable to cough, speak, or breathe. The nursing assistant panics and shouts, "Oh no, you're choking! Hold still so I can get my arms around you!"

Was the nursing assistant's communication appropriate? If not, what would have been more appropriate?

_____

_____

_____

_____

_____

_____

_____

_____

_____

INTERPERSONAL COMMUNICATION

Write T or F to indicate if the statement is true or false.

_____ Stay with the injured resident while you call for the nurse.

_____ It is not necessary to report a brief seizure to the nurse.

_____ Your calmness is a reassuring form of communication.

_____ If your resident has a seizure, attempt to restrain the violent movements by holding the resident's body with your hands.

_____ Ask the choking resident if he or she can cough.

OBSERVING, REPORTING, AND RECORDING

A life-threatening emergency occurs at work. The nurse directs you to call EMS. List the information you need to give over the telephone.

_____

_____

_____

_____

_____

_____

_____

_____

_____

EXPLORE MEDIALINK

Check out www.prenhall.com/grubbs for additional chapter-specific interactive study and review activities.

8

THE RESIDENT'S UNIT

OBJECTIVES

1. List ten guidelines for maintaining a restorative environment.
2. List six pieces of equipment that might be found in the resident's unit.
3. List six guidelines for care and use of equipment.

4. List six guidelines for cleaning equipment.
5. Explain the responsibility of the nursing assistant in maintaining the resident's unit.

VOCABULARY

The following words or terms will help you to understand this chapter:

Restorative environment
Emesis basin
Emesis

Urinal
IV (Intravenous) fluids

Disinfection
Sterile

The resident's unit is the room or area that contains the resident's furniture and belongings. It is a private space—a retreat. The resident lives in the unit. When you enter the resident's unit, you are entering a home. Demonstrate the same courtesies when you enter the resident's unit that you would use as a guest in any home. You are a guest in the resident's room.

$\mathcal{A}$ RESTORATIVE ENVIRONMENT

A **restorative environment** is one that promotes independence. It is arranged in a way that allows as much self-care as possible. Adequate lighting is provided, with switches or controls that are within the resident's reach. A call signal is available that allows the resident to call staff members with a minimum of effort.

Safety is very important. Emergency signals and safety bars are provided in the bathroom. A person who does not have to depend on others for safety feels more secure. A feeling of security promotes independence.

Privacy is protected in a restorative environment. Maintaining privacy increases the resident's feeling of self-worth.

Cleanliness and neatness are important to a restorative environment. Housekeepers clean the unit daily and as needed. Maintenance employees keep the furniture and equipment repaired. The use of aseptic practices helps to keep the resident healthy and free from disease, making it easier to maintain independence.

A restorative environment is familiar and homelike to the resident. The resident is encouraged to bring family pictures and mementos from home. A favorite afghan or cushion might be placed on the bed. When space permits, the resident may want to have a rocking chair, chest of drawers, or other personal furniture. The resident should be able to look around the unit and recognize familiar objects. It is comforting to awaken at night and see a picture of a loved one on the bedside table.

The Effects of a Restorative Environment

A restorative environment improves self-esteem, motivation, and independence. These positive

---

GUIDELINES

MAINTAINING A RESTORATIVE ENVIRONMENT

- Safety is the most important consideration in caring for the resident's unit.
- Wash your hands upon entering and leaving the resident's room.
- Keep furniture arranged to promote resident independence, convenience, and safety.
- Always place the call signal within the resident's reach.
- Leave the bed close to the floor when you leave the room to ensure ease and safety so that the resident can get in and out of it independently.
- Keep the bed wheels locked.
- Protect the resident's privacy by closing window coverings, doors, and privacy screens or curtains during personal care.
- Knock at the door before entering the resident's room.
- Noise and temperature should be kept at a level that is comfortable for the resident.
- Keep the unit neat and use aseptic practices to prevent infection.
- Extra linen should not be stored in the resident's room.
- The overbed table is a clean area. Do not place bedpans, urinals, soiled linen, or other soiled supplies on it.
- Report broken items immediately and remove them from use until they are repaired. Use of broken equipment can be unsafe.
- Handle the resident's personal belongings with care.
- Do not discard supplies or equipment that are soiled with body fluids or body substances in the resident's room. These should go to the proper utility room for disposal.
- Remove the food tray as soon as the resident has finished a meal.
- Provide privacy for the resident's visits with friends and family.
- Ask to look in the resident's drawers before doing so.
- Store the personal belongings where the resident wishes.

GUIDELINES (Continued)

- Keep fresh drinking water available and within reach if the resident is allowed to drink.
- Check the comfort of the resident before leaving the room.
- To promote independence, assistive equipment should be kept within the resident's reach when it is not being used.

feelings support and promote each other. A resident with high self-esteem feels more motivated. The motivated resident strives for independence, and being independent improves self-esteem. A restorative environment protects dignity and privacy. Having personal belongings helps to maintain the resident's identity. It creates a home-like atmosphere as well as a sense of ownership and control.

𝓕URNITURE AND EQUIPMENT

The resident's unit contains furniture and equipment to help meet the resident's basic needs (see Figure 8-1 ■). The furniture is designed to promote health and wellness. Although the facility furnishes all the necessary furniture and equipment, some items may belong to the resident. Furniture that is provided for the resident includes a bed, an overbed table, a bedside table, and a chair. Some rooms also might have a chest of drawers or a desk. Closets and storage space are provided for each unit.

The Overbed Table

The overbed table is considered a clean area. The resident may use it for meals or personal care and grooming. It also is used for some treatments and procedures. Contaminated linens or equipment (such as bedpans) should not be placed on it.

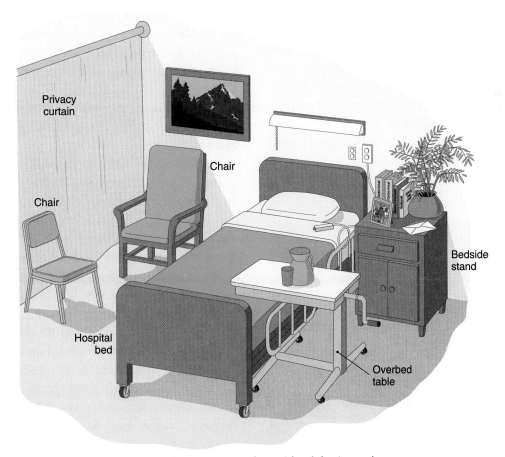

FIGURE 8-1 ■ Furniture is provided in each unit to meet the resident's basic needs.

The Bedside Table

The bedside table provides storage for personal care equipment such as wash basins and bedpans. It also provides a convenient place for small personal items such as a toothbrush, denture cup, toothpaste, hairbrush, comb, hearing aid, and eyeglasses. The water pitcher and cup often are found on top of the bedside table. Personal mementos also may be placed there.

The Call Signal

The facility provides a call signal for each unit. This allows the resident to call for assistance as needed. The call signal may be a light or a bell that is connected to an intercom at the nurses' station. When the resident pushes a button, a light will go on outside the door and at the nurses' station. Sometimes an alarm also will ring. The nurse may be able to talk to the resident through the intercom. It is important to keep the call signal always within the resident's reach and to answer all call lights promptly (see Figure 8-2 ■).

Bathrooms

Bathrooms are located conveniently for all residents. The bathroom may be located in each room or between two rooms. Other bathrooms are located off main hallways for residents who are out of their rooms. In addition to typical equipment, the bathrooms also contain call signals and handrails.

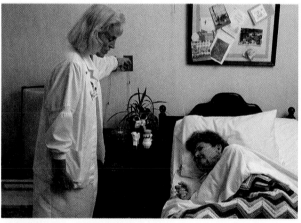

FIGURE 8-2 ■ The call signal allows the resident to call for assistance as needed.

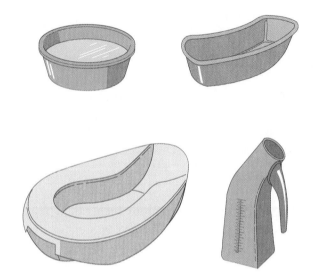

FIGURE 8-3 ■ Examples of standard equipment that will be in the resident's unit.

Equipment

Standard equipment that usually is provided in a resident's unit includes a wash basin, emesis basin, bedpan, and urinal (see Figure 8-3 ■). These items are used for personal care. An **emesis basin** is a small kidney-shaped pan into which the resident spits or vomits (**emesis** is vomitus). The curved edge of the basin is designed to fit the curve of the resident's chin. The emesis basin also may be used for mouth care. A **urinal** is a container that the male resident uses when urinating. It is used for the resident who cannot go into the bathroom.

A water container and cup also may be furnished. Most residents bring their own toothbrush, toothpaste, comb, brush, and other personal care items. Although some residents may have their own bar of soap, most facilities provide liquid soap in dispensers. The facility also will provide lotion for residents who do not bring their own.

Sometimes a resident will require special equipment to be used for administering oxygen, tube feedings, or **IV (intravenous) fluids** administered through a needle into the vein (see Figure 8-4 ■). This type of equipment is returned to the appropriate storage area when not in use. Wheelchairs are available for residents who need them. However, some residents may have their own. Canes, walkers, and crutches usually belong to the individual resident. It is your responsibility to

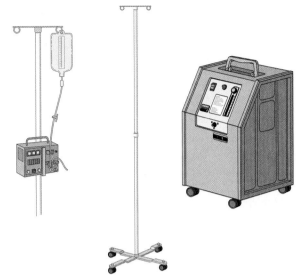

FIGURE 8-4 ■ Examples of special equipment that might be needed.

GUIDELINES (Continued)

- Ask the nurse to explain if you do not know how to use a piece of equipment.
- Personal equipment and supplies should not be shared by residents.
- Discard disposable equipment in the proper container in the dirty utility room (see Figure 8-5 ■). Do not discard used equipment in an open waste container.
- Do not attempt to perform a procedure with equipment that you do not know how to use.
- Check equipment before you use it and report defects immediately.
- Do not use equipment that is defective or damaged (see Figure 8-6 ■).
- Follow the guidelines for cleaning of equipment.

know which equipment belongs to the resident and which is the property of the facility.

CARE AND USE OF EQUIPMENT

Using and caring for equipment is an important responsibility of the nursing assistant. Using equipment correctly prevents infection or injury to the resident or yourself. The proper care of equipment prevents waste and helps to hold down the cost of health care.

Correct Use of Equipment

You will be taught the correct method for using many pieces of equipment during your training program. The use of some equipment is explained during orientation to the long-term care facility.

GUIDELINES

THE CARE AND USE OF EQUIPMENT

- Refer to the procedure book or instruction manuals for instructions on the use of equipment.
- Always follow the correct steps when using equipment.
- Do not take shortcuts because they can lead to accidents.

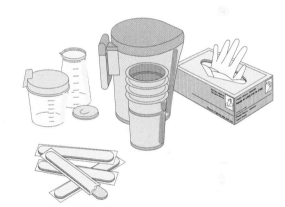

FIGURE 8-5 ■ Examples of disposable equipment.

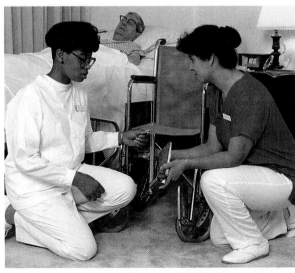

FIGURE 8-6 ■ Report defective equipment immediately.

Nondisposable Equipment

Larger and more expensive equipment usually is not disposable and must be cleaned before reuse. Cleaning reduces the number of microorganisms on the equipment. Some equipment must be disinfected or sterilized. **Disinfection** (see Figure 8-7 ■) is the use of chemicals to destroy pathogens. It does not kill all microorganisms. An object that is **sterile** is free of all microorganisms.

GUIDELINES

CLEANING EQUIPMENT

- Wear gloves and follow standard precautions.
- Wash with soap and hot water.
- Use a brush if necessary.
- Rinse equipment in cold water and dry.
- Disinfect or sterilize.
- Keep disinfectants out of the residents' reach because they may be harmful.

Preventing Waste

Medical equipment is expensive. This is one of the reasons that health care costs so much. Buying and replacing equipment contributes to the cost of health care. Waste costs money.

Cost containment is an important issue in health care today. You can do your part in keeping costs

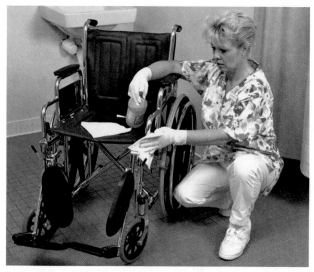

FIGURE 8-7 ■ Disinfectants are used to destroy pathogens.

down by the correct care and use of equipment. All of us bear the burden of the high cost of health care.

RESPONSIBILITIES IN MAINTAINING THE RESIDENT'S UNIT

Nursing assistants in long-term care have many responsibilities regarding the resident's unit. They help to keep it clean and neat. After providing care to the resident, they clean and put away equipment. The rules of safety and asepsis must be followed. One of your most important responsibilities is to maintain a restorative environment.

CHAPTER HIGHLIGHTS

1. Treat the resident's belongings with respect and care.
2. A restorative environment increases the resident's self-esteem.
3. The overbed table is considered a clean area.
4. It is important to keep the call signal always within the resident's reach and to answer lights promptly.
5. Using equipment correctly prevents injury to the resident and yourself.
6. If you do not know how to use a piece of equipment, ask the nurse to explain.
7. Always discard disposable equipment in the proper container.
8. Immediately report equipment that is defective or damaged.
9. Maintain a restorative environment for the residents.

VOCABULARY REVIEW

Fill in the blanks with the vocabulary term that best completes the sentence.

1. _____ is the use of chemicals to destroy pathogens.

2. A container that the male resident uses when urinating is a/an _____.

3. A _____ is an environment that promotes independence.

4. Another name for vomitus is _____.

5. _____ are administered through a needle into a vein.

6. An object that is _____ is free of all microorganisms.

7. A/an _____ is a small kidney-shaped pan into which the resident spits or vomits.

8. An item that is _____ has been exposed to microorganisms.

9. _____ means being able to care for yourself and being in control of your life.

10. Microorganisms that cause disease or infection are _____.

CHECK YOUR UNDERSTANDING

The following questions cover the highlights of this chapter. Choose the best answer for each question.

1. Which of the following does *not* contribute to a restorative environment?
   A. The overbed table is placed in the resident's closet.
   B. The unit is clean, neat, and peaceful.
   C. The environment promotes independence.
   D. The call signal is within the resident's reach.

2. What is your best response if you are not sure how to use a piece of equipment?
   A. Do the best you can.
   B. Ask the nurse to explain.
   C. Ask the administrator to explain.
   D. Don't use the equipment.

3. What is the *first* step in cleaning soiled equipment?
   A. Wash it with hot, soapy water.
   B. Disinfect or sterilize it.
   C. Wash it with plain hot water.
   D. Rinse it with cold water.

4. Used disposable supplies and equipment should be discarded in
   A. the resident's wastebasket
   B. the proper container
   C. the clean-utility room
   D. the bathroom wastebasket

5. The footrest on the resident's wheelchair is broken. What should you do?
   A. Tell the nurse when you finish using it.
   B. Report it immediately.
   C. Put it aside and get another one.
   D. Continue to use it carefully.

6. The nursing assistant's most important consideration in caring for the resident's unit is
   A. resident safety
   B. making the bed
   C. the amount of time used
   D. keeping the bathroom clean

7. Where should the wheelchair be kept while the resident is in bed?
   A. In the closet
   B. At the foot of the bed
   C. Folded up in the hallway
   D. Next to the bed within the resident's reach

8. Which of the following may the nursing assistant place on the overbed table?
   A. clean linen
   B. soiled linen
   C. the bedpan
   D. medication

AGE-SPECIFIC TIP

The call signal provides a communication lifeline for the elderly resident with limited mobility. Be sure it is within the resident's reach.

CULTURALLY SENSITIVE TIP

Communicate respect for cultural differences by handling the resident's personal belongings carefully.

EFFECTIVE PROBLEM SOLVING

The resident complains that conversation outside his door at night disturbs his sleep. The nursing assistant replies, "I'm sorry, but we have to communicate with each other."

Was the nursing assistant's communication appropriate? If not, what would have been more appropriate?

_____
_____
_____
_____
_____
_____
_____
_____
_____
_____
_____
_____
_____

INTERPERSONAL COMMUNICATION

Which communications support a restorative environment? Check the examples that are appropriate.

_____ Knocking on the door before entering
_____ Asking the resident before opening the blinds
_____ Telling the resident to clean up her messy closet
_____ Answering the call signal when it's convenient

OBSERVING, REPORTING, AND RECORDING

What would you observe in a room that contributed to a restorative environment? Make a list.

_____
_____
_____
_____
_____
_____
_____
_____
_____
_____
_____
_____
_____
_____

EXPLORE MEDIALINK

Check out www.prenhall.com/grubbs for additional chapter-specific interactive study and review activities.

$\mathcal{B}$EDMAKING

$\mathcal{O}$BJECTIVES

1. Maintain the physical safety and emotional comfort of the resident when making a bed.
2. Use correct body mechanics when making a bed.
3. Apply the rules of asepsis when making beds.

4. Identify four restorative guidelines to follow while making beds.
5. Explain the use of communication and observation during bedmaking.
6. Demonstrate the procedures described in this chapter.

$\mathcal{V}$OCABULARY

The following words or terms will help you to understand this chapter:

Body alignment

Pressure sore

Draw sheet
Comatose

Bedmaking is important because it helps promote rest and sleep for the resident. Rest and sleep are essential to health and well-being. A well-made bed promotes comfort, ensures resident safety, and offers a pleasing, professional appearance. A bed will be more comfortable if the linen is clean and free from wrinkles (see Figure 9-1 ■). Privacy is maintained by using a bath blanket to avoid exposing the resident's body during procedures. A neat, clean bed can also improve the resident's mood and increase self-esteem.

SAFETY

As in all tasks, the most important concern is resident safety. The following safety factors should be considered when making a bed:

Body Mechanics

Always use correct body mechanics while making a bed. Raise the bed to a height that is comfortable for you. Stand with your feet apart and your back straight. Bend at your knees, not at your waist. Avoid twisting motions by turning your whole body at once when you change directions. Make as much of one side of the bed as possible before be-

ginning the other side. This technique uses less of your energy, and is faster and more efficient. Review the guidelines for using correct body mechanics in Chapter 6.

Body Alignment

Body alignment means maintaining a normal or correct anatomical position. This helps the resident look and feel more comfortable. Use pillows, pads, and other special equipment to support the body and prevent bony areas, such as the knees, from rubbing together. When positioning a resident on the side, use pillows to support the upper arm and leg. Another pillow rolled against the back helps keep the resident's body in proper alignment.

Skin Protection and Prevention of Pressure Sores

A **pressure sore** is a breakdown of tissue that occurs when blood flow is interrupted. It is sometimes called a "decubitus" or "bedsore." Correct bedmaking helps to prevent pressure sores. Anything that might cause pressure on the resident's skin should be avoided. Keep the linen free of wrinkles, small objects, or crumbs. Change a wet or dirty bed immediately because it also can cause skin problems. Pressure sores are discussed in detail in Chapter 12.

Most facilities use mattresses with a waterproof covering. If protective pads are used, they must be changed as soon as they become wet or dirty. Avoid excessive padding because it causes pressure.

Furniture and Equipment

Before you leave the room, return the bed to its lowest position and lock the wheels. The gatch handles should be positioned out of the way so that no one will be injured. A gatch handle is a crank that is used to change the position of the bed. Be sure the call signal is within the resident's reach. If the resident is out of the room, fasten the call signal to the bedding or place it where it is readily available.

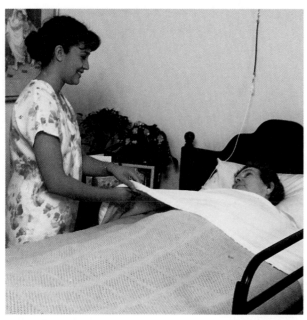

FIGURE 9-1 ■ A bed will be more comfortable if the linen is clean and free from wrinkles.

GUIDELINES

HANDLING USED LINEN

- Wear gloves and follow standard precautions when handling linen contaminated with body fluids or substances. Gloves may be worn for handling all soiled linen.
- Do not shake used linen.
- Hold used linen away from your uniform.
- When removing linen from the bed, roll it away from you with the side that touched the resident on the inside.
- Never place used linen on the overbed table or the floor. Use bags, if provided.
- Take used linen directly to the linen hamper.
- Wash your hands after handling used linen.
- Keep the used-linen hamper away from food and medicine carts and clean linen storage. Hallway linen hampers should not be taken into residents' rooms.
- Keep linen hampers covered and empty them regularly.
- Check used linen for personal items such as glasses, dentures, or hearing aids.

HANDLING CLEAN LINEN

- Place clean linen on the overbed table or another clean surface.
- Do not place clean linen on another resident's furniture.
- Carry clean linen away from your uniform.
- When changing a pillow case, do not hold the pillow against your body or truck it under your chin.
- Avoid shaking clean linen.
- Wash your hands before handling clean linen.
- Keep the clean-linen cart covered.
- Always position the clean-linen cart away from used-linen hampers, housekeeping carts, and trash containers.
- Take only what you need into the resident's room. Unused linen that is in the room is contaminated and must be taken to the used-linen hamper. It may not be used for another resident.
- Clean linen that touches the floor is contaminated.

$\mathcal{A}$SEPSIS AND INFECTION CONTROL

Following standard precautions and the rules of asepsis helps to prevent the spread of infection.

Handwashing

You may need to wash your hands several times during the bedmaking procedure. Remember, handwashing is the best way to prevent the spread of infection. Always wash your hands before you begin, before handling clean linen, after handling soiled linen, and before leaving the room. Hands must be washed before applying and after removing gloves.

$\mathcal{T}$YPES OF BEDS

There are many types of beds in long-term care facilities. Some are electric and some are manual (operated by hand). The electric controls (see Figure 9-2 ■) may be located so that the resident can operate them, or they may be at the foot of the bed, out of the resident's reach.

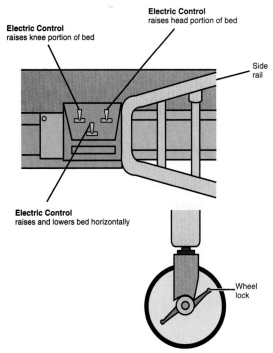

FIGURE 9-2 ■ Electric controls for a bed may be located where the resident can operate them or they may be at the foot of the bed. The bed wheels have locks.

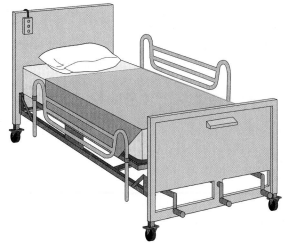

FIGURE 9-3 ■ The manually operated bed has gatch handles to change the position of the bed.

Manual beds are equipped with gatch handles (see Figure 9-3 ■) to change the position of the bed. Usually, there are three controls. One raises and lowers the entire bed. The second handle operates the head of the bed, and the third one operates the foot of the bed. Handles or cranks must be folded under the bed or positioned out of the way to prevent injuries.

Most beds are on wheels to allow them to be moved as needed. Always lock the wheels when you finish moving the bed. A bed on wheels will move very easily and quickly.

Side Rails

There are many kinds of side rails. Although they may not look alike or work the same way, they all have the same purpose—to protect the resident. It is not correct to raise the side rails on all residents' beds because side rails are a form of restraint. Familiarize yourself with facility policies, and identify residents requiring the use of side rails.

Mattresses

Mattresses tend to slide toward the foot of the bed. This can make the resident uncomfortable when the head of the bed is raised. Before you make the bed, slide the mattress to the top of the bed. You may need to do this several times a day for a bedbound resident. If necessary, ask a coworker to help. A mattress pad

may be used between the mattress and the bottom sheet to make the resident more comfortable.

LINEN

Organization of linen is important when you make a bed. Collect the linen in the order in which it will be used. The first piece of linen you pick up should be the first piece you will be putting on the bed (either a mattress pad or a bottom sheet if a mattress pad is not used). Stack the linen on your arm in the following order:

* Mattress pad
* Bottom sheet
* Draw sheet
* Top sheet
* Blanket
* Bedspread
* Pillowcase

Carry the linen to the resident's unit, holding it away from your uniform. Place the linen on a clean surface, turning the entire stack over so that the linen is in the order in which it will be used (see Figure 9-4 ■). The mattress pad will now be on top.

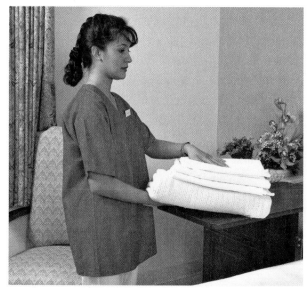

FIGURE 9-4 ■ Stack the linen in the order that it will be used.

Draw Sheets

A **draw sheet** is a small sheet that is placed across the middle of the bottom sheet. It also is known as a "pull sheet" or "turning sheet." When the draw sheet is tucked in, it helps keep the bottom sheet in place and free of wrinkles. When it is not tucked in, it can be used to move and position the resident. Usually a draw sheet is about one-half the size of a regular sheet. If no draw sheet is available, you can make one by folding a regular sheet to the size needed. The procedures for using a draw sheet to move and position a resident will be explained in Chapter 11.

Use of Linen

Because facilities differ in their use of linen, it is important to learn the policy of your facility. Some facilities use draw sheets, while others use disposable or nondisposable pads. Although fitted bottom sheets are used in many places, others may use flat sheets. Many facilities remove the bedspread when the resident is in bed.

Linen is used for bedmaking and bathing. It also may be used for comfort or to position the resident. Sheets are not to be used as restraints. Special lightweight blankets called "bath blankets" are available to use when bathing residents or performing other personal care procedures. A bath blanket provides the resident with privacy, warmth, and comfort.

Linen Changes

A complete change of linen may not be necessary every day. Most of the residents are up and about during the day and use their beds only at night. Beds are changed more often for residents who spend most of their time in bed. All beds are changed immediately if they become wet or dirty.

STRIPPING A BED

Before clean linen is placed on a bed, the used linen must be removed. This procedure is called "stripping a bed." Many times, the bed is stripped as soon as the resident gets out of bed. If the bed linens are dirty or wet, apply gloves before stripping. Follow the guidelines for handling dirty linen. Remove gloves and wash your hands. Wipe the bed with disinfectant before applying clean linen. Let the nurse know if the mattress is damaged.

Check carefully for personal items that may be in the bed. Residents sometimes put jewelry, glasses, or dentures under their pillows or in the linens. These items may be lost or ruined if they go through the laundry.

A CLOSED BED

A closed bed is fully made with a blanket and bedspread in place. It is made for the resident who is up for the day. A closed bed also is made when the bed will not be in use.

AN OPEN BED

An open bed is made with the linen turned down. Open beds are made for residents who will be returning to the bed after being up for a short while. The bed is made while the resident is out of it. The linen is turned down, and the bed is ready for the resident. An open bed also may be prepared for a new admission. Usually, a bedspread is not used on an open bed.

AN OCCUPIED BED

Making a bed with the resident in it is called "making an occupied bed." This is done when a resident is not able to get out of bed. Critically ill or **comatose** (unconscious) residents are residents for whom you may need to make an occupied bed.

A bedspread may not be needed for this procedure. It usually is folded and put away when the resident is in bed.

Always use the restorative approach when making an occupied bed. This technique encourages the resident to participate as much as possible. Always explain what you are going to do, even if the resident is confused or unconscious. A resident who is very ill may be able to cooperate if you explain first.

PROCEDURE

Stripping a Bed

■ Beginning Steps

Before any procedure, you always must follow the five basic steps: wash your hands, collect the equipment, identify the resident, explain the procedure, and protect privacy.

✋ Follow Standard Precautions

1. Raise the bed to a comfortable working height and lock the wheels.
2. Wear gloves if the linen is wet or soiled, and follow the guidelines for handling used linen.
3. Loosen the linen all around the bed.
4. Remove the pillow from the pillowcase.
5. If the bedspread and blanket are dirty, roll them up with the rest of the linen. If they are to be reused, fold them separately, using the following steps:

   a. Grasp the bedspread at the top center edge and the corner nearest you. Fold it by bringing the top edge of the spread to the bottom edge of the spread.
   b. Grasp the center of the folded edge with one hand and the corner nearest you with the other hand. Fold the bedspread again by bringing the folded edge to the bottom edge of the spread.
   c. Fold the spread by grasping the edges nearest you and bringing these edges to the edges of the spread on the other side of the bed.
   d. Fold the spread over the back of the bedside chair.
   e. Repeat the steps for the blanket.
6. Roll or fold the rest of the linen away from you with the side that touched the resident inside the roll (see Figure 9-5 ■).
7. Place the used linen in the used-linen hamper immediately.
8. If the mattress is wet, wipe it with disinfectant and observe for damage.

■ Ending Steps

To complete the procedure, perform the following steps:

Make the resident comfortable, positioning in good body alignment. Make the resident safe, placing the call signal within reach, lowering the bed, and raising the side rails, if appropriate. Wash your hands. Record and report the procedure as required.

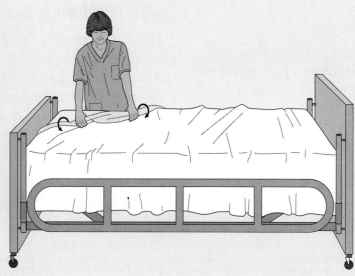

FIGURE 9-5 ■ Roll the soiled linen away from you, with the side that touched the resident inside the roll. ■

PROCEDURE

Making a Closed Bed

■ **Beginning Steps**

Before any procedure, you always must follow the five basic steps: wash your hands, collect the equipment, identify the resident, explain the procedure, and protect privacy.

Follow Standard Precautions

1. Place the clean linen, in the order in which it will be used, on a clean surface in the resident's room.
2. Raise the bed to a comfortable working height and lock the wheels.
3. If you have not stripped the bed, you must do so at this time.
4. Slide the mattress to the top of the bed.

Working from one side of the bed, use the following steps:

5. Put the mattress pad on the bed.
6. Place the bottom sheet in the center of the bed.
7. Check to see how the sheet is folded. If you are using a flat sheet, unfold the sheet and place the narrow hem at the bottom, even with the foot of the mattress. The wide hem will be at the top (see Figure 9-6 ■) and the rough side of the hem should be face down on the mattress.
8. Smooth the side nearest you.
9. Tuck the sheet under the top of the mattress at the head of the bed on the side nearest you.

10. Make a mitered corner (see Figure 9-7 ■).
    a. Grasp the edge of the sheet 10 to 12 inches from the top of the bed and fold it onto the mattress (see Figure 9-7A ■).
    b. Tuck the part of the sheet that is hanging down under the mattress (see Figure 9-7B ■).
    c. Bring the folded part down over the edge of the mattress (see Figure 9-7C ■).
    d. Tuck the entire side of the sheet under the mattress (see Figure 9-7D ■).
11. If a draw sheet is to be used, place it on top of the sheet, about 12 inches from the top edge of the mattress (see Figure 9-8 ■).
12. Tuck the draw sheet under the mattress on the side nearest you.
13. Put the top sheet on the center of the bed.
14. Unfold the sheet with as little movement as possible.
15. Center the top sheet with the wide hem even with the top of the mattress and the stitched or seamed side up. Keep the rough edges away from the resident's body.
16. Smooth the side of the bed nearest you. Do not tuck the bottom of the top sheet under the mattress yet.
17. Place the blanket over the top sheet as follows:
    a. Unfold and center it.
    b. The top of the blanket should be about 6 to 8 inches below the top edge of the top sheet.
    c. Smooth the blanket on the side nearest you.
    d. Fold the top sheet down over the top of the blanket to make a cuff.

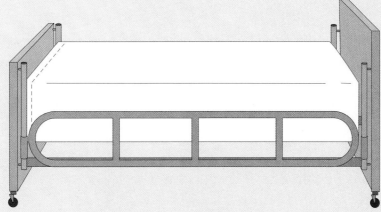

FIGURE 9-6 ■ The bottom sheet is placed on the bed with the narrow hem at the bottom, even with the foot of the mattress.

(continued)

Making a Closed Bed (Continued)

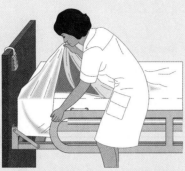

A Grasp the edge of the sheet 10 to 12 inches from the top of the bed and fold it onto the mattress.

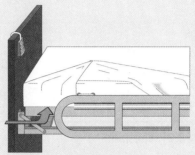

B Tuck the part of the sheet that is hanging down under the mattress.

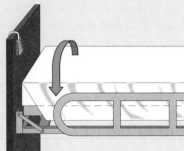

C Bring the folded part down over the mattress.

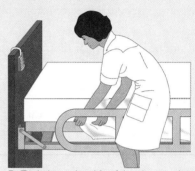

D Tuck the entire side of the sheet under the mattress.

FIGURE 9-7 ■ Miter the corners of the sheet to make the bed look neat.

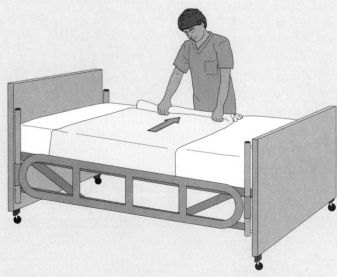

FIGURE 9-8 ■ The draw sheet is placed on top of the bottom sheet. It should be pulled tight and tucked under the mattress.

(continued)

18. Place the bedspread over the blanket as follows:
    a. Unfold and center it.
    b. Place the bedspread so that about 18 inches extend over the head of the bed (this will be used to cover the pillow).
    c. Smooth the bedspread on the side nearest you.
    d. Turn about 24 to 25 inches of the bedspread back from the head of the bed.
19. Tuck in the top sheet, the blanket, and the bedspread all at the same time at the foot of the bed on this side, and make a mitered corner.

👆 **Go to the other side of the bed to finish the procedure as follows:**

20. Tuck in the bottom sheet at the head of the bed (see Figure 9-9 ■).
    a. Make a mitered corner and pull the bottom sheet tight as you tuck it under the entire length of the mattress on this side.
    b. Smooth it to remove wrinkles.

21. Pull the draw sheet tight and tuck it under the mattress.
22. Straighten the top linen, working from the top to the foot of the bed.
23. Tuck the top linen under the foot of the mattress. After smoothing and tightening it, make a mitered corner.
24. Finish turning the top of the bedspread down about 24 to 25 inches. Turn the top of the sheet over the top of the blanket.

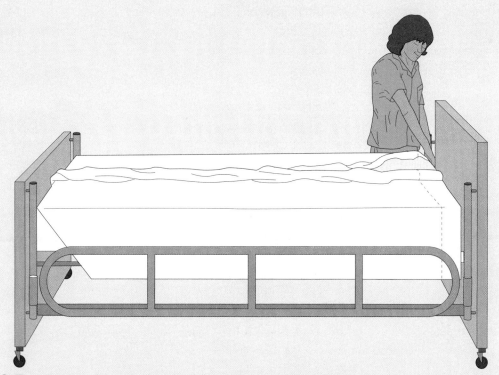

FIGURE 9-9 ■ Go to the other side of the bed and tuck in the bottom sheet at the head of the bed.

(continued)

Making a Closed Bed (Continued)

25. Place the pillow on the bed, and put it into the pillow-case, using the following steps (see Figure 9-10 ■).

   a. With one hand, grasp the clean pillowcase at the center of the seamed end (see Figure 9-10A ■).

   b. Turn the pillowcase back over that hand with your free hand (see Figure 9-10B ■).

   c. Grasp the pillow at the center of one end with the hand that is inside the pillowcase (see Figure 9-10C ■).

   d. Pull the pillowcase down over the pillow with your free hand (see Figure 9-10D ■). Line up the seams of the pillowcase with the edge of the pillow.

   e. Straighten the pillowcase, making sure that the corners of the pillow are in the corners of the pil-lowcase (see Figure 9-10E ■).

   f. Fold the extra material of the pillowcase under the pillow.

26. Place the pillow on the bed so that the open edge of the pillowcase is facing away from the door.

27. Cover the pillow with the bedspread.

28. Attach the call signal to the bed if the resident is out of the room, and tidy the room.

■ Ending Steps

To complete the procedure, perform the following steps:

Make the resident comfortable, positioning in good body alignment. Make the resident safe, placing the call signal within reach, lowering the bed, and raising the side rails, if appropriate. Wash your hands. Record and report the procedure as required.

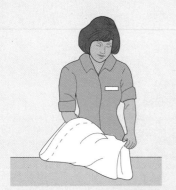

A With one hand, hold the pillowcase at the center of the seamed end.

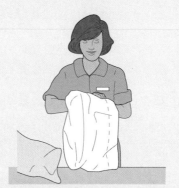

B Turn the pillowcase back over that hand with your free hand.

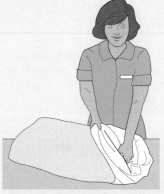

C Grasp the pillow at the center of one end with the hand that is inside the pillowcase.

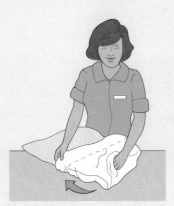

D Pull the pillowcase down over the pillow with your free hand.

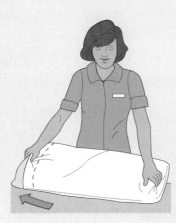

E Straighten the pillowcase.

FIGURE 9-10 ■ The nursing assistant is putting the pillow into the pillowcase.

PROCEDURE

Making an Open Bed

■ Beginning Steps

Before any procedure, you always must follow the five basic steps: wash your hands, collect the equipment, identify the resident, explain the procedure, and protect privacy.

Follow Standard Precautions

1. Place the clean linen, in the order in which it will be used, on a clean surface in the resident's room.
2. Raise the bed to a comfortable working height and lock the wheels.
3. If you have not stripped the bed, you must do so now.
4. Slide the mattress to the top of the bed.

Working from one side of the bed, use the following steps:

5. Put the mattress pad on the bed.
6. Place the bottom sheet in the center of the bed.
7. Check to see how the sheet is folded. Unfold the sheet and place the narrow hem at the bottom, even with the foot of the mattress. The wide hem will be at the top (see Figure 9-6) and the rough side of the hem should be face down on the mattress.
8. Smooth the side nearest you.
9. Tuck the sheet under the top of the mattress at the head of the bed on the side nearest you.
10. Make a mitered corner (see Figure 9-7).
11. If a draw sheet is to be used, place it on top of the sheet, about 12 inches from the top edge of the mattress (see Figure 9-8).
12. Tuck the draw sheet under the mattress on the side nearest you.
13. Put the top sheet on the center of the bed.
14. Unfold the sheet with as little movement as possible.
15. Center the top sheet with the wide hem even with the top of the mattress and the stitched or seamed side up.
16. Smooth the side of the bed nearest you. Do not tuck the bottom of the top sheet under the mattress yet.
17. Place the blanket over the top sheet as follows:
    a. Unfold and center it.
    b. The top of the blanket should be about 6 to 8 inches below the top edge of the top sheet.
    c. Smooth the blanket on the side nearest you.
    d. Fold the top sheet down over the top of the blanket to make a cuff.
18. Tuck in top sheet and blanket all at the same time, at the foot of the bed on this side, and make a mitered corner.

Go to the other side of the bed to finish the procedure as follows:

19. Tuck in the bottom sheet at the head of the bed (see Figure 9-9).
    a. Make a mitered corner and pull the bottom sheet tight as you tuck it under the entire length of the mattress on this side.
    b. Smooth the sheet to remove wrinkles.
20. Pull the draw sheet tight and tuck it under mattress.
21. Straighten the top linen, working from the top to the foot of the bed.
22. Tuck the top linen under the foot of the mattress. After smoothing and tightening it, make a mitered corner.
23. Turn the top of the sheet over the top of the blanket.
24. Place the pillow on the bed, and put it into the pillowcase, using the steps shown in Figure 9-10.
25. Place the pillow on the bed so that the open edge of the pillowcase is facing away from the door.
26. Grasp the top of the sheet and blanket, and fold it to the foot of the bed (see Figure 9-11 ■).
27. Tidy the room.

■ Ending Steps

To complete the procedure, perform the following steps:

Make the resident comfortable, positioning in good body alignment. Make the resident safe, placing the call signal within reach, lowering the bed, and raising the side rails, if appropriate. Wash your hands. Record and report the procedure as required.

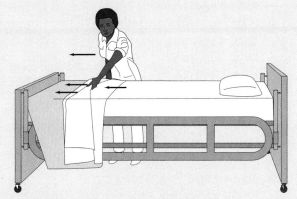

FIGURE 9-11 ■ Grasp the top of the sheet and blanket and fold them to the foot of the bed.

PROCEDURE

Making an Occupied Bed

■ Beginning Steps

Before any procedure, you always must follow the five basic steps: wash your hands, collect the equipment, identify the resident, explain the procedure, and provide privacy.

Follow Standard Precautions

1. Place the clean linen, in the order in which it will be used, on a clean surface in the resident's room.
2. Pull the curtain around the bed and/or close the door.
3. Raise the bed to a comfortable working height and lock the wheels.
4. Lower the head of the bed, being sure to maintain a height that is safe and comfortable for the resident.
5. Lower the side rail on the side of the bed nearest you. Be sure the rail is up on the opposite side of the bed.
6. Loosen the top linen at the foot of the bed.
7. Remove the blanket.
   a. If it is dirty, remove it by rolling or folding it away from you, with the side that touched the resident inside the roll.
   b. If it is to be reused, fold it over the back of the chair.
8. To be sure that the resident is covered at all times cover the resident with a bath blanket, using the following steps:
   a. Unfold the bath blanket over the top sheet.
   b. Ask the resident to grasp the top of the bath blanket or tuck the top edge under the resident's shoulders to keep it in place (see Figure 9-12 ■).
   c. Grasp the sheet under the bath blanket and slide it out at the foot of the bed, rolling it with the side that touched the resident on the inside. Place it with the used linen.
   d. If you do not have a bath blanket, leave the top sheet in place over the resident or use a clean top sheet. The resident must be kept covered for warmth and privacy.
9. Move the mattress to the top of the bed.
10. Assist the resident to turn away from you to the far side of the bed (see Figure 9-13 ■).
    a. Help the resident to maintain correct body alignment.
    b. Adjust the pillow as needed.
    c. Be sure the resident is not too close to the side rail.

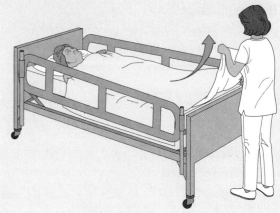

FIGURE 9-12 ■ Tuck the top edge of the bath blanket under the resident's shoulders to hold it in place while you slide the top sheet out from under the blanket.

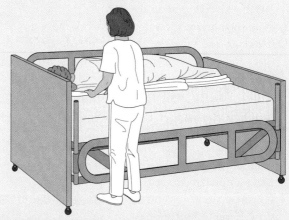

FIGURE 9-13 ■ The used bottom linen is folded to the resident's body and tucked under to hold it in place.

11. Loosen the bottom linen on this side of the bed and fold it to the resident's body. Tuck it under the resident's body (see Figure 9-13).

Working from the side of the bed nearest you, use the following steps:

12. Put the mattress pad on the bed.
13. Place the bottom sheet in the center of the bed, next to the resident.

(continued)

14. Check to see how the sheet is folded. Unfold the sheet and place the narrow hem at the bottom, even with the foot of the mattress (see Figure 9-6) with the rough side of the hem face down on the mattress.
15. Smooth the side nearest you, and tuck the sheet under the top of the mattress at the head of the bed.
16. Make a mitered corner (see Figure 9-7).
17. If a draw sheet is to be used, place it on top of the sheet about 12 inches from the top edge of the mattress (see Figure 9-8).
18. Tuck the draw sheet under the mattress.
19. Fold the clean linen toward the resident, next to the used linen (see Figure 9-14 ■).
20. Raise the side rail on this side.
21. Ask the resident to turn or move toward you to the clean side of the bed. Assist as necessary.
    a. Explain that the resident will roll across the folded linen.
    b. Be sure the resident is not too close to the rail.
    c. Adjust the pillow.

🖐 Go to the opposite side of the bed.

22. Lower the rail on this side.
23. Loosen the used bottom linen, roll it away from you with the side that touched the resident on the inside, and place it with the other used linen.
24. Unfold the clean linen that is in the center of the bed.
25. Straighten the bottom sheet, and tuck it in at the head of the bed.
    a. Make a mitered corner.
    b. Tuck the sheet under the mattress while pulling it tight.
26. Straighten the draw sheet, and tuck it under the mattress while pulling it tight (see Figure 9-15 ■).

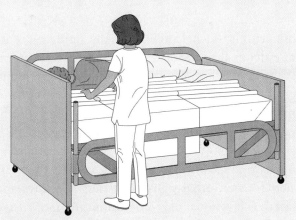

FIGURE 9-14 ■ The clean linen is folded toward the resident, next to the used linen.

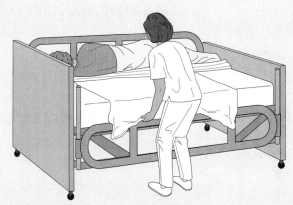

FIGURE 9-15 ■ The draw sheet is straightened, pulled tight, and tucked under the mattress.

27. Assist the resident to a comfortable position.
28. Put the top sheet on the center of the bed.
29. Unfold the sheet with as little movement as possible.
30. Center the top sheet so that the wide hem is even with the top of the mattress and the stitched or seamed side is up.
31. Smooth this side of the bed. Do not tuck the bottom of the top sheet under the mattress yet.
32. Place the blanket over the top sheet as follows:
    a. Unfold and center it.
    b. The top of the blanket should be about 6 to 8 inches below the top edge of the top sheet with the top sheet folded down over it.
    c. Smooth the blanket on this side.
33. Ask the resident to hold the clean top sheet and blanket as you remove the used sheet or bath blanket by pulling it from under the clean linen at the foot of the bed. Roll the used linen with the side that touched the resident to the inside.
    a. If the resident cannot hold the clean sheet, you may tuck it beneath the shoulders.
    b. Place the used sheet or bath blanket with the used linen that has already been removed.
34. Tuck the top linen under the bottom of the mattress on this side of the bed and make a mitered corner.
35. Put the side rail up on this side of the bed. Go to the other side of the bed and lower the side rail.

(continued)

Making an Occupied Bed (Continued)

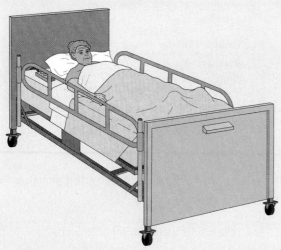

FIGURE 9-16 ■ The top linen is straightened and tucked in at the bottom of the mattress.

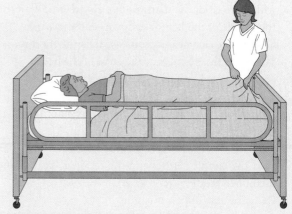

FIGURE 9-17 ■ Pull up on the top linen to loosen it over the resident's feet.

36. Complete the bed by straightening the top linen and tucking it in at the bottom of the mattress (see Figure 9-16 ■) and making a mitered corner.
37. Raise the side rail.
38. Make sure the top linen is not too tight over the resident's toes. Loosen it by pulling up the top linen or making a pleat (see Figure 9-17 ■).
39. Place the pillow on the bed, and put it into the pillowcase (see Figure 9-10).
40. Place the pillow on the bed so that the open edge of the pillowcase is facing away from the door.
41. Tidy the room.

42. Pull the curtain from around the bed and/or open the door.
43. Dispose of the linen in the used-linen hamper if you have not already done so.

■ Ending Steps

To complete the procedure, perform the following steps:

Make the resident comfortable, positioning in good body alignment. Make the resident safe, placing the call signal within reach, lowering the bed, and raising the side rails, if appropriate. Wash your hands. Record and report the procedure as required.

$\mathcal{A}$ RESTORATIVE APPROACH TO BEDMAKING

There are many opportunities to use restorative measures when making a resident's bed. This is especially true when you are making an occupied bed. The following guidelines will help you protect the resident's safety and promote independence during the bedmaking procedure.

Communication and Observation

Bedmaking provides an excellent time for communicating with the resident. You will have the perfect opportunity to help maintain the resident's sense of individuality and self-esteem. Talk about current events and ask questions. Show your interest and give encouragement. You may hear verbal complaints and problems that cannot be observed otherwise. Remember how important it is to be a good listener. Your visual observations of movements and posture are possible at this time. Be alert for nonverbal signs of distress. Gestures and facial expressions may communicate more than words. Remember that touch is a form of communication, so be gentle and confident.

GUIDELINES

A RESTORATIVE APPROACH TO BEDMAKING

- Talk to the resident and encourage communication.
- Explain the procedure step by step to all residents.
- Encourage residents to get out of bed when possible.
- Encourage the resident to help in turning and moving.
- Protect the resident's privacy at all times.

GUIDELINES (Continued)

- Handle the resident gently and confidently.
- Leave the bed at a safe, low level with the call signal within reach.
- Observe and report any changes in the resident's condition.
- Make sure the linen is not too tight over the resident's toes by pulling up the top linen or making a pleat.

CHAPTER HIGHLIGHTS

1. Bedmaking is important because it helps promote rest and sleep for the resident.
2. Always protect the resident's privacy while making the bed.
3. The most important concern in all tasks is resident safety.
4. Raise the bed to a comfortable working height, and use correct body mechanics.
5. As much as possible, make one side of the bed at a time.
6. Keep the bed wrinkle-free and smooth.
7. Change linen immediately if it is soiled.
8. Follow standard precautions and wear gloves when appropriate.
9. Don't shake clean or used linen.
10. Never place used linen on a clean surface or on the floor.
11. Collect the clean linen in the order in which it will be used.
12. Carry clean linen away from your uniform.
13. Handle the resident gently, and position him or her in correct body alignment.
14. Always use the restorative approach to bedmaking.
15. Communicate with the resident during bedmaking.
16. Raise the side rails when appropriate.
17. Leave the call signal within the resident's reach.

VOCABULARY REVIEW

Fill in the blank with the vocabulary term that best completes the sentence.

1. A breakdown of skin tissue that occurs when blood flow is interrupted is called a/an _____.

2. A/An _____ is made with the linen turned down, ready for the resident's return to bed.

3. A small sheet placed across the middle of the bottom sheet to help secure the bottom linen is a/an _____.

4. A/An _____ is a crank used to change the position of the bed.

5. _____ is the absence of pathogens.

6. If the resident is not able to get out of bed, you will need to make a/an _____ _____.

7. _____ means maintaining a normal or correct anatomical body position.

8. An item that has been used or exposed to germs is considered _____.

9. _____ means that the resident is unconscious.

10. Correct _____ means using the body in a careful and efficient manner.

CHECK YOUR UNDERSTANDING

The following questions cover the highlights of t his chapter. Choose the best answer for each question.

1. Which is the most efficient way to make a bed?
   A. Make one side of the bed before beginning the other side.
   B. Secure each sheet on both sides as you go.
   C. Make the bottom half of the bed first.
   D. Make the top half of the bed first.

2. Which of the following bedmaking techniques does *not* help prevent skin breakdown?
   A. Keep the linen free from wrinkles.
   B. Remove crumbs from the linens.
   C. Place two pads under the resident's body.
   D. Change a wet bed immediately.

3. How do you remove soiled linen from the bed without contaminating your uniform?
   A. Fold the side that touched the resident on the outside.
   B. Fold the linen away from you.
   C. Fold the linen toward you.
   D. Cover the linen with plastic before you begin.

4. You are making a bed with an unconscious resident in it. Which of the following is most appropriate?
   A. Be quiet and concentrate on your work.
   B. Don't explain because the resident can't hear you.
   C. Explain what you are doing to the resident.
   D. Talk to your coworker while you make the bed.

5. You are making an occupied bed. Which of the following is the most restorative approach?
   A. Do everything for the resident.
   B. Encourage the resident to help in turning and repositioning.
   C. Tell the resident to get out of bed.
   D. Lower both side rails.

6. What is the correct way to place a clean pillowcase on a pillow?
   A. Tuck the pillow under your chin and pull the pillowcase up over the pillow.
   B. Drop the pillow into the pillowcase and shake it vigorously.
   C. Hold the pillow against your body and pull the pillowcase over the pillow.
   D. Lay the pillow on the bed and pull the pillowcase down over the pillow.

AGE-SPECIFIC TIP

The elderly bedbound resident may not feel like talking. During bedmaking, observe for nonverbal communications such as facial expression and body movement.

CULTURALLY SENSITIVE TIP

The resident who speaks another language may have difficulty understanding what you are saying. Remember that touch is a form of communication and handle the resident gently.

EFFECTIVE PROBLEM SOLVING

The nursing assistant is making an occupied bed for an unconscious resident. Assuming that the resident cannot hear, the nursing assistant talks to the resident's roommate instead of to the unconscious resident.

    Was the nursing assistant's communication appropriate? If not, what would have been more appropriate?

_____

_____

_____

_____

_____

_____

_____

_____

_____

_____

INTERPERSONAL COMMUNICATION

The following statements are nursing assistant responses to a resident's daughter who wants to help make her father's bed. Check the examples that are appropriate.

_____ "No, thank you. I don't need any help."

_____ "Why don't you get some coffee while I make the bed."

_____ "I would appreciate your help. Can you straighten his pillow?"

_____ "Go ahead and finish it. I'll be next door."

OBSERVING, REPORTING, AND RECORDING

List four observations that you might make during bedmaking that should be reported to the nurse.

_____

_____

_____

_____

_____

_____

_____

_____

_____

_____

_____

_____

_____

_____

EXPLORE MEDIALINK

Check out www.prenhall.com/grubbs for additional chapter-specific interactive study and review activities.

10

ADMISSION, TRANSFER, AND DISCHARGE

OBJECTIVES

1. Describe the emotional impact of admission to the long-term care facility.
2. List four responsibilities of the nursing assistant in the admission process.
3. List four responsibilities of the nursing assistant in transferring a resident.
4. List four responsibilities of the nursing assistant in the discharge process.
5. List seven guidelines for restorative admission, transfer, and discharge.
6. Demonstrate the procedures described in this chapter.

VOCABULARY

The following terms will help you to understand this chapter:

Orient   **Discharge planning**

Approaches for providing emotional support and procedures for assisting in admissions, transfers, and discharges of residents are provided in this chapter.

THE EMOTIONAL IMPACT OF ADMISSION

Residents who are admitted to a long-term care facility may feel stressed, anxious, and frightened. Many have suffered losses such as loss of health, spouse, home, or possessions. The loss of independence and the ability to care for oneself can be devastating. Giving up one's home with familiar routines for a new environment filled with uncertainty can be very frightening. Imagine how you would feel if you had to move, without your friends and family, to an unfamiliar place.

Events prior to admission may have been stressful for residents and family members. The confused resident who wanders may have been unsafe at home (see Figure 10-1 ■). Most families prefer to care for relatives at home, but sometimes this isn't possible. When needs can no longer be met at home, admission to a long-term care facility may be necessary. Family members may feel angry or guilty because they believe they have failed.

Nursing assistants play a very important role in easing the emotional stress for the resident and family. Your attitude can reduce many fears and provide a more comfortable beginning for the new resident. First impressions are lasting, so it is important to make a positive impression on both the resident and the family.

ADMITTING THE RESIDENT

The admission process begins in the business office, where information about the facility is provided. Plans and arrangements for admission are made, and paperwork is completed. Among other duties, the nursing assistant is responsible for preparing the room, welcoming the resident, completing the belongings list, and orienting the resident to the facility. Before the resident's arrival, prepare the room with all the necessary items. Be sure to check with the nurse for information such as the resident's abilities and disabilities and whether food or fluids are allowed. Prepare the room to be comfortable and welcoming.

Warmly greeting the new resident by name will help create a feeling of welcome and comfort. Call the resident by his or her proper name and title unless directed to do otherwise. For example, you might say, "Good morning, Mr. Smith." Introduce yourself by name and title. Accompany the resident to the room. Greet the family in a friendly manner and encourage them to accompany the resident. Remember that they may also be uncomfortable or nervous about the admission.

The Belongings List

The nurse will provide you with a form to list the resident's valuables and personal belongings. Describe each item and list quantities. Jewelry must be described by color of metal and stones. What appears to be precious metal or stones may not be. For example, jewelry that the resident calls

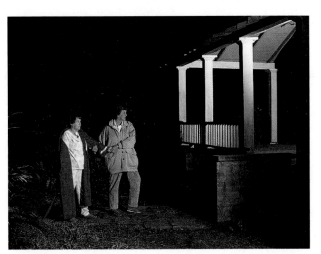
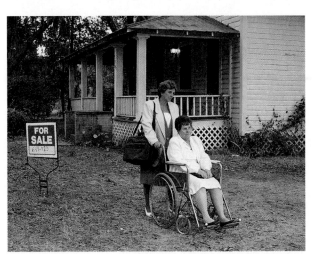

FIGURE 10-1 ■ Prior to admission, the new resident and his or her family may have experienced many stressful events.

a gold and diamond ring would be described as "a yellow metal ring with a clear stone." If medications are found in the belongings, tell the nurse. Always handle the resident's belongings with care and respect.

Belongings are marked according to facility policy. Family members should be instructed to advise the staff when they bring in additional items. Items that are taken from the facility must be deleted from the list.

FAMILIARIZING THE RESIDENT WITH THE FACILITY

Orient (familiarize) the resident to the facility. Explain mealtimes, dining locations, visiting hours, and smoking rules. Show the resident how to find the nurses' desk, rest rooms, water fountains, TV rooms, recreation areas, and the chapel. Identify the areas of the room and the furniture that will be used by the resident. Provide a general idea of daily schedules and ask about preferences. Introduce the resident to other residents and staff members (see Figure 10-2 ■).

Before leaving, assure the resident that you will be nearby and available. Explain the use of the call signal and intercom. Leave the call signal within reach. Be sure to check back frequently. Help to make it comfortable and safe.

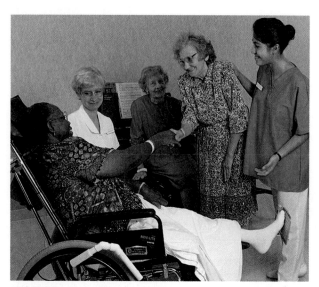

FIGURE 10-2 ■ Introduce the new resident to other residents and staff members.

TRANSFERRING THE RESIDENT

The nursing assistant plays a very important role in transferring a resident. The transfer may be from room to room or from one nursing unit to another. Transfers can be very upsetting to the resident. Even a healthy resident, who is willing to move, may find that moving is both physically and emotionally distressful. The resident will need emotional support from staff members to make the transfer successful. You can maintain a restorative attitude during the transfer by offering support and encouragement. Remember to be a good listener, as the resident may want to express feelings about the move. The nursing assistant's responsibilities in transferring a resident include collecting the resident's belongings, transporting him to the new area, introducing him to the new staff, and ensuring his comfort in the new area.

DISCHARGING THE RESIDENT

Discharge can be a stressful event, even in the most positive circumstances. We expect the resident to be happy to have recovered enough to return home. But the resident may have doubts about being able to function adequately at home. Or he may be sad at leaving friends and caregivers he has learned to trust. Sometimes a resident is discharged to a hospital or another long-term care facility. That can cause fear and anxiety. Emotional support and reassurance can help the resident calm these fears and adjust to the discharge.

Discharge cannot take place until the doctor has written an order and financial arrangements have been made. The nurse will inform you of the time of discharge, after notification by the doctor and the business office. If a resident attempts to leave and you have not been informed of the discharge, notify the nurse immediately.

Discharge planning (the plans and arrangements for care of the resident after discharge) is the responsibility of nurses. The plan begins on admission to the facility and follows through the actual discharge. It includes resident and family education for the resident's care at home. Nursing assistants can help by reinforcing the nurse's instructions. Let the nurse know if the family seems to

PROCEDURE

Admitting a Resident

■ Beginning Steps

Before any procedure, you always must follow the five basic steps: wash your hands, collect the equipment, identify the resident, explain the procedure, and protect privacy.

✋ Follow Standard Precautions

1. Assemble equipment on the overbed table.
2. Adjust the bed to the correct height and turn down the linen to open the bed.
3. Place the hospital gown or pajamas on the foot of the bed.
4. Introduce yourself to the resident and family.
5. Provide privacy and show the family where they can wait.
6. Assist the resident to change clothes if necessary.
7. Help the resident unpack. List clothes and belongings according to facility policy.
8. Measure the resident's height and weight.
9. Assist the resident to the bed or a chair.
10. Measure the resident's vital signs.
11. Notify the nurse immediately if the resident complains of pain or dyspnea.
12. Collect specimens if ordered.
13. Collect information and complete the admission checklist.
14. Provide water if allowed.
15. Orient the resident to facility routines such as mealtimes and visiting hours. Identify the location of the nurses' station, restrooms, and dining room.

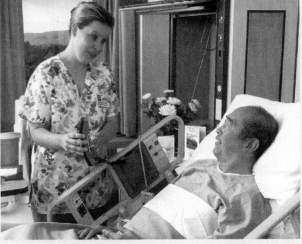

FIGURE 10-3 ■ Explain and demonstrate the call signal to the resident.

Demonstrate the bed controls and call signal (see Figure 10-3 ■).
16. Identify and encourage the use of safety bars and rails.

■ Ending Steps

To complete the procedure, perform the following steps:

Make the resident comfortable, positioning in good body alignment. Make the resident safe, placing the call signal within reach, lowering the bed, and raising the side rails. if appropriate. Wash your hands. Record and report the procedure as required.

need more information. This may indicate that they do not fully understand the plan.

The nursing assistant's responsibilities in discharging a resident include assisting the resident to dress, packing her belongings, transporting her to the discharge vehicle, and returning equipment to the proper area. In some facilities you may be responsible for stripping the bed and cleaning the unit. You may be asked to take the resident to the discharge area. Most residents are transported in wheelchairs. Never leave the resident unattended. Help load the resident's belongings and assist the resident into the discharge vehicle (see Figure 10-4 ■).

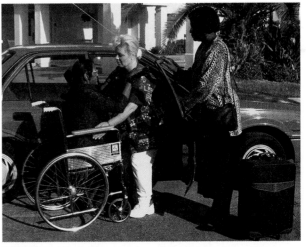

FIGURE 10-4 ■ Assist the resident into the vehicle.

PROCEDURE

Transferring a Resident

■ **Beginning Steps**

Before any procedure, you always must follow the five basic steps: wash your hands, collect the equipment, identify the resident, explain the procedure, and protect privacy.

Follow Standard Precautions

1. Get a report from the nurse that includes the resident's destination and method of transport. Arrange for help if necessary.
2. Carefully place the resident's belongings and supplies on a utility cart for transport. Check closets and drawers carefully.
3. Assist the resident to a wheelchair or stretcher. Sometimes the entire bed is transported with the resident in it.
4. Acknowledge the resident's fears and distress while maintaining a positive, supportive attitude.
5. Transport the resident to the new unit.
6. Assist the resident to the bed or chair as needed.
7. Introduce the resident to his or her roommate and the staff.

8. Put away the resident's belongings respectfully and carefully.
9. Demonstrate the bed controls and call signal. Make sure the resident is comfortable and safe.
10. Record and report to the nurse on the new unit when you have completed the transfer.
11. Return the wheelchair, utility cart, or other equipment to the storage area and return to your own unit.
12. Report to your supervisor when you return to your unit.
13. Strip the bed and remove supplies and equipment from the unit. In some facilities, this is the responsibility of the housekeeping staff.

■ **Ending Steps**

To complete the procedure, perform the following steps:

Make the resident comfortable, positioning in good body alignment. Make the resident safe, placing the call signal within reach, lowering the bed, and raising the side rails, if appropriate. Wash your hands, Record and report the procedure as required.

PROCEDURE

Discharging a Resident

■ **Beginning Steps.**

Before any procedure, you always must follow the five basic steps: wash your hands, collect the equipment, identify the resident, explain the procedure, and protect privacy.

Follow standard precautions.

1. Assist the resident to dress.
2. Assist the resident to pack. Check drawers and closets carefully. Place the resident's belongings on a utility cart.
3. Complete the inventory list according to facility policy.

4. Check with the nurse to make sure the resident has received discharge instructions.
5. Assist the resident into a wheelchair.
6. Transport the resident to the discharge area and assist her into the discharge vehicle.
7. Make sure the resident is buckled in safely and comfortably.
8. Return the wheelchair and cart to the storage area.
9. Strip the bed and clean the unit unless this is the responsibility of the housekeeping staff.
10. Wash your hands. Report the procedure as required.

USING A RESTORATIVE APPROACH FOR ADMISSION, TRANSFER, AND DISCHARGE

A restorative approach to care begins upon admission to a long-term care facility. Because it is not normal to give up independence, home, and individual lifestyle, the resident will need to be reassured and encouraged. Restorative care must be continued throughout residence. The primary restorative goal is to return the resident to a normal life at home. The following guidelines will help you provide a restorative approach.

GUIDELINES

RESTORATIVE ADMISSION, TRANSFER, AND DISCHARGE

- Provide restorative care every day on every shift.
- Offer encouragement and praise.
- Provide frequent reassurance.
- Be courteous, friendly, and helpful.
- Use empathy and think about the resident's and family members' feelings.
- Encourage resident independence.

GUIDELINES (Continued)

- Support the resident's efforts to express individuality.
- Be aware of and respect cultural differences.
- Encourage the resident to express feelings.
- Encourage the resident to help plan and prepare for the move.
- Allow the resident to help organize and arrange the environment (see Figure 10-5 ■).
- Maintain a supportive attitude.
- Be aware of the resident's fears and anxieties.

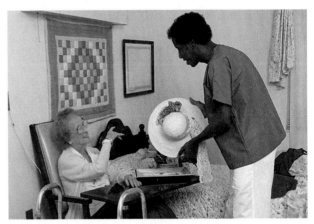

FIGURE 10-5 ■ Involve the resident in arranging her room.

CHAPTER HIGHLIGHTS

1. Admission to a long-term care facility is stressful for both the resident and family.
2. Nursing assistants play an important role in easing the emotional stress for residents and family members.
3. Greet the resident by name and introduce yourself.
4. List valuables and label clothing according to facility policy.
5. Orient the new resident to the facility, and introduce residents and staff members.
6. Maintain a restorative attitude during transfer by offering support and encouragement to the resident.
7. Listen while the resident expresses feelings about moving.
8. Discharge can be a stressful event even in the most positive circumstances.
9. A restorative approach to care begins upon admission and continues through discharge.
10. A friendly, helpful, and reassuring attitude can reduce the stress of admission, transfer, or discharge.
11. Emotional support is necessary during any kind of move within a health care facility.

VOCABULARY REVIEW

Fill in the blanks with the vocabulary term that best completes the sentence.

1. A/an _____ is a form that lists the resident's valuables and personal belongings.

2. Mental and physical strain or tension is _____.

3. A/an _____ provides health care to people who are unable to care for themselves at home but are not sick enough to be in a hospital.

4. To _____ is to familiarize the resident with the new surroundings.

5. Being able to care for oneself and being in control of one's life is _____.

6. A _____ is the plans and arrangements for care of the resident after discharge.

7. Infection control practices designed to protect health care workers from exposure to blood, body fluids, and body substances are called _____.

8. _____ is nursing care that assists each resident to function at the highest possible level of independence.

9. Understanding how you would feel if it were your mother who was being admitted to the facility is _____.

10. Undressing the new resident without pulling the privacy curtain is _____ of _____.

CHECK YOUR UNDERSTANDING

The following questions cover the highlights of this chapter. Choose the best answer for each question.

1. Which of the following statements about admission is *false*?
   A. Most families prefer to care for elderly relatives at home.
   B. Some elderly people are unsafe at home.
   C. Most people prefer to put elderly relatives in a long-term care facility.
   D. Family members may be unable to care for elderly relatives at home.

2. An elderly woman is being admitted to your unit. What is the best way to greet her?
   A. "Hello, Mrs. Smith. I'm Janet, your nursing assistant."
   B. "Well, hello! What's your name?"
   C. "Hey, Grannie. You're new here, aren't you?"
   D. "Hi there. I'm Janet, your nursing assistant."

3. During admission, the resident tells you that her ring is real gold and diamonds. How should you describe it on the belongings list?
   A. A real gold and diamond ring.
   B. A yellow metal ring with a clear stone.
   C. A yellow ring with a glass stone.
   D. A yellow metal ring with a diamond stone.

4. Which of the following statements about transferring is most supportive?
   A. "Don't worry. I'm sure you'll like the new room."
   B. "Don't complain. You're lucky to get such a nice room."
   C. "I can see you're upset. You ought to call your doctor."
   D. "I can see you're upset. How can I help you?"

5. A resident who has not been discharged insists that she is going home. What should you do?
   A. Restrain her immediately.
   B. Notify the nurse immediately.
   C. Tell her that she cannot leave without a doctor's order.
   D. Tell her that she can leave if she wants to.

6. You have just admitted a new resident. Which of the following is the most restorative approach?
   A. Unpack all his clothes and put them away for him.
   B. Tell him he'll need to unpack for himself.
   C. Encourage a family member to unpack for him.
   D. Encourage the resident to participate in unpacking.

AGE-SPECIFIC TIP

Most elderly residents are slow to adapt to change. Give them time to adjust to the new environment and encourage them to express their feelings.

CULTURALLY SENSITIVE TIP

The feeling of failure regarding the admission of a loved one to a long-term care facility is more pronounced in some cultures. Help the family to cope by communicating in a warm, friendly manner.

EFFECTIVE PROBLEM SOLVING

Mr. Charro is nervous and upset about his admission to the nursing home. In an attempt to make him more comfortable, the nursing assistant begins to tease him and tell him jokes. Was the nursing assistant's communication appropriate? If not, what would have been more appropriate?

_____
_____
_____
_____
_____
_____
_____
_____
_____
_____
_____
_____
_____

INTERPERSONAL COMMUNICATION

Which statements reflect a restorative approach to admission, transfer, or discharge? Check the examples that are appropriate.

_____ "Don't cry. You're going to love it here."

_____ "Where would you like to put this photograph?"

_____ "I know you don't want to move, and I'll miss you."

_____ "You can't put that statue on the bedside table because there isn't room."

_____ "You should be happy that you're going home."

OBSERVING, REPORTING, AND RECORDING

List four observations you would record while admitting a resident.

_____
_____
_____
_____
_____
_____
_____
_____
_____
_____

EXPLORE MEDIALINK

11

$\mathcal{M}$OVING AND EXERCISING RESIDENTS

$\mathcal{O}$BJECTIVES

1. Identify ten benefits of physical activity.
2. Identify ten complications of limited activity.
3. List six guidelines for restorative activity techniques.
4. Identify four rules of body mechanics to be used while moving and positioning residents.
5. Explain the importance of body alignment.
6. Demonstrate four basic body positions.
7. List three advantages of using a gait/transfer belt.
8. Identify six guidelines for using a mechanical lift.
9. Describe five guidelines for transporting a resident in a wheelchair.
10. List six guidelines for assisting a resident to ambulate.
11. Identify five safety guidelines for performing range-of-motion exercises.
12. Demonstrate the procedures described in this chapter.

$\mathcal{V}$OCABULARY

The following words or terms will help you to understand this chapter:

Contracture
Paralysis
Muscle atrophy
Constipation
Fecal impaction
Extremities
Edema

Hypostatic pneumonia
Disoriented
Body mechanics
Body alignment
Supine position
Prone position
Lateral position

Fowler's position
Dangling
Geri-chair
Ambulate
Range-of-motion exercises
Abduction
Adduction

SECTION 1 The Restorative Approach to Activity

Section one explains the principles of activity and how the body works.

THE IMPORTANCE OF EXERCISE AND ACTIVITY

Exercise is good for elderly residents. Physical activity helps maintain the well-being of all body systems. Some of the benefits of physical activity are included in the following table.

THE BENEFITS OF PHYSICAL ACTIVITY
Increased muscle strength and tone
Increased respiratory rate and depth
Improved circulation
Increased immune function
Improved elimination (removal of body waste)
Improved digestion
Improved physical and emotional well-being
Increased independence and self-esteem
Improved mental function
Increased longevity

COMPLICATIONS OF LIMITED EXERCISE AND ACTIVITY

Lack of exercise causes problems that may affect all body systems. The following table includes some of the many complications of limited activity.

A pressure sore (decubitus) is a breakdown in skin tissue that occurs when blood flow is interrupted. If a resident lies or sits in one position too long or is positioned incorrectly, pressure will cause skin damage.

A **contracture** is a permanent shortening of a muscle due to lack of use or lack of exercise. A contracture results when a part of the body is not moved and exercised enough. Have you ever noticed a person with a weak arm holding it against the chest? If it is kept in this position for a period of time, a contracture may develop (see Figure 11-1 ■).

COMPLICATIONS OF LIMITED ACTIVITY
Pressure sores
Contractures
Muscle atrophy
Constipation
Fecal impaction
Edema
Blood clots
Urinary tract infection (UTI)
Kidney stones
Pneumonia
Confusion
Depression

One form of contracture is called "foot drop." Foot drop occurs when the foot is not supported in natural alignment. A contracture may be the result of **paralysis** (the inability to move a body part) or a spastic condition. However, most contractures can be prevented by exercise, proper positioning, and other restorative techniques.

Muscle atrophy is wasting or a decrease in the size of a muscle. Atrophy occurs when the muscle is not used or exercised.

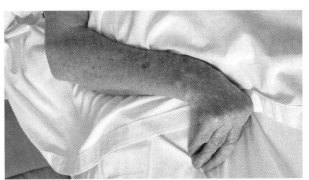

FIGURE 11-1 ■ Keeping the arm in one position for a long period of time can cause a contracture.

Decreased activity may slow digestion. When this happens, the large intestine absorbs too much water from the stool, which becomes dry and hard. **Constipation** is the passage of hard, dry stool. One complication of constipation is a **fecal impaction** (a large amount of hard, dry stool). When constipation is not relieved, an impaction can fill the rectum. The impaction must be removed before the person can have a normal bowel movement. Nursing assistants do not remove impactions.

Inactivity causes circulation to slow down and become sluggish. When blood flow to the **extremities** (the arms and legs) slows, fluid collects in the tissues. This accumulation of fluid causes swelling and is called **edema**. Poor circulation is the major factor contributing to blood clots. It also plays a role in the development of pneumonia, urinary tract infections, and kidney stones.

Hypostatic pneumonia is a type of pneumonia that occurs when a person remains too long in one position. Gravity causes blood and other fluids to pool in one part of the lung, where infection can easily occur.

Limited activity can affect the resident's mental and emotional status. The lack of stimulation, combined with slowed circulation, may cause the resident to become **disoriented** (confused as to person, place, or time). Inactive people easily can become depressed. They may feel helpless and without hope. An active life is a healthy life. Inactivity damages the body and dulls the spirit.

$\mathcal{R}$ESTORATIVE TECHNIQUES

Restorative nursing care can prevent most of the complications of limited activity. Assisting the resident to move and exercise will give you many opportunities to use restorative techniques. Always encourage the resident to do as much as possible. This promotes the resident's mobility and increases body strength. It also helps to build his or her independence and self-esteem.

Remember the principles of restorative care that were described in Chapter 4 of this text:

- Treat the whole person.
- Start rehabilitation early.
- Stress ability—not disability.
- Encourage activity.
- Maintain a restorative attitude.

GUIDELINES

RESTORATIVE ACTIVITY TECHNIQUES

- Follow the principles of restorative care.
- Determine the resident's abilities and disabilities.
- Be aware of the resident's sense of balance.
- Know what special equipment will be needed.
- Be aware of the resident's motivation and ability to follow directions.
- Keep directions simple and consistent.
- Allow time for independent self-care.
- Watch for signs of fatigue or frustration.
- Use praise and encouragement frequently (see Figure 11-2 ■).
- Emphasize the positive and focus on success.

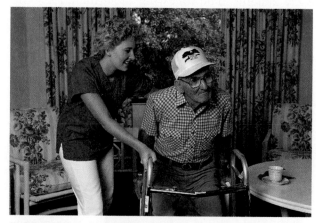

FIGURE 11-2 ■ Praise and encouragement are great motivators.

BODY MECHANICS AND BODY ALIGNMENT

Body Mechanics

The use of the body to move is **body mechanics**. Always use correct body mechanics when assisting the resident in moving and exercising. Posture is important. Stand with your feet apart for a wide base of support. Tighten your abdominal muscles and keep your back straight. Bend your knees (squat) and use the large muscles of your thighs. Turn your body, without twisting, in the direction in which you are moving the resident. Stand close to the resident and use smooth, co-ordinate movements. If two staff members are lifting, coordinate the lift by counting out loud, "1, 2, 3." Body mechanics is explained in more detail in Chapter 6.

When positioning the resident or assisting with exercises, bring the bed to a comfortable working height and lock the wheels. The bed should be as flat as the resident can tolerate. Keep the side rail up on the opposite side while providing care. Use a turning sheet (draw sheet) if needed, and get help when necessary.

Body Alignment

It is important that the resident is positioned in correct **body alignment** (maintaining a normal or correct anatomical position). When the resident is lying down, the trunk of the body should be in a straight line. The extremities should be positioned for comfort and supported with pillows as necessary (Figure 11-3A ■). Correct body alignment prevents stress on the musculoskeletal system and promotes comfort. Look at the resident when you are finished. If he doesn't look comfortable, he may not be in correct body alignment.

Body alignment also is important when sitting in a chair. The resident should sit straight, with the back against the back of the chair (see Figure 11-3B ■). The feet should either touch the floor or be propped on a stool or footrest. A person who is slumped over in a chair or leaning to the side is not

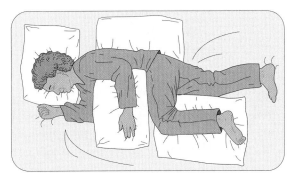

A The trunk of the body should be in a straight line.

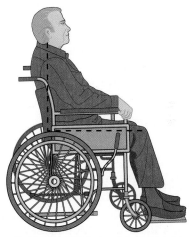

B The resident should sit straight, with his back against the back of the chair.

FIGURE 11-3 ■ Correct body alignment promotes comfort and helps to prevent complications.

in proper body alignment and soon will become tired and uncomfortable.

Restorative Equipment

Equipment designed to help the resident maintain correct body alignment includes foot supports, bed cradles and splints (see Figure 11-4 ■). Foot supports are used to keep the feet and ankles in alignment and prevent foot drop. A bed cradle keeps the top linen from pressing on the toes.

Hand and wrist splints are designed individually for the person who needs them and are used to prevent contractures of the hands or wrists. Pillows and linens are commonly used as positioning devices to help maintain correct body alignment.

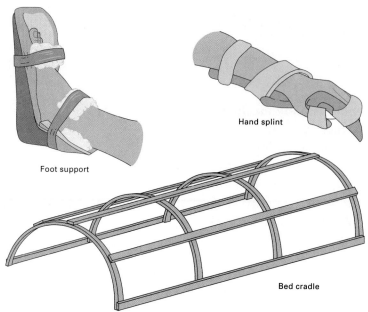

Foot support

Hand splint

Bed cradle

FIGURE 11-4 ■ Special equipment used to help the resident maintain correct body alignment.

SECTION *2* Moving and Positioning Residents

Section two shows the practical aspects of moving residents.

ASSISTING THE RESIDENT IN POSITIONING AND TURNING

It is very important that the resident changes position frequently when in bed or sitting for any length of time. Although some residents will be able to do this for themselves, others will need your assistance. A person who is very ill or comatose needs to be turned at least every 2 hours. Changing positions promotes comfort, stimulates circulation, and helps to prevent complications.

Basic Body Positions

Although there are many ways of positioning the body, there are four basic positions: supine, prone, lateral, and Fowler's.

A person in a **supine position** is lying on the back (see Figure 11-5A ■). This position sometimes is called "horizontal recumbent." In this position, the person is flat on the back. For correct body alignment, the resident's head and shoulders are supported on a pillow. The arms are at the sides and also may be supported by pillows. A weak or paralyzed arm may be positioned on a pillow to prevent edema.

In the **prone position**, the resident is lying on the abdomen (see Figure 11-5B ■). The arms may be at the sides or flexed upward by the head. The head is turned to the side and may be supported by a small pillow. The bed should be flat. Most residents cannot tolerate this position for 2 hours.

A person in the **lateral position** is lying on the side. The upper arm and upper leg are supported on pillows. A pillow against the back helps the resident to maintain correct body alignment. If possible, bring the upper leg forward and support it with a pillow (see Figure 11-5C ■).

Fowler's position is a sitting or semisitting position (see Figure 11-5D ■). The head of the bed is elevated, and sometimes the foot of the bed is raised slightly. To maintain correct body alignment, the resident should sit with the spine straight. The head and arms may be supported by pillows. You might be asked to place the resident in a high-Fowler's or a semi-Fowler's position. These terms refer to the degree of elevation of the head of the bed. Residents with respiratory problems and those with feeding tubes may need to be in a Fowler's position.

There are other positions that may be used occasionally. Semisupine and semiprone positions may be used because there is less pressure on bony prominences (see Figures 11-5E ■ and Figures 11-5F ■). Sims' position is a lateral position in which the lower arm is behind the resident and the upper leg is bent or flexed in a knee-chest position (see Figure 11-6A ■). Elderly residents with limited mobility may have difficulty assuming this position.

The orthopneic position often is used by residents who have respiratory problems. The person sits straight up in bed, or on the side of the bed, and leans forward in an attempt to breath more easily. The arms are raised and supported by an overbed table (see Figure 11-6B ■). A pillow placed on the table helps to cushion and support the body. If the resident is sitting on the side of the bed, a stool or chair should be placed under the feet to provide support.

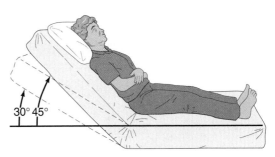

D Fowler's position (45°), and
Semi-Fowler's position (30°)

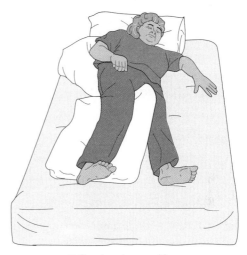

E Semisupine position

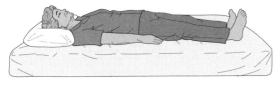

A Supine position

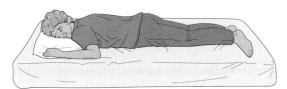

B Prone position

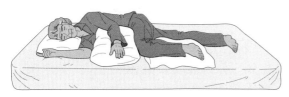

C Lateral position

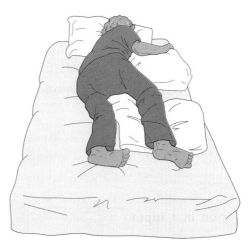

F Semiprone position

FIGURE 11-5 ■ Basic body positions

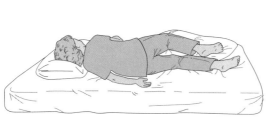

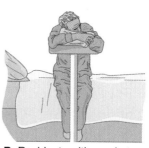

A Sims' position

B Residents with respiratory disease often use the orthopneic position.

FIGURE 11-6 ■ Special body positions

Assisting a Resident to Move Up in Bed

A person tends to slide down in bed when the head is elevated. That causes stress on the musculoskeletal system and makes the resident uncomfortable. Sliding also causes friction and leads to skin damage.

It may be necessary to assist the resident up in bed several times during a shift. Encourage the resident to help as much as possible. To protect yourself and the resident, get help when necessary.

ℙROCEDURE

Assisting the Resident to Move Up in Bed

■ Beginning Steps

Before any procedure, you always must follow the five basic steps: wash your hands, collect the equipment, identify the resident, explain the procedure, and protect privacy.

👋 Follow Standard Precautions

1. Raise the bed to a comfortable working height and lock the wheels.
2. Adjust the bed to as flat a position as possible.
3. Raise the side rail on the opposite side and lower the side rail on your working side.
4. Place the pillow against the headboard.
5. Facing the head of the bed, stand with your feet apart (one in front of the other), bend your knees, and keep your back straight.
6. Place one arm under the resident's shoulders and the other under the thighs.
7. Ask the resident to bend the knees and brace the feet against the bed. The arms may be at the side, elbows bent, and hands braced against the bed (see Figure 11-7A ■).
8. Explain that on the count of "3" the resident should push with the hands and feet at the same time that you lift.

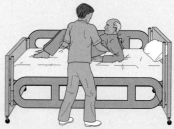

A Ask the resident to bend his knees and brace his feet; he also should bend his elbows and brace his hands, if possible.

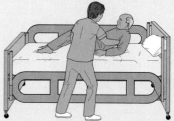

B Shift your weight from your back leg to your front leg as you move the resident up in bed.

FIGURE 11-7 ■ Assisting the resident up in bed

9. On the count of "3," shift your weight from your back leg to your front leg as you move the resident up in bed (see Figure 11-7B ■).
10. Replace the pillow and straighten the linen.

(continued)

■ **Ending Steps**

To complete the procedure, perform the following steps:

Make the resident comfortable, positioning in good body alignment. Make the resident safe, placing the call signal within reach, lowering the bed, and raising the side rails, if appropriate. Wash your hands. Record and report the procedure as required.

■

𝒫ROCEDURE

Moving the Resident Up in Bed with a Lift Sheet

■ **Beginning Steps**

Before any procedure, you always must follow the five basic steps: wash your hands, collect the equipment, identify the resident, explain the procedure, and protect privacy.

🖐 **Follow Standard Precautions**

1. Arrange for a coworker to help you.
2. Raise the bed to a comfortable working height and lock the wheels.
3. Adjust the bed to as flat a position as possible.
4. Lower the side rail on your working side. Your assistant on the other side will do the same.
5. Place the pillow against the headboard.
6. Facing the head of the bed, stand with your feet apart (one in front of the other), bend your knees, and keep your back straight.
7. Roll the lift sheet close to the side of the resident's body (see Figure 11-8 ■) and straighten the linens.
8. Grasp the lift sheet with one hand at the resident's shoulder and the other hand at hip level.
9. On the count of "3" shift your weight from one foot to the other as you and your assistant move the resident up in bed.
10. Replace the pillow, unroll the lift sheet.

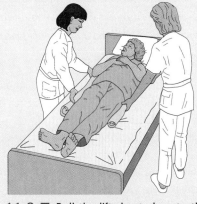

FIGURE 11-8 ■ Roll the lift sheet close to the sides of the resident's body when moving her up in bed.

■ **Ending Steps**

To complete the procedure, perform the following steps:

Make the resident comfortable, positioning in good body alignment. Make the resident safe, placing the call signal within reach, lowering the bed, and raising the side rails, if appropriate. Wash your hands. Record and report the procedure as required.

■

Moving a Resident Up in Bed With a Lift Sheet

Some residents, such as those who are helpless, critically ill, or comatose, will not be able to help move themselves up in bed. The easiest way to assist them is with a lift sheet (draw sheet). This procedure requires two people, one on either side of the bed (see Figure 11-8). A lift sheet supports body alignment and pro-

tects the resident's skin from friction. Lower the bed as flat as possible to make the procedure easier.

Moving the Resident to the Side of the Bed

It may be necessary to move the resident to one side of the bed when turning. The resident also will need to be moved to the side of the bed when being assisted to get up. Move the resident's body in segments (sections), beginning with the head and shoulders. Then move the waist and thighs, followed by the legs and feet (see Figure 11-9).

A lift sheet may be necessary if the resident is difficult to move. Get help if necessary.

Assisting the Resident to Turn

You may assist the resident to turn to either side (see Figures 11-10 and 11-11). The lateral (side-lying) position is a comfortable position and helps to relieve pressure on the bony areas of the back. A lift sheet will make this procedure easier. Get help if necessary.

𝒫ROCEDURE

Moving the Resident to the Side of the Bed

■ Beginning Steps

Before any procedure, you always must follow the five basic steps: wash your hands, collect the equipment, identify the resident, explain the procedure, and provide privacy.

Follow Standard Precautions

1. Raise the bed to a comfortable working height and lock the wheels.
2. Adjust the bed as flat as possible.
3. Raise the side rail on the opposite side and lower the side rail on your working side.
4. Stand with your feet apart (one in front of the other), your knees bent, and your back straight.
5. Place the resident's arms across the chest.
6. Place your arms under the neck and shoulders and move the upper section of the body toward you (see Figure 11-9A ■) as you shift your weight from one leg to the other.

7. Place your arms under the resident's waist and thighs and move the middle of the body toward you in the same manner (see Figure 11-9B ■).
8. Place your arms under the legs and move the lower part of the body toward you (see Figure 11-9C ■).
9. Reposition the pillow and check for correct body alignment.
10. Begin the positioning or transfer procedure, or go on to the next step of this procedure.
11. If you are going to leave the resident in this position, straighten the linens.

■ Ending Steps

To complete the procedure, perform the following steps:

Make the resident comfortable, positioning in good body alignment. Make the resident safe, placing the call signal within reach, lowering the bed, and raising the side rails, if appropriate. Wash your hands. Record and report the procedure as required.

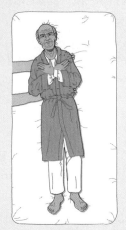 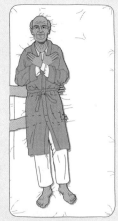 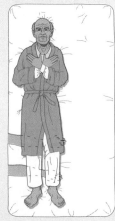

A Place your arms under the resident's neck and shoulders to move the upper part of the body toward you.

B Place your arms under the resident's waist and thighs as you move the middle of the body.

C Place your arms under the legs to move the lower part of the body.

FIGURE 11-9 ■ Moving the resident to the side of the bed

𝒫ROCEDURE

Assisting the Resident to Turn Away from You

■ Beginning Steps

Before any procedure, you always must follow the five basic steps: wash your hands, collect the equipment, identify the resident, explain the procedure, and provide privacy.

🖐 Follow Standard Precautions

1. Raise the bed to a comfortable working height and lock the wheels.
2. Adjust the bed as flat as possible.
3. Raise the side rail on the opposite side and lower the side rail on your working side.
4. Move the resident to the side of the bed nearest you, following the correct procedure.
5. Flex the resident's farther arm next to the head and place the other arm across the chest. Cross the resident's leg that is nearest you over the other leg (see Figure 11-10A ■).
6. Place one hand on the resident's near shoulder and the other on the near hip, and turn the resident away from you, onto the side (see Figure 11-10B ■).

7. Reposition the pillow under the resident's head.
8. Place a pillow under the upper arm to support the elbow, wrist, and hand. Place a pillow under the upper leg, supporting the knee, ankle, and foot (see Figure 11-10C ■).
9. Raise the side rail.
10. Go to the other side of the bed and lower the side rail.
11. Adjust the bottom shoulder and hip for comfort.
12. Place a pillow at the resident's back for comfort and support.
13. Straighten the linen.

■ Ending Steps

To complete the procedure, perform the following steps:

Make the resident comfortable, positioning in good body alignment. Make the resident safe, placing the call signal within reach, lowering the bed, and raising the side rails, if appropriate. Wash your hands. Record and report the procedure as required.

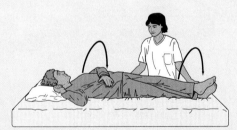

A Bend the resident's farther arm next to her head and place the other arm across her chest. Cross her near leg over her other leg.

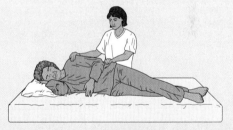

B Place one hand on the resident's shoulder and the other on her hip. Turn her away from you onto her side.

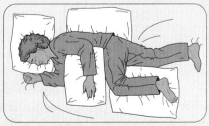

C Place pillows under her upper arm and leg for support.

FIGURE 11-10 ■ Assisting the resident to turn away from you

PROCEDURE

Assisting the Resident to Turn Toward You

■ Beginning Steps

Before any procedure, you always must follow the five basic steps: wash your hands, collect the equipment, identify the resident, explain the procedure, and protect privacy.

Follow Standard Precautions

1. Raise the bed to a comfortable working height and lock the wheels.
2. Adjust the bed as flat as possible.
3. Raise the side rail on the opposite side and lower the side rail on your working side.
4. Move the resident to the side of the bed nearest you, following the correct procedure.
5. Raise the side rail that is nearer to you. Go to the other side of the bed and lower the side rail.
6. Flex the resident's nearer arm next to the head, and place the other arm across the chest. Cross the leg

that is farther from you over the other leg (see Figure 11-11A ■).
7. Place one hand on the resident's far shoulder and the other on the far hip, and turn the resident toward you, onto the side (see Figure 11-11B ■).
8. Reposition the pillow under the resident's head.
9. Place a pillow under the upper arm to support the elbow, wrist, and hand. Place a pillow under the upper leg, supporting the knee, ankle, and foot.

■ Ending Steps

To complete the procedure, perform the following steps:

Make the resident comfortable, positioning in good body alignment. Make the resident safe, placing the call signal within reach, lowering the bed, and raising the side rails, if appropriate. Wash your hands. Record and report the procedure as required.

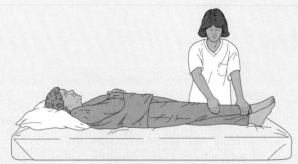

A Place the resident's arm across her chest. Cross the far leg over the near leg.

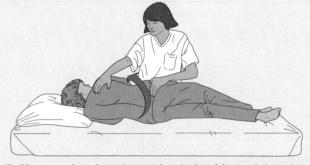

B Place one hand on the resident's shoulder and the other on her hip and turn her toward you onto her side.

FIGURE 11-11 ■ Assisting the resident to turn toward you

Assisting the Resident to a Sitting Position

There are times when you will assist the resident to sit up in bed (see Figure 11-12). This procedure can be used for personal care, for positioning, as a comfort measure, or to assist a resident out of bed. Sometimes, you will only need to raise the resident's head and shoulders to straighten linens or a pillow.

Assisting the Resident to Sit on the Side of the Bed (Dangle)

Sitting on the side of the bed is called **dangling** (see Figure 11-13). It may be used as a form of

restorative exercise or it may be a part of the procedure to assist the resident to get out of bed. Provide a footstool if the resident's feet do not reach the floor. *Never* leave a resident alone while dangling.

You always should allow the resident to dangle for a few minutes before standing. Dangling for a few minutes helps prevent dizziness. Observe the resident carefully while dangling. Observe the color of the skin for paleness or perspiration. Take the pulse and respirations. The resident who complains of pain or dizziness should be laid back down immediately. Notify the nurse.

PROCEDURE

Assisting the Resident to a Sitting Position

■ Beginning Steps

Before any procedure, you always must follow the five basic steps: wash your hands, collect the equipment, identify the resident, explain the procedure, and protect privacy.

🖐 Follow Standard Precautions

1. Raise the bed to a comfortable working height and lock the wheels.
2. Lower the side rail on your working side.
3. Stand facing the head of the bed.
4. Place your arm under the resident's near arm and grasp the shoulder.
5. Ask the resident to grasp your shoulder (see Figure 11-12A ■).
6. Place your free arm under the resident's neck and shoulders (see Figure 11-12B ■).
7. On the count of "3," assist the resident to a sitting position (see Figure 11-12C ■).

8. Continuing to lock arms, use the arm that was supporting the resident's neck and shoulders to straighten the linens and pillow. Pull the pillow down so that the shoulders will be supported.
9. Continue the procedure:
   a. If the resident wants to remain in this position for a while, ensure comfort and support.
   b. If the resident wants to return to the supine position, use the locked-arm procedure to assist.

■ Ending Steps

To complete the procedure, perform the following steps:

Make the resident comfortable, positioning in good body alignment. Make the resident safe, placing the call signal within reach, lowering the bed, and raising the side rails, if appropriate. Wash your hands. Record and report the procedure as required.

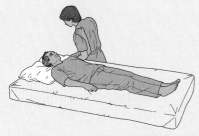

A Place your arm under the resident's arm and grasp his shoulder. Ask the resident to place his arm under your arm and grasp your shoulder.

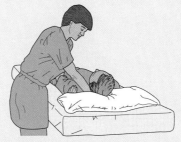

B Place your free arm under the resident's neck and shoulder.

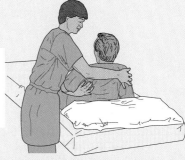

C Assist the resident to a sitting position.

FIGURE 11-12 ■ Assisting the resident to a sitting position

PROCEDURE

Assisting the Resident to Sit on the Side of the Bed (Dangle)

■ Beginning Steps

Before any procedure, you always must follow the five basic steps: wash your hands, collect the equipment, identify the resident, explain the procedure, and provide privacy.

🖐 Follow Standard Precautions

1. Lower the bed as much as possible and lock the wheels.
2. Assist the resident to a sitting position, following correct procedure.

(continued)

3. Place one arm behind the resident's neck and shoulders, and place your other arm under the resident's knees (see Figure 11-13A ■).

4. On the count of "3," turn the resident toward you so that the legs hang over the side of the bed (see Figure 11-13B ■).

5. Assist the resident to a position of correct body alignment.

6. Ask the resident to push with the hands against the mattress to help to maintain an upright position.

7. Keep your arm behind the resident's neck and shoulders for support until you are sure the resident has gained balance (see Figure 11-13C ■).

8. Check the pulse and respirations.

9. Continue the procedure:
   a. Allow the resident to dangle for 15 to 20 minutes while you remain nearby. *Never* leave a resident alone while dangling.
   b. Return the resident to bed by reversing the procedure.

10. If you have assisted the resident back to bed, straighten the linen.

■ Ending Steps

To complete the procedure, perform the following steps:

Make the resident comfortable, positioning in good body alignment. Make the resident safe, placing the call signal within reach, lowering the bed, and raising the side rails, if appropriate. Wash your hands. Record and report the procedure as required.

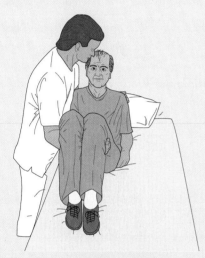

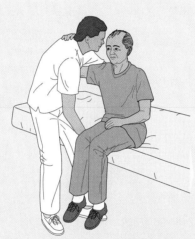

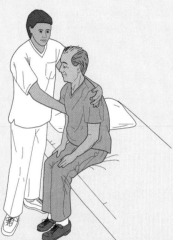

A Place one hand behind the resident's neck and shoulders; place your other arm under his knees.

B Turn the resident toward you so that his legs hang over the side of the bed.

C Keep your hand behind the resident's neck and shoulders to support him until you are sure he has gained his balance.

FIGURE 11-13 ■ Assisting the resident to dangle.

𝒫ROCEDURE

Assisting the Resident to Transfer from the Bed to a Wheelchair

■ Beginning Steps

Before any procedure, you always must follow the five basic steps: wash your hands, collect the equipment, identify the resident, explain the procedure, and protect privacy.

🖐 Follow Standard Precautions

1. Position the chair at the head of the bed on the resident's strong side. Place a pad or blanket on the seat of the wheelchair (see Figure 11-14A ■).

(continued)

2. Lock the wheels and fold up the footrest of the wheelchair.
3. Place the bed in its lowest position and lock the wheels.
4. Be sure the resident is wearing nonskid shoes.
5. Assist the resident to sit on the side of the bed and dangle for a few minutes (see Figure 11-14B ■).
6. Assist the resident to put on a robe if he is not already dressed.
7. Assist the resident to a standing position using the following steps:
    a. Stand facing the resident, bend your knees, and keep your back straight.
    b. Place your arms under the resident's arms, with your hands supporting the resident's back.
    c. Brace your knees against the resident's knees and block the feet with yours (see Figure 11-14C ■).
    d. If possible, the resident should brace with the hands against the mattress and push up as you lift.
    e. On the count of "3," straighten your knees as you bring the resident to a standing position (see Figure 11-14D ■).
8. Ask the resident to take small steps as both of you turn toward the chair.

9. Ask the resident to back up until the back of the legs touch the front of the chair.
10. Ask the resident, if able, to grasp the arms of the chair (see Figure 11-14E ■). If not, the resident can place his hands on your forearms.
11. On the count of "3," bend your knees as you lower the resident into the chair (see Figure 11-14F ■).
12. Use pillows for support if necessary (see Figure 11-14G ■).
13. Cover the resident's legs with a lap robe for warmth and privacy. Be sure the feet touch the floor or are otherwise supported.

■ Ending Steps

To complete the procedure, perform the following steps:

Make the resident comfortable, positioning in good body alignment. Make the resident safe, placing the call signal within reach, lowering the bed, and raising the side rails, if appropriate. Wash your hands. Record and report the procedure as required.

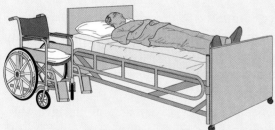

A Position the chair with the back even with the head of the bed.

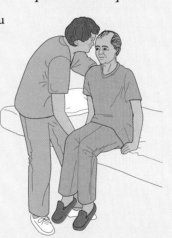

B Assisst the resident to dangle.

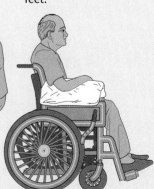

C Brace your knees against the resident's knees and block his feet with your feet.

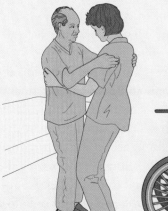

D Bring the resident to a standing position.

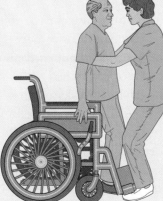

E Ask the resident to grasp the chair as you support him.

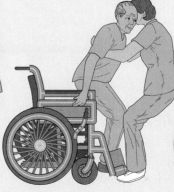

F Bend your knees as you lower the resident to the chair.

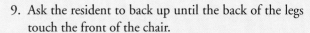

G Use pillows as necessary to position the resident in correct body alignment.

FIGURE 11-14 ■ Assisting the resident to transfer from the bed to a chair.

Report to the nurse after you have completed the procedure. Include the following in your report: the length of time the resident was dangling, how well the procedure was tolerated, vital signs, and any other observations you made.

ASSISTING THE RESIDENT TO TRANSFER

Assisting the resident to transfer safely (move from one place to another) is an important responsibility of the nursing assistant. Follow the rules of body mechanics and the guidelines for restorative activity techniques. Encourage the resident to do as much as possible. Before you begin the transfer, arrange for help if needed, and prepare any supplies or equipment that you will use. Make sure the resident is wearing safe shoes. One of the safest types of footwear is laced-up athletic shoes. Be sure to brace the resident's knees with your own and block his feet with your feet. This helps prevent falls if the resident's knees buckle or his feet slip. Be sure that wheels on beds, stretchers, and wheelchairs are locked during the transfer. Get help if you are not able to move a resident by yourself.

Determine if the resident has a weak side and remember that the strong side leads. This means that the resident should step out with the strong foot first, place his weight on the strong side, and let the weak side follow. When possible, place the wheelchair at the head of the bed, on the strong side, facing the foot of the bed.

Much of the information you need to assist the resident to transfer will be found on your assignment sheet or on the care plan. However, the circumstances may vary from time to time. Check with the nurse if you are not sure what to do.

Assisting the Resident to Transfer from the Bed to a Chair or Wheelchair

Assist the resident (see Figure 11-14) to sit up in a chair when possible. This helps to prevent the complications of bedrest. Body organs are in natural alignment and function more effectively in an upright position. Check that the resident's hips are at

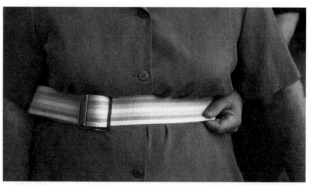

FIGURE 11-15 ■ The gait/transfer belt protects the resident and you.

the back of the seat and that the spine is against the back of the chair.

Using a Gait/Transfer Belt

A gait/transfer belt is used to assist unsteady residents to transfer or walk. This includes residents who are weak or prone to falling. It is made of a strong, washable material and has a safety buckle (see Figure 11-15 ■). The belt is applied around the resident's waist, over the clothing. It should fit snugly and not slide up over the ribs or down over the hips. The buckle is fastened off center, in the front, to prevent discomfort or injury.

There are several advantages in using a gait/transfer belt. It reduces the chance of injury to the resident and the nursing assistant. It helps prevent falls and provides a sense of security. Because you have the belt to hold on to, you will feel more in control of the situation. The gait/transfer belt allows you to use correct body mechanics.

The gait/transfer belt is not appropriate for all residents. It is not used on an unconscious resident or one who has had recent rib fractures. It is seldom used with a resident who has abdominal tubes or has had recent surgery. A belt might feel suffocating to a resident who has trouble breathing. A confused resident might misunderstand and think the belt is a restraint. Always explain that the belt is used only for safety reasons and that it will be removed as soon as the procedure is completed.

Many long-term care facilities have made the use of gait/transfer belts mandatory for any

PROCEDURE

Using a Gait/Transfer Belt to Assist the Resident in Transferring from the Bed to a Chair

■ Beginning Steps

Before any procedure, you always must follow the five basic steps: wash your hands, collect the equipment, identify the resident, explain the procedure, and protect privacy.

Follow Standard Precautions

1. Position the chair at the head of the bed on the resident's strong side. Place a pad or blanket on the seat of the wheelchair.
2. Lock the wheels and fold up the footrest of the wheelchair.
3. Place the bed in its lowest position and lock the wheels.
4. Be sure the resident is wearing nonskid shoes.
5. Assist the resident to sit on the side of the bed and dangle for a few minutes.
6. Assist the resident to put on a robe if she is not already dressed.
7. Place a gait/transfer belt on the resident so that it fits snugly. Leave enough room for your fingers to slip under the belt. Fasten the buckle off-center, in the front (see Figure 11-16A ■).
8. Assist the resident to a standing position using the following steps:
   a. Stand facing the resident, bend your knees, and keep your back straight.
   b. The resident should brace with the hands against the mattress and push as you lift. If this is not possible, the resident's hands should be placed on your forearms.
   c. Grasp the gait/transfer belt from underneath, in the back. Your hands should be spaced wide apart for leverage (see Figure 11-16B ■).
   d. Brace your knees against the resident's knees and block the feet with your feet.
   e. On the count of "3," straighten your knees as you bring the resident to a standing position.
9. Assist the resident to move in front of the chair and ask her to take small steps backward until the backs of her legs touch the front of the chair.
10. On the count of "3," bend your knees as you assist the resident into the chair. Hold on to the gait/transfer belt as you do this (see Figure 11-16C ■).
11. Remove the gait/transfer belt.
12. Check to see that the resident is comfortable and in correct body alignment. Use pillows for support if necessary.
13. Cover the resident's legs with a lap robe for warmth and privacy. Be sure the feet touch the floor or are otherwise supported.

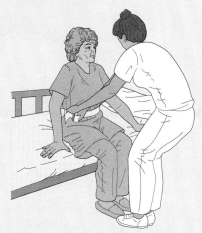

A The gait/transfer belt should fit snugly, and the buckle should be fastened off-center, in the front.

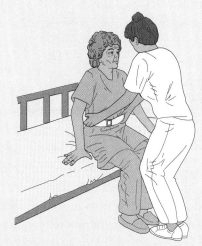

B Grasp the gait/transfer belt from underneath with both hands.

FIGURE 11-16 ■ Using a gait/transfer belt to assist the resident in transferring from the bed to a chair.   (continued)

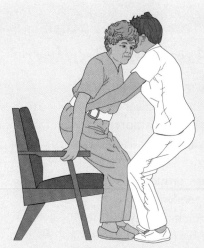

C Holding on to the gait/transfer belt, lower the resident into the chair as you bend your knees.

14. The chair may be positioned so that the resident can be observed by the staff.

■ Ending Steps

To complete the procedure, perform the following steps:

Make the resident comfortable, positioning in good body alignment. Make the resident safe, placing the call signal within reach, lowering the bed, and raising the side rails, if appropriate. Wash your hands. Record and report the procedure as required.

hands-on assistance. This means you must use the belt whenever it is appropriate. When you are not using the gait/transfer belt, wear it around your own waist. That way, it will be available whenever you need it. The resident will become used to seeing it on you and will be reassured that it is not a form of restraint. The gait/transfer belt is a useful tool that will help make your job easier and safer.

Using a Gait/Transfer Belt to Assist the Resident in Transferring from the Bed to a Chair

It is easier and safer to use a gait belt when transferring the resident (see Figure 11-16).

USING A MECHANICAL LIFT

Many types of mechanical lifts are available, so the procedure varies (see Figure 11-17 ■). There are mechanical lifts that operate with a hydraulic pump and electronic lifts that are battery operated. Many facilities have two or more types to meet individual needs. Be sure to read the instructions in the procedure book and know how to use each type of lift in your facility.

The mechanical lift is used to help transfer residents who are very heavy or who are unable to move. Using a lift protects residents and staff members. The

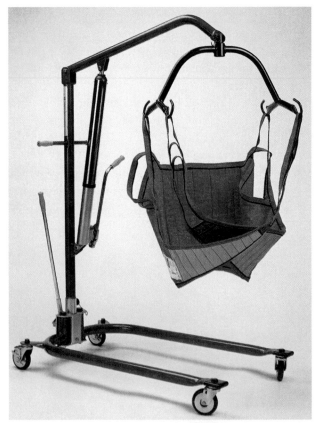

FIGURE 11-17 ■ A portable mechanical lift. *Photo courtesy of Guardian Products, a division of Sunrise Medical.*

mechanical lift usually is portable and can be taken to the resident's bedside. The following guidelines will help you safely use a mechanical lift.

GUIDELINES

USING A MECHANICAL LIFT

- It is safer to have assistance when using the lift. One person operates the lift, while the other guides the resident's body and the chains or straps.

- Know how to operate the lift. The first few times you use the lift, be certain to get someone who is experienced with the equipment to assist you.

- Explain the procedure and reassure the resident frequently. Speak to the resident before beginning the transfer.

- Check to see that the resident is positioned correctly and that the equipment is working properly *before* moving the lift away from the bed.

- Stabilize the resident and the frame throughout the procedure.

- Do not transport the resident out of the room with the lift unless it is specifically designed for that purpose.

- Position the resident's arms over the chest or in the lap while in the lift.

- If hooks are used to secure chains or straps, the open end of the hook should face away from the resident (see Figure 11-18 ■).

- The battery of an electronic lift should be placed on the charger when not in use.

- Never leave a resident suspended in a lift. If an emergency occurs, return the resident to the bed quickly and safely.

*U*SING A WHEELCHAIR

A wheelchair may be used to transport a resident who is unable to walk. The resident may be an amputee, paralyzed, weak, or recovering from surgery.

A wheelchair allows the resident to maintain a normal sitting position. For the resident who can't walk, a wheelchair increases mobility. It provides opportunities for socializing. It creates hope and motivation, which leads to increased self-esteem and independence.

A wheelchair may be manual or motorized. A manual chair is moved by turning the wheels by hand or by someone pushing it. Some residents will need assistance in moving the wheelchair, but many will be able to operate it by themselves. A motorized wheelchair is battery-operated and can be moved with little effort on the part of the resident. Wheelchairs come in different styles and sizes to accommodate individual needs.

One type of wheelchair that often is used in long-term care is a geri-chair (geriatric chair). A **geri-chair** is a recliner on wheels. It has a high back and is well padded and comfortable. A tray, which can be used for eating and other activities, fits on the front (see Figure 11-19 ■). The following guidelines will help you assist the resident in using a wheelchair.

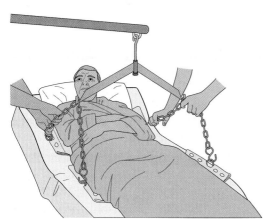

FIGURE 11-18 ■ The open end of the hooks should face away from the resident.

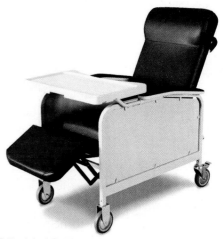

FIGURE 11-19 ■ A geri-chair is often used in long-term care. *Cliner, Winco, Inc. Ocala, FL*

GUIDELINES

USING A WHEELCHAIR

- Make sure the wheelchair is in good repair.
- Use the right size wheelchair. Use pillows to support the resident if necessary.
- Speak to the resident before moving the wheelchair. Make sure the resident knows what you are going to do so that he won't be startled.
- Lock the brakes when the chair is stopped.
- To prevent injury, make sure the resident's hands are away from the wheels when the wheelchair is being pushed. His hands should be in his lap.
- Be careful of the resident's legs and feet when pushing the wheelchair. The feet can get caught under the chair.
- Don't push the wheelchair too fast. This can frighten the resident or cause an accident.
- Clean the chair on a regular basis. Clean it immediately if it becomes soiled with food or body waste.
- Check to see that the resident in a wheelchair is in good body alignment. The resident's back, from hip to shoulder, should be positioned against the back of the chair.
- Use a pad in the chair seat to protect the resident's skin and for repositioning.
- The resident in a wheelchair should be repositioned frequently. Encourage the resident to lean from side to side in the chair to promote circulation.
- To take a resident in a wheelchair down a ramp, stand behind the chair and pull it down the ramp (see Figure 11-20 ■).
- To take a resident in a wheelchair through a doorway or into an elevator, go in first and pull the chair in behind you.

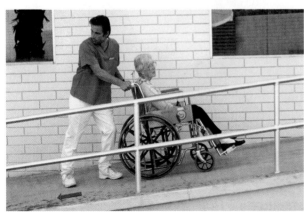

FIGURE 11-20 ■ Stand behind the wheelchair and pull it after you when going down a ramp.

Repositioning the Resident in a Wheelchair

The resident in a wheelchair should be repositioned at least every 2 hours. Repositioning may be necessary more frequently if the resident slides down in the chair. Two people may be required for this procedure, with one lifting from either side. Use the seat pad to lift if one is in place. Do not pull the resident up by the arms. This can result in a dislocated shoulder or other injury. Lock the brakes and move the footrests aside before you begin.

USING A STRETCHER

A resident who is not able to sit up in a chair or who is very ill may need to be transported by stretcher. Three or four people are needed to perform this procedure safely. A drawsheet makes the transfer easier and safer. If a draw sheet is not available, loosen the bottom sheet all the way around and use it as a lift sheet (see Figure 11-21).

Reverse the following procedure to transfer the resident from the stretcher to a bed.

GUIDELINES

USING A STRETCHER

- At least three people are needed to safely transfer the resident.
- Raise the bed to the same level as the stretcher.
- Lock the wheels of both the stretcher and the bed.
- Follow the rules of correct body mechanics.
- Fasten the safety straps across the resident who is on a stretcher.
- Keep the stretcher's side rails up while transporting a resident.
- Two people are needed to transport a resident on a stretcher, one at the resident's head and the other at the feet.
- Move the stretcher feet first. The staff member in front guides the stretcher, while the staff member in back watches the resident.
- When entering an elevator, one staff member should back into the elevator, pulling the stretcher. The same procedure is used to go through a doorway.
- Never leave a resident alone on a stretcher. You are responsible for the resident's safety until someone else takes over.

PROCEDURE

Moving the Resident from the Bed to a Stretcher

■ Beginning Steps

Before any procedure, you always must follow the five basic steps: wash your hands, collect the equipment, identify the resident, explain the procedure, and protect privacy.

🖐 Follow Standard Precautions

1. Arrange for coworkers to help you.
2. Raise the bed to a comfortable working height and lock the wheels.
3. Remove the top linen after covering the resident with a bath blanket. Loosen the draw sheet.
4. Lower the side rail on your side.
5. Using the draw sheet, move the resident toward you.
6. Your assistant on the other side of the bed lowers the rail and holds the resident to prevent a fall.
7. Position the stretcher against the near side of the bed and lock the wheels. Adjust the height of the bed even with the stretcher (see Figure 11-21A ■).
8. Two assistants will stand at the side of the stretcher. You and an assistant will stand beside the bed.
9. Roll the draw sheet close to the sides of the resident's body.
10. On the count of "3," move the resident from the bed to the stretcher (see Figure 11-21B ■).
11. Center the resident on the stretcher and place a pillow under the head and shoulders, if allowed.
12. Check for correct body alignment and cover the resident with the bath blanket.
13. Fasten the safety straps and raise the side rails (see Figure 11-21C ■).
14. Unlock the wheels and transport the resident with the help of one assistant.
15. Stay with the resident until someone else takes over.

■ Ending Steps

To complete the procedure, perform the following steps:

Make the resident comfortable, positioning in good body alignment. Make the resident safe, placing the call signal within reach, lowering the bed, and raising the side rails, if appropriate. Wash your hands. Record and report the procedure as required.

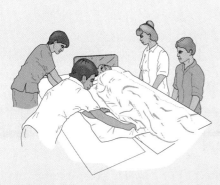 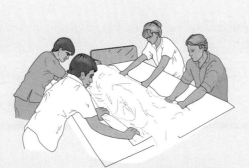 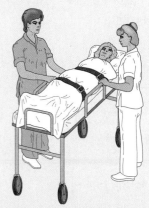

A Position the stretcher even with the bed.

B On the count of "3" move the resident from the bed to the stretcher.

C Fasten the safety straps and raise the side rails when you have the resident properly positioned.

FIGURE 11-21 ■ Moving the resident from a bed to a stretcher.

SECTION 3 Ambulation and Exercise

Section three explains how to help residents move.

ASSISTING THE RESIDENT TO WALK

The ability to **ambulate** (walk) allows a person to move about and go from place to place. Ambulation is an excellent form of exercise. It builds strength and stamina. Body functions are more efficient when a person is in an upright position. Ambulation provides independence and leads to increased self-esteem. It is a satisfying feeling to be able to stand up and walk.

Ambulation opens opportunities to explore the environment, to join in activities, and to make social contacts. The inability to walk is a severe loss to most people. Feelings of frustration, anger, or sadness may cause withdrawal. The isolation that results can lead to depression.

A resident may be unable to walk as a result of disease or injury. An injury to the head or back may result in paralysis that is not always permanent. A broken leg or hip will interfere with ambulation until it heals. A stroke may leave the resident unable to walk. Arthritis may make walking painful and difficult.

A restorative exercise program, ordered by the doctor, helps to prepare the resident for ambulation. These exercises can begin while the resident is still bedbound. The purpose of this program is to increase muscle strength and improve circulation. Dangling can be used as an exercise. It not only helps strengthen, it also helps the resident to gain balance. The resident may need to practice standing. This can be done in physical therapy or at the resident's bedside.

Some residents will need special assistive equipment to help them ambulate. Braces,

---

GUIDELINES

ASSISTING A RESIDENT TO AMBULATE

- Offer whatever assistance the resident needs to ambulate safely.
- Use praise and encouragement frequently.
- Provide opportunities to walk.
- Encourage the resident to do as much as possible independently.
- Reinforce physical therapy instructions.
- Be familiar with the equipment the resident needs.
- Use a gait/transfer belt whenever possible.
- Walk at the resident's side and slightly behind.
- Remind the resident to use the safety handrails in the hallway. Handrails help prevent falls.

PROCEDURE

Using a Gait/Transfer Belt to Assist the Resident to Ambulate

■ Beginning Steps

Before any procedure, you always must follow the five basic steps: wash your hands, collect the equipment, identify the resident, explain the procedure, and provide privacy.

Follow Standard Precautions

1. Assist the resident in dangling for a few minutes to gain balance.

2. Apply the gait/transfer belt around the waist.
3. Bring the resident to a standing position using the correct procedure (see Figure 11-22A ■).
4. Keep your hands on the gait/transfer belt until balance is regained.
5. While holding on to the gait/transfer belt, change the position of your hands. Hold the belt in the back and on one side (see Figure 11-22B ■).

(continued)

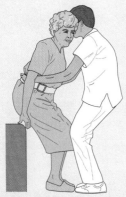

A Holding the gait belt with both hands, bring the resident to a standing position.

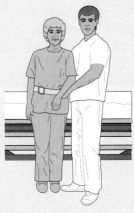

B Change the position of your hands so that one hand is holding the belt on the side and the other is holding the belt in the back.

FIGURE 11-22 ■ Using a gait/transfer belt to assist resident with ambulation

6. Assist the resident to walk. Walk at the resident's side, and slightly behind, while holding the belt with both hands (see Figure 11-22C ■).

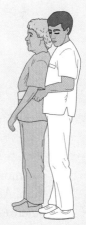

C Stand at the resident's side and slightly behind her, holding onto the belt with both hands.

7. Encourage the resident to stand straight and walk as normally as possible. If the resident is weak, a coworker can follow behind with a wheelchair.
8. Return the resident to the chair or bed and remove the belt.
9. Note the distance the resident has walked and how well the procedure was tolerated.

■ Ending Steps

To complete the procedure, perform the following steps:

Make the resident comfortable, positioning in good body alignment. Make the resident safe, placing the call signal within reach, lowering the bed, and raising the side rails, if appropriate. Wash your hands. Record and report the procedure as required.

crutches, canes, and walkers are used for this purpose. The physical therapist, working with the resident's doctor, will decide what type of equipment is appropriate. The physical therapist will provide the equipment, teach the resident how to use it, and evaluate the resident at regular intervals.

Protecting a Falling Resident

The resident may become weak or dizzy while being assisted to ambulate. If the resident begins to fall, pull the resident close to your body with the gait/transfer belt (see Figure 11-23A ■). Let the resident slide slowly down your leg to the floor (see Figure 11-23B ■). This helps you to control the direction of the fall and to prevent head injuries. Bend your knees as you lower the resident to the floor, and keep your back straight. Do not attempt to prevent the fall by trying to hold the resident off the floor. You could hurt both the resident and yourself. Report this incident to the nurse immediately.

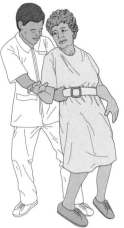
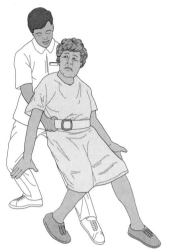

A If the resident begins to fall, pull her close to your body with the gait/transfer belt.

B Ease her to the floor by letting her slide down your leg.

FIGURE 11-23 ■ Protecting a falling resident

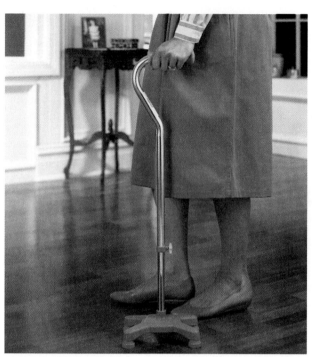

FIGURE 11-24 ■ A quad cane provides more support than a single-tip cane but is more difficult to move. *Sammons, Preston, Rolyan–U.S.A.*

ASSISTING THE RESIDENT TO WALK WITH A CANE, WALKER, OR CRUTCHES

The use of canes, walkers, and crutches allows independence for residents who are weak or have poor balance. These devices are recommended by the occupational therapist or physical therapist, who also teaches the residents to use them properly. The therapist teaches staff members about the use of assistive devices and should be consulted anytime a question arises. Discuss your concerns with the nurse. Frequently check the tips of canes, walkers, and crutches to ensure that the rubber is intact.

Canes

Canes provide balance and support when one side of the body is weak. Canes usually are held on the strong side of the body. Single-tip, three-point (tripod), and four-point (quad) (see Figure 11-24 ■) canes are available.

When the resident's hand is on the cane grip, the shoulders should be at a normal level. The cane grip should be level with the resident's hip, and the tip is placed 6 to 10 inches to the side of the resident's foot. The arm is flexed slightly as the cane is moved forward about 12 inches. A step forward is then taken with the opposite (weak) leg. This foot is moved to a position even with the cane. The strong leg then is moved forward beyond the weak leg and cane. This sequence is repeated throughout ambulation.

Walkers

Most walkers have four legs that rest on the floor. They may have wheels to help residents who are unable to lift the walker to move it forward. A basket (see Figure 11-25 ■), tray, and/or pouch may be added to allow the resident to carry belongings.

Use the information provided in the following guidelines to assist the resident with a walker.

GUIDELINES

ASSISTING THE RESIDENT WITH A WALKER

- Be sure the walker is the correct size. The walker handgrip should be at hip level, and the elbow should be flexed at a 20 degree angle.
- Check the tips on the walker legs to be sure the rubber is intact. A missing tip causes the walker to be unbalanced.

(continued)

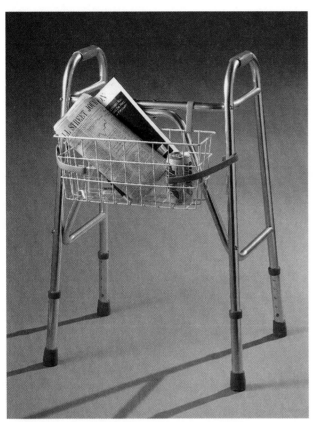

FIGURE 11-25 ■ One type of walker. *Sammons, Preston, Rolyan–U.S.A.*

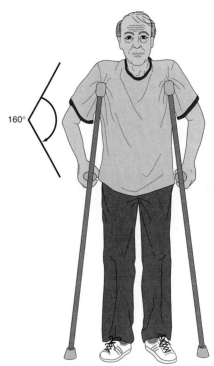

FIGURE 11-26 ■ It is important that crutches fit correctly.

GUIDELINES (Continued)

- Ask the resident to step into the walker with the affected (weak) foot first. This provides a frame of support for the weak leg, while the strong leg is left behind.

- Ask the resident to bring the strong foot forward next to the weak foot to complete the step. Each step should move the resident forward about 6 inches.

- Do not use the walker as a support to raise the body from a sitting position. The walker could slip and cause a fall.

Crutches

A resident who is unable to use one leg, or has only one leg, may use crutches. Crutches must be fitted correctly according to the resident's height. Handgrips and underarm braces also must fit (see Figure 11-26 ■).

Although it is the therapist's responsibility to teach the resident to use walkers, canes, and crutches, you play an important role in observing incorrect use. Make the resident aware of the problem. If incorrect use continues, report this to the nurse.

RANGE-OF-MOTION AND OTHER RESTORATIVE EXERCISES

Restorative Exercises

Restorative exercise programs contribute to the resident's physical and emotional well-being. They help to prevent contractures and other complications of inactivity. Some examples of restorative exercises include walking, dancing, and aerobic exercises (see Figure 11-27 ■). A rocking chair provides exercises for those who are unable to take part in other physical activities. Comatose and other bedridden residents also need exercise. One of the most helpful types of restorative exercises is range-of-motion exercises.

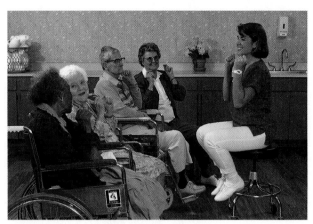

FIGURE 11-27 ■ Excercise helps to prevent contractures and other complications of inactivity.

Range-of-Motion Exercises

"Range of motion" refers to the distance a joint will move comfortably. **Range-of-motion exercises** are exercises that are performed to take each joint through its normal area of movement. These exercises are done to prevent loss of movement or to regain full range of motion after an illness. Range-of-motion exercises are one of the best measures to prevent contractures.

Range-of-motion exercises may be active, assisted, or passive. Active exercises are those that the resident does without assistance. Assisted exercises are performed with residents who need some help. Passive exercises are done by someone else for the resident. The resident's physical and mental condition determines which type of exercise is to be done. Some of the exercises may be combined, and the exact exercises may vary. This information will be included in the resident's care plan.

Plan range-of-motion exercises as a part of self-care or ADLs. Brushing the hair, taking a bath, and walking provide opportunities for range-of-motion exercises. Encourage the resident to do as much as possible. Report any increase or decrease in range of motion to the nurse. Do not be discouraged if the range-of-motion is limited. Exercise within those limitations. A small amount of mobility is better than none.

You will need to be familiar with some of the terms that are used to describe body movement and direction. Some of the more common terms are found in the following table.

GUIDELINES

RANGE-OF-MOTION EXERCISES

- Follow the resident's plan of care.
- Check with the nurse to find out which exercises are to be done and how many times the exercises are to be repeated.
- While providing range-of-motion exercise, use both hands to support the joints.
- Use slow, rhythmic motions.
- Stop at the point of resistance or if a resident complains of pain.
- Watch the resident's face for signs of pain or discomfort.

BODY MOVEMENTS AND DIRECTIONS	
Term	Description
Extension	Straightening and extending
Flexion	Bending
Abduction	Moving away from the midline of the body ("Absent")
Adduction	Moving toward the midline of the body ("Add to")
External rotation	Rolling away from the body
Pronation	Turning down
Supination	Turning up
Hyperextension	Extending beyond a straight line
Internal rotation	Rolling in toward the body
Radial deviation	Moving the hand toward the thumb
Ulnar deviation	Moving the hand toward the little finger
Plantar flexion	Bending the foot downward
Dorsal flexion	Bending the foot upward

PROCEDURE

Performing Range-of-Motion Exercises

■ Beginning Steps

Before any procedure, you always must follow the five basic steps: wash your hands, collect the equipment, identify the resident, explain the procedure, and provide privacy.

Follow Standard Precautions

1. Raise the bed to a comfortable working height, lock the wheels, and lower the side rails.
2. Exercise the resident's neck gently. Support the head with both hands.
   a. Move the head down, up, and back; then straighten the neck and head (see Figure 11-28A ■).

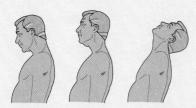

Extension Flexion Hyperextension

FIGURE 11-28A

   b. Turn the head to the right side, straighten it, turn to the left side, and straighten (see Figure 11-28B ■).

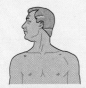

Right rotation Left rotation

FIGURE 11-28B

c. Move the head toward the right shoulder, straighten it, move the head toward the left shoulder, and straighten the head again (see Figure 11-28C ■).

Right lateral flexion Left lateral flexion

FIGURE 11-28C

3. Exercise the shoulder: Place one hand under the resident's elbow. Grasp the resident's hand with your other hand.
   a. Raise the resident's arm over the head and down again while keeping the elbow straight (see Figure 11-28D ■).

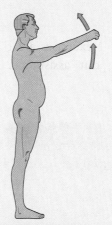 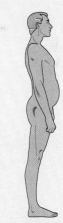
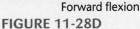

Forward flexion Extension

FIGURE 11-28D

(continued)

b. Raise the resident's arm out to the side and bring it back to the side, keeping the elbow straight (see Figure 11-28E ■).

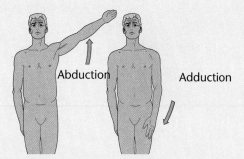

Abduction Adduction

FIGURE 11-28E

c. Bring the arm out to the side, bend the elbow, and rotate the forearm and hand downward and then upward (see Figure 11-28F ■).

External rotation Internal rotation

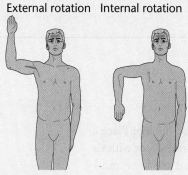

FIGURE 11-28F

4. Exercise the elbow and the forearm: Place one hand under the elbow and grasp the resident's hand with your other hand.
   a. Bend the resident's elbow toward the shoulder and then straighten the elbow (see Figure 11-28G ■).

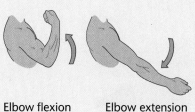

Elbow flexion Elbow extension
FIGURE 11-28G

b. Turn the forearm so that the palm of the hand faces down. Then turn the forearm so that the hand faces up (see Figure 11-28H ■).

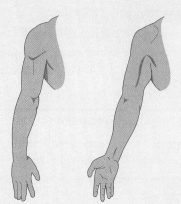

Forearm pronation Forearm supination
FIGURE 11-28H

5. Exercise the wrist: Both of your hands should support the resident's wrist and hand.
   a. Bend the wrist up and then down (see Figure 11-28I ■).

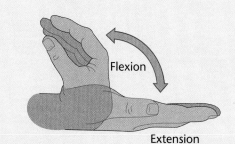

Flexion

Extension

FIGURE 11-28I ■

(continued)

b. Keeping the fingers together, bend the wrist from side to side (see Figure 11-28J ■).

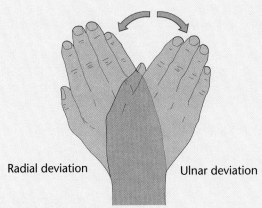

Radial deviation   Ulnar deviation

FIGURE 11-28J

6. Exercise the fingers: Support the hand at the wrist and above each joint that you are exercising.
   a. Bend and straighten each finger separately. Then make a fist and open it with the fingers together (see Figure 11-28K ■).

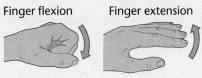

Finger flexion   Finger extension

FIGURE 11-28K

b. Bring the fingers together and then spread them apart (see Figure 11-28L ■).

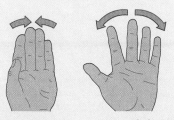

Finger adduction   Finger abduction

FIGURE 11-28L

c. Bring the thumb across the palm of the hand and then bring the thumb away from the hand (see Figure 11-28M ■).

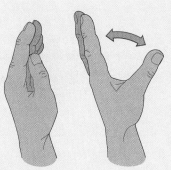

Thumb adduction   Thumb abduction

FIGURE 11-28M

d. Touch the thumb to the tip of each finger (see Figure 11-28N ■).

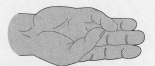

Finger/thumb opposition

FIGURE 11-28N

7. Exercise the hip: Place one hand below the knee and support the foot with the other hand.
   a. Bend the knee and bring it up toward the chest. Straighten the knee as you lower the leg to the bed (see Figure 11-28O ■).

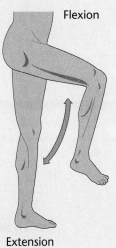

Flexion

Extension

FIGURE 11-28O

(continued)

b. Raise the leg up off the bed, keeping the knee straight. Lower the leg to the bed again (see Figure 11-28P ■).

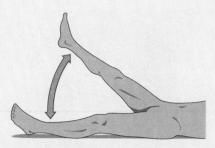

Straight leg raising

FIGURE 11-28P

c. Keeping the knee straight, bring the leg away from the body, then bring the leg back to the body (see Figure 11-28Q ■).

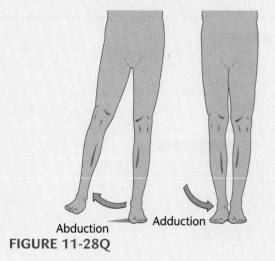

Abduction   Adduction

FIGURE 11-28Q

d. Rotate the hip in, so that the toes point toward the other leg. Then rotate the hip out, so that the toes point away from the other leg (see Figure 11-28R ■).

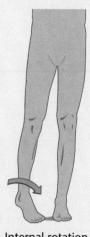

Internal rotation   External rotation

FIGURE 11-28R

8. Exercise the knee: Place your hands under the knee and the ankle to support the joints.
   a. Bend the knee; then straighten it (see Figure 11-28S ■).

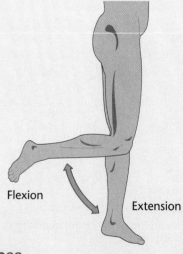

Flexion   Extension

FIGURE 11-28S

(continued)

9. Exercise the ankle: Place your hands under the foot and ankle to support the joint.

   a. Bend the foot down. Then bend the foot up toward the head (see Figure 11-28T ■).

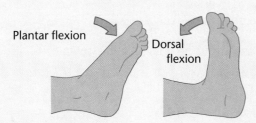

Plantar flexion   Dorsal flexion

FIGURE 11-28T

10. Exercise the toes: Support the foot with one hand as you exercise the toes with the other hand.

    a. Bend and straighten the toes separately. Then bend and straighten the toes together (see Figure 11-28U ■).

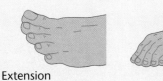

Extension

FIGURE 11-28U

b. Bring the toes together and then separate them (see Figure 11-28V ■).

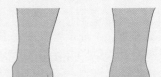
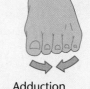
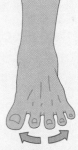

Adduction   Abduction

FIGURE 11-28V

■ **Ending Steps**

To complete the procedure, perform the following steps:

Make the resident comfortable, positioning in good body alignment. Make the resident safe, placing the call signal within reach, lowering the bed, and raising the side rails, if appropriate. Wash your hands. Record and report the procedure as required.

Chapter Highlights

1. Physical activity is necessary to maintain the well-being of all body systems.
2. Restorative nursing care can prevent most of the complications of inactivity.
3. Encourage the resident to be as independent as possible.
4. Use correct body mechanics when assisting the resident in moving and transferring.
5. Correct body alignment promotes comfort and prevents stress on the musculoskeletal system.
6. Changing body positions promotes comfort, stimulates circulation, and helps to prevent complications.
7. Using a lift sheet makes moving and transferring the resident easier and safer.
8. Keep the side rail up on the opposite side of the bed when you are working with the resident.
9. Return the bed to its lowest position when you are finished working with it.
10. Dangling on the side of the bed helps the resident to gain balance.
11. Lead with the resident's strong side when moving and transferring him or her.
12. Using a gait/transfer belt reduces the risk of injury to the resident and the nursing assistant.

CHAPTER HIGHLIGHTS (Continued)

13. The mechanical lift is used to help transfer residents who are very heavy or who are unable to move.

14. Always lock the brakes when the wheelchair is stopped.

15. Never leave a resident alone on a stretcher.

16. Ambulation provides exercise that leads to independence and increased self-esteem.

17. Range-of-motion exercises are one of the best restorative measures to prevent contractures.

VOCABULARY REVIEW

Fill in the blank with the vocabulary term that best completes the sentence.

1. A person who is confused as to person, place, or time is _____.

2. To _____ is to walk.

3. A breakdown in skin tissue that occurs when blood flow is interrupted is a _____ _____.

4. _____ means moving away from the body.

5. The accumulation of fluid in body tissue is _____.

6. A _____ is a permanent shortening of a muscle due to lack of exercise or use.

7. _____ is the inability to move a body part.

8. _____ is the passage of hard, dry stool.

9. The arms and legs are the _____.

10. The person in a _____ position is lying on his back.

CHECK YOUR UNDERSTANDING

The following questions cover the highlights of this chapter. Choose the best answer for each question.

1. Which of the following statements about the elderly is true?
   A. Most elderly people are not able to exercise.
   B. Exercise is good for elderly people.
   C. Elderly people do not need to exercise.
   D. Elderly people do not benefit from exercise.

2. A resident you are assisting to ambulate starts to fall. What should you do?
   A. Hold the resident up as long as you can.
   B. Slide the resident down your leg to the floor.
   C. Stand back so that the resident doesn't fall on you.
   D. Fall down with the resident.

3. While performing range-of-motion exercises, the resident complains of pain when you have barely moved his arm. What will you do?
   A. Stop at that point and exercise a different joint.
   B. Tell him it will stop hurting in a minute.
   C. Tell him it has to hurt to get better.
   D. Exercise the joint more slowly.

4. How can you help the resident maintain correct body alignment while she is lying on her side?
   A. Support her head with two pillows.
   B. Support her upper arm and upper leg with pillows.
   C. Support her lower arm and lower leg with pillows.
   D. Support her head and knees with pillows.

5. The most important reason for using a lift sheet when moving a resident up in bed is to
   A. prevent friction on the resident's skin
   B. prevent contractures of the resident's joints
   C. make your job easier
   D. get the job done faster

6. The resident has a weak right side. What is the best way to assist him out of a chair?
   A. Have him lead with his left foot first.
   B. Have him lead with his right foot first.
   C. Let him lead with whichever foot he wants.
   D. Lift him up with a mechanical lift.

7. How can you prevent the resident's knees from buckling when you assist him to stand?
   A. Tell him to lock his knees.
   B. Tell him to bend his knees.
   C. Stand away from him so that he can move easily.
   D. Block his knees with your knees.

8. You have to use a mechanical lift to get a resident out of bed and you are not sure how to use the equipment. What should you do?
   A. Use it and hope you remember all the steps.
   B. Leave the resident in the bed.
   C. Ask the nurse to show you how to use the lift.
   D. Get the resident up without using the lift.

AGE-SPECIFIC TIP

Some elderly residents are unable to stand. Talk to residents at eye level rather than standing over them and looking down.

CULTURALLY SENSITIVE TIP

Independence is important to individuals of many cultural groups. Be supportive of the resident's efforts to be independent.

EFFECTIVE PROBLEM SOLVING

The weak elderly resident is trying to exercise by himself. The nursing assistant says, "You're too old and frail to do those exercises. I'm afraid you'll hurt yourself. You need to get more rest." Was the nursing assistant's communication appropriate? If not, what would have been more appropriate?

_____

_____

_____

_____

_____

_____

_____

_____

_____

_____

_____

INTERPERSONAL COMMUNICATION

Write a T or F to indicate if the statement is true or false.

_____When two staff members are transferring or lifting a resident, moving on the count of "3" helps coordinate movement and prevent injury.

_____When two staff members are transferring or lifting a resident, nodding your head at your coworker when it's time to lift helps coordinate movement and prevent injury.

_____Keep directions simple and consistent when helping the resident to move.

_____If the resident complains of pain during range-of-motion exercises, stop as soon as you have completed all the exercises.

OBSERVING, REPORTING, AND RECORDING

List four complications of limited activity that should be observed, reported, and recorded.

_____

_____

_____

_____

_____

_____

_____

_____

_____

_____

EXPLORE MEDIALINK

12

RESTORATIVE SKIN CARE: PREVENTION OF PRESSURE SORES

OBJECTIVES

1. List six changes of aging that occur in the skin.
2. Identify three types of injury to the skin.
3. List six guidelines for providing foot care.
4. Identify the two causes of pressure sores.
5. Identify the four possible beginning signs of a pressure sore.
6. List six guidelines for restorative skin care.

VOCABULARY

The following words or terms will help you to understand this chapter:

Integument
Nutrients
Petechiae
Bruise
Laceration

Incision
Pressure sore
Shearing
Incontinence
Hydration

Bony prominence
Obese
Coccyx
Sacrum

Risk factors for skin problems of the elderly are described and guidelines for skin care are included in this chapter.

STRUCTURE AND FUNCTION OF THE SKIN

The skin serves as a barrier to protect the body from infection, loss of fluid, and loss of body heat. Keeping the resident's skin healthy and intact (unbroken) is an important responsibility of nursing assistants. Healthy skin is clean, soft, and moist. Use creams and lotions to help keep it that way (see Figure 12-1 ■).

The skin is composed of two layers, the epidermis (outer layer) and dermis. A layer of subcutaneous fat supports the skin from underneath. Functions of the skin include protection, regulation of body temperature, and sensory reception.

A more detailed description of the skin is provided in Chapter 22.

SKIN CONDITIONS

Changes of Aging

The first visible signs of aging often occur in the **integument** (skin). Many of the changes that occur with aging increase the risk of injury and skin damage for the elderly person. They include:

- Dry, thin, fragile skin that tears easily
- Loss of fatty tissue that normally provides padding and insulation

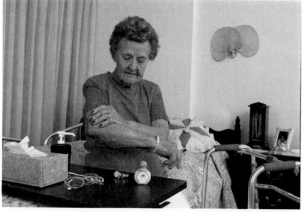

FIGURE 12-1 ■ Using creams and lotions help keep skin clean, soft, and moist.

- Decreased sensitivity to heat and cold
- Loss of skin tone and elasticity leading to wrinkles
- Increased risk of infection and slow healing

To be healthy, the cells of the skin must receive a constant and adequate supply of **nutrients** (food elements) and oxygen. Poor circulation may decrease the delivery of nutrients and oxygen to the skin. Decreased circulation also prevents the removal of waste products and toxins. Healing slows and infection may result.

Observe the resident's skin carefully and report any changes immediately. Bleeding or a change in the size or color of a mole may be a sign of skin cancer. **Petechiae** (patches of surface bleeding due to fragile blood vessels) are covered with extremely fragile skin. Dryness and skin sensitivity may lead to rashes and skin breakdown.

Injuries

The skin is the body's first line of defense against the environment. Injured skin cannot protect the body from the invasion of micro-organisms. Slight injuries may lead to major problems. A **bruise** is an injury that discolors but does not break the skin. A **laceration** is a rough tear, and an **incision** is a clean, smooth cut.

Foot Care

Because the feet and legs are especially at risk, due to poor circulation, they must be protected from injury. This is especially true for diabetics who often develop circulatory complications. Observe the feet carefully while you are providing care and report any problems to the nurse. The following guidelines will help you provide good foot care.

> ## GUIDELINES
> ### PROVIDING FOOT CARE
> - Examine the feet at least once daily, and observe for and report any problems such as discoloration, injury, or edema (see Figure 12-2 ■).
> - Wash the feet daily and dry them thoroughly, especially between the toes.

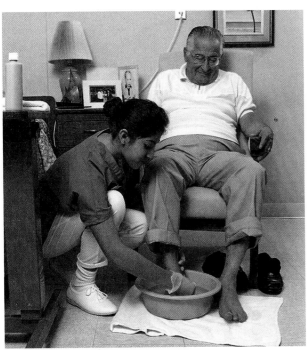

FIGURE 12-2 ■ The feet and legs must be observed carefully.

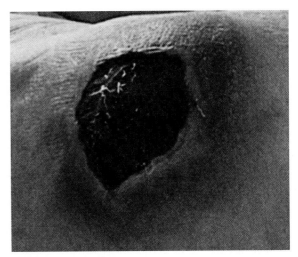

FIGURE 12-3 ■ A pressure sore can result in pain and infection.

GUIDELINES (Continued)

- Let the nurse know if the toenails need to be trimmed. In many areas, nursing assistants are not allowed to trim toenails.

- Encourage regular exercise.

- Keep bed linen over the resident's feet loose to prevent pressure.

- When transferring a resident who uses a wheelchair, move the footrests out of the way to prevent injury.

- Check to see that shoes and socks fit well.

- Inspect shoes and socks for tears or objects that might injure the foot.

CAUSES AND PREVENTION OF PRESSURE SORES

A **pressure sore** is a breakdown of skin tissue that occurs when blood flow is interrupted (see Figure 12-3 ■). When blood flow cannot deliver nutrients and oxygen, or remove waste products and toxins, tissue dies and a pressure sore forms. Pressure and shearing cause pressure sores. **Shearing** is a force upon the skin that stretches it between the bone

inside and a surface outside the body. Excessive perspiration, **incontinence** (the inability to control urine or feces), poor nutrition, and inadequate **hydration** (supply of fluids) all contribute to the development or worsening of pressure sores.

Pressure

You may see how pressure stops blood flow by pressing your thumbs against a plate of clear plastic or glass. Observe, through the glass, the skin color that results during this pressure. As soon as you have released the pressure, the color will return to normal.

Pressure causes problems over **bony prominences** (places where bones are near the surface of the skin). Figure 12-4 ■ indicates the bony prominences of the body where pressure sores are likely to develop. The skin in these areas is thin enough that the blood vessels can be pinched closed. The vessels are pinched between the bony prominence and the surface upon which it rests.

Pressure sores are the most challenging skin problems that may affect the elderly, paralyzed, comatose (unconscious), malnourished, or **obese** (overweight) resident. Obese residents may develop pressure sores in skin folds. Pressure from casts, braces, or traction also can cause pressure sores. The paralyzed or comatose resident is unable to move in a normal manner and may not experience skin sensations that encourage movement.

A paralyzed or comatose resident may not realize the need to reposition and may not feel the

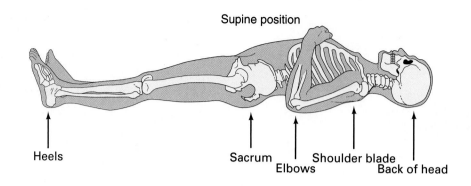

Supine position

Heels   Sacrum   Elbows   Shoulder blade   Back of head

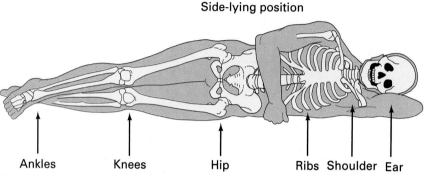

Side-lying position

Ankles   Knees   Hip   Ribs   Shoulder   Ear

FIGURE 12-4 ■ Pressure sores form most often over bony prominences.

discomfort of pressure from objects that are against the skin. Without frequent position changes and movement, pressure sores will develop. A malnourished resident has less subcutaneous fat and therefore is at increased risk of pressure sore formation. The skin must be well nourished and have adequate hydration to be healthy.

Shearing

In addition to pressure, shearing also can cause pressure sores. As the skin is stretched under pressure (see Figure 12-5 ■), the small surface blood vessels are pulled at an angle and become pinched or twisted closed. This blocks the blood flow and skin tissue dies. Shearing takes place when the body slides on a surface, as it does when the head of the bed is raised. As the body slides toward the foot of the bed, the skin is stretched and the blood vessels over the sacrum and coccyx are pinched. The **coccyx** is located at the base of the spine and often is referred to as the "tail bone." The **sacrum** is the bone directly above the coccyx. This is the most common location for pressure sores to occur.

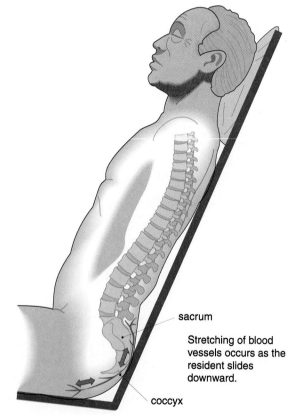

sacrum

Stretching of blood vessels occurs as the resident slides downward.

coccyx

FIGURE 12-5 ■ When the skin is stretched by shearing, blood vessels are pulled at an angle.

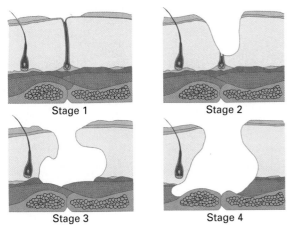

FIGURE 12-6 ■ Pressure sores are classified by the depth of tissue destruction.

Signs and Stages of Pressure Sores

The first sign of a pressure sore is a reddened area that stays red even after the pressure is relieved. Sometimes the skin will be pale or darkened. Pressure sores are classified into stages according to the depth of tissue damage (see the following description and Figure 12-6 ■).

Stage 1: Reddened area on the skin; heat, pain numbness, and tingling may occur.
Stage 2: Blisters with possible broken skin.
Stage 3: Skin in destroyed; deep sore; possible infection and scarring.
Stage 4: Deep sore that spreads into surrounding tissues; muscle or bone is exposed.

At any stage the resident may experience pain, and treatment is lengthy and very expensive. Pressure sores progress rapidly and are much easier to prevent than to treat. Early reporting of signs of pressure sores may prevent the progress from a stage 1 to a stage 4.

RESTORATIVE SKIN CARE

As a nursing assistant, you will play an important role in the prevention of pressure sores. While prevention requires much attention and time, curing a pressure sore is much more time-consuming and stressful. Most pressure sores can be prevented.

Preventing long-lasting, painful, and costly skin problems depends upon your careful observation and commitment to preventive care. One of the best ways to prevent pressure sores is to keep the skin clean, dry, and healthy. Following the guidelines for restorative skin care will help protect the resident from skin damage.

Sometimes you will need to use pressure relieving equipment. This equipment includes devices that are designed to relieve pressure and friction on the resident's skin and to prevent shearing. Items as ordinary as pillows may be used to position the body in a way that relieves pressure. Other pressure-relieving equipment is pictured and described in Figure 12-7 ■. Remember that this equipment only provides additional protection for the skin. It does not replace skin care.

GUIDELINES

RESTORATIVE SKIN CARE

- Follow the resident's plan of care.
- Reposition the resident at least every two hours to keep pressure off areas at risk.
- Cleanse the skin of urine and feces immediately. Urine and feces contain chemicals and bacteria that quickly cause skin breakdown. Dry well after cleansing.
- Massage gently *around*—not *on*—reddened areas with lotion. Additional skin breakdown may occur if the damaged area is massaged.
- Keep linen clean, dry, and free from wrinkles.
- Be sure the bed is free of small objects that might injure the skin.
- Maintain good nutrition and hydration.
- Position tubes to avoid pressure on the skin.
- Observe carefully for pressure that may be caused by braces, splints, casts, traction, or shoes.

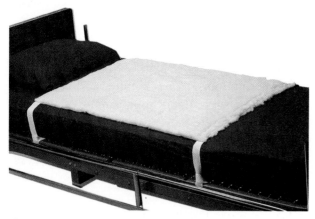

Sheep skin or fleece. *Posey Corp.*

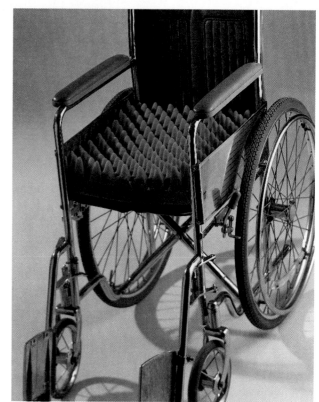

Egg crate. *Posey Corp.*

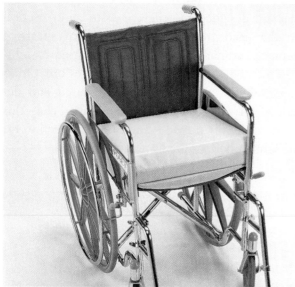

Gel foam cushion. *Sammons, Preston, Rolyann-U.S.A. Inc.*

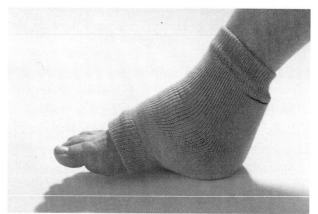

Heel/elbow protector. *Posey Corp.*

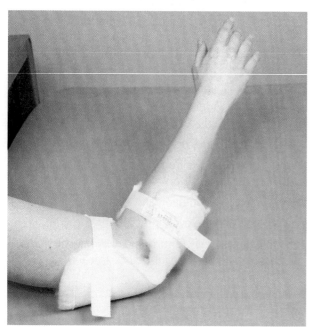

Heel/elbow protector. *Posey Corp.*

FIGURE 12-7 ■ Pressure-relieving devices help to protect the skin.

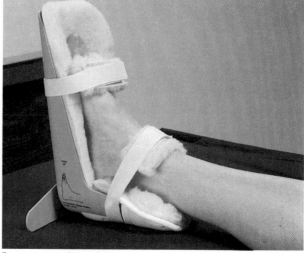

Foot support. *Posey Corp.*

CHAPTER HIGHLIGHTS

1. Changes of aging increase the risk of injury and skin damage for the elderly.

2. The feet and legs are at greatest risk due to poor circulation.

3. Observe the resident's skin carefully and report any changes immediately.

4. Pressure sores result from obstructed blood flow, which causes tissue death.

5. Bony prominences of the body are common pressure points where pressure sores develop.

6. Residents who are at higher risk of developing pressure sores include the elderly, immobilized, malnourished, debilitated, and obese.

7. Signs of pressure sores include pale or darkened skin, redness, and heat.

8. The nursing assistant plays an important role in the prevention of pressure sores.

9. Reposition the resident every 2 hours to keep pressure off areas at risk.

10. Cleanse the resident's skin immediately after an episode of incontinence.

11. Massage gently around—not on—a reddened area on the skin.

VOCABULARY REVIEW

Fill in the blanks with the vocabulary term that best completes the sentence.

1. _____ is the inability to control urine.

2. A breakdown of skin tissue that occurs when blood flow is interrupted is a/an _____ _____.

3. A/An _____ is an injury that discolors but does not break the skin.

4. The correct name for skin is _____.

5. _____ is the supply of fluids in the body.

6. A rough tear in the skin is a/an _____.

7. A/An _____ is a clean, smooth cut in the skin.

8. A/An _____ person is overweight.

9. The end of the spine, often called the "tail bone," is the _____.

10. _____ are patches of surface bleeding due to fragile blood vessels.

CHECK YOUR UNDERSTANDING

The following questions cover the highlights of this chapter. Choose the best answer to each question.

1. Which of the following is a guideline for providing foot care?
   A. Examine the resident's feet at least once a month.
   B. Keep the area between the toes moist.
   C. Cut the resident's toenails as needed.
   D. Encourage regular exercise.

2. Which of the following is *not* a change of aging in the integumentary system?
   A. The skin becomes thinner.
   B. The skin becomes dryer.
   C. The skin loses padding.
   D. The skin becomes oily.

3. You observe a reddened area on the skin. What should you do?
   A. Nothing. It is not your responsibility.
   B. Massage it. The nurse probably will notice it later.
   C. Report it to the nurse immediately.
   D. Call the resident's doctor immediately.

4. You are assigned to care for an elderly resident who is bedbound. How often should this resident be turned and repositioned?
   A. every hour
   B. every 2 hours
   C. every 4 hours
   D. every 8 hours

5. A beginning sign of a pressure sore is
   A. a rash
   B. perspiration
   C. discolored skin
   D. incontinence

6. Which of the following statements about pressure sores is *not* true?
   A. Treatment is lengthy and very expensive.
   B. Incontinence can make pressure sores worse.
   C. Pressure sores are much easier to prevent than to treat.
   D. Paralyzed residents do not get pressure sores.

AGE-SPECIFIC COMMUNICATION TIP

You may need to touch the elderly resident to get his or her attention before you speak. Extra time may be needed for the resident to become focused before he or she can participate in communication.

CULTURALLY SENSITIVE TIP

There are cultural differences that affect the resident's response to touch. Explain that you are going to massage the resident before you touch his or her skin.

EFFECTIVE PROBLEM SOLVING

While positioning Mr. Arnold in the bed, the nursing assistant notices that the hip he has been lying on is red and the skin feels warm. He complains that the hip feels sore and he thinks the doctor should be called. The nursing assistant responds, "I told the nurse about this yesterday. I'm sure she called the doctor about it."

Was the nursing assistant's communication appropriate? If not, what would have been more appropriate?

_____

_____

_____

_____

_____

_____

_____

_____

_____

_____

_____

_____

INTERPERSONAL COMMUNICATION

Fill in the blank.

An alert and oriented resident sits in a wheelchair most of the day. Remind him or her to change _____ frequently to prevent skin damage and other complications.

OBSERVING, REPORTING, AND RECORDING

Elderly residents' skin may be dry, fragile, and easily damaged. List four signs and symptoms of pressure sores that should be observed, reported, and recorded.

_____

_____

_____

_____

_____

_____

_____

_____

_____

_____

EXPLORE MEDIALINK

Check out www.prenhall.com/grubbs for additional chapter-specific interactive study and review activities.

13

PERSONAL CARE AND HYGIENE

OBJECTIVES

1. Describe the effect of personal care on self-esteem.
2. Identify five important observations to make during oral hygiene.
3. Identify ten guidelines for assisting and providing oral care.
4. List three steps to be taken to protect dentures during denture care.
5. Identify ten guidelines for bathing.
6. List two aseptic principles of perineal care.
7. Identify ten guidelines for assisting with a shower or tub bath.
8. List eight guidelines for nail care.
9. Identify ten guidelines for assisting the resident to dress.
10. Identify six guidelines for changing the resident's clothing.
11. Describe the effect that independence in personal care and dressing has upon the resident's self-esteem.
12. Perform the procedures described in this chapter.

VOCABULARY

The following words or terms will help you to understand this chapter:

Incontinence	Toothettes	Perineal care (peri-care)
Oral hygiene	Comatose	Defecation
Emesis basin	Dentures	Intravenous IV
Expectorate	Axillae	

Routines and restorative measures, as well as guidelines and procedures for providing personal care and hygiene, are described in this chapter.

PERSONAL CARE CHOICES

Personal care includes bathing; care of the mouth, nails, and hair; shaving; dressing; and for women, applying makeup. This care is provided whenever it is needed. Attending to personal care helps to improve the resident's self-esteem and maintain health. Grooming and personal hygiene involve choices that the resident may make. These choices include whether to bathe in the tub or shower, when and how often to perform hygiene, and what products to use.

Many residents depend upon the nursing assistant for help with personal hygiene. Some are totally dependent for maintaining healthy skin, cleanliness, and grooming. **Incontinence**, (inability to control urine or feces), immobility, illness, and confusion increase the time and effort required for maintaining hygiene. Encourage the resident to be involved and to do as much as possible. If you are not sure what personal care is required for each resident, check the care plan or ask the nurse.

DAILY CARE ROUTINES

In the long-term care facility there usually are some routines that are followed for daily hygiene of residents. These are often referred to as "A.M. care" and "H.S." or "P.M. care." A.M. care is usually performed in the morning before breakfast is served. H.S. (hour of sleep or bedtime) or P.M. care is performed at bedtime when the resident is preparing to go to sleep.

A.M. Care

It is important to assist residents before breakfast in order to awaken them and help them prepare for a pleasant meal. Most residents may go to the dining room to eat, while others may eat in their rooms, in bed or in a chair.

Awakening the resident and ensuring comfort may improve the appetite. A freshly washed face and clean mouth will make breakfast more pleasant. The activity of performing this self-care will help provide exercise, improve the appetite, and maintain independence. Residents should always do as much self-care as possible with your assistance as needed.

Although A.M. care for some residents may not be completed until after breakfast, all residents should be assisted to toilet, perform **oral hygiene** (mouth care), wash their face and hands, comb their hair, and dress. The resident's unit and linen should be straightened prior to breakfast. Bathing may be done at any time of day but is most often completed during the morning.

Other personal care that may be accomplished includes toileting, peri-care, care of hair and nails, shaving, backrubs, and dressing. After this care is provided, the bed is made and the room is left in a neat condition for the day.

H.S. Care

H.S. care is performed at bedtime when the resident is preparing to go to sleep. The purpose of this care is to help the resident relax. At bedtime, the resident should toilet and perform peri-care. Oral hygiene also is performed, and the face and hands should be washed. Linen should be changed or straightened. Night clothes are provided and the unit is tidied at this time (see Figure 13-1 ■). A backrub at bedtime is very helpful in promoting relaxation and a good night's sleep.

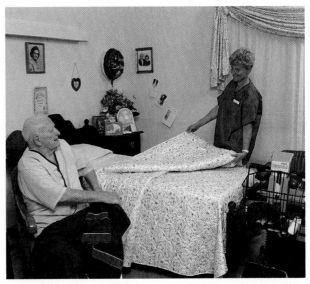

FIGURE 13-1 ■ H.S. care refreshes the resident and promotes relaxation for sleep.

PROCEDURE

Assisting with Oral Hygiene

■ Beginning Steps.

Before any procedure, you always must follow the five basic steps: wash your hands, collect the equipment, identify the resident, explain the procedure, and protect privacy.

Follow standard precautions.

1. Place equipment and supplies on paper towels on the overbed table.
2. Raise the bed to a comfortable working height and lock the wheels.
3. Raise the head of the bed if allowed.
4. Place a bath towel across the resident's chest.
5. Place the overbed table across the bed in front of the resident.
6. Put on gloves.
7. Allow the resident to rinse the mouth with water or diluted mouthwash. You may hold the emesis basin to the chin for expectoration (see Figure 13-2 ■).
8. Place toothpaste on the wet toothbrush and encourage the resident to do the brushing.
9. Assist the resident to rinse the mouth and expectorate into the emesis basin. Help the resident clean any water or toothpaste off the face.
10. Clean and put away equipment; discard disposables.
11. Wipe off the overbed table.
12. Remove your gloves and wash your hands.
13. Open the privacy curtain.

■ Ending Steps

To complete this procedure, perform the following steps:

Make the resident comfortable, positioning in good body alignment. Make the resident safe, placing the call signal within reach, lowering the bed, and raising the side rails, if appropriate. Wash your hands. Record and report the procedure as required.

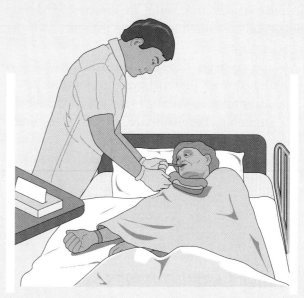

FIGURE 13-2 ■ The emesis basin may be used for expectoration.

ORAL HYGIENE

Oral care includes brushing the teeth and tongue. Conditions of the mouth and lips that should be observed and reported include the following:

- Cracked, blistered, or swollen lips
- Unpleasant mouth odor
- Swelling, redness, sores, bleeding, white patches, or coating of the mouth
- Loose, broken, or chipped teeth
- Resident complaints

Some residents may need mouth care every 2 hours or more frequently because of excessive dryness, sores, or a bad taste that develops. These may result from the presence of a tube in the nose, oxygen administration, illness, unconsciousness, medications, or lack of fluid intake. An uncomfortable mouth or a bad taste can result in a poor appetite and inadequate fluid intake.

GUIDELINES

ASSISTING AND PROVIDING ORAL HYGIENE

- Encourage residents to perform oral hygiene as independently as possible and assist as needed.
- Protect the resident's clothing by placing a towel across the chest before brushing. (continued)

GUIDELINES (Continued)

- Some residents, including those who are unconscious, will depend upon you to perform oral hygiene for them.

- Reminding and assisting confused or forgetful residents may be necessary.

- Check to be sure that oral care has been completed satisfactorily by the resident.

- When gathering supplies for oral hygiene, check the care plan for assistive equipment that should be used.

- Provide an **emesis basin** (a small curved basin) if oral hygiene will be performed in bed. This may be used for the resident to **expectorate** (spit).

- Provide mouthwash, dental floss, and **Toothettes** (sticks with small sponges used for oral care).

- Wear gloves for any contact with body fluids, including saliva.

- Always communicate with the **comatose** (unconscious or unresponsive) resident. Explain each step prior to performing it, and talk to the resident throughout care.

- Turn the comatose resident to the side.

- Toothpaste and water are not used when a resident is unable to swallow. Lemon-glycerine swabs, applicators moistened with mouthwash, or Toothettes (see Figure 13-3 ■) may be used.

- Use the principles that follow for thorough tooth brushing.

Remember that poor oral health can cause tooth loss, discomfort, loss of appetite, low self-esteem, and a decline in general health.

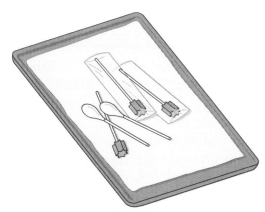

FIGURE 13-3 ■ Lemon-glycerine swabs and Toothettes are commercial products for oral care.

Principles for Thorough Tooth Brushing

- Wear gloves.
- Use a soft- to medium-bristled brush.
- Brush in a circular motion while holding the brush at a 45° angle.
- Brush the inner, outer, and then chewing surfaces of the upper teeth.
- Brush the lower teeth in the same manner.
- Brush the tongue and gums.

Denture Care

Dentures (false teeth) should be cleaned as often as natural teeth. Ask the resident if he would prefer to clean his own dentures.

GUIDELINES

PROVIDING DENTURE CARE

- Wear gloves to provide denture care.

- Always check linen and clothing pockets for dentures that may have been placed there. Be sure to check the pillow case thoroughly.

- Rinse the resident's mouth while the dentures are out. This will remove food, bacteria, and seeds that may have collected on mouth surfaces.

- Always carry dentures in a denture cup or emesis basin to prevent dropping them.

- Hold dentures over a basin filled with water or lined with a towel to prevent damage if they slip from your hands while you brush them (see Figure 13-5 ■).

- Store dentures in cool water when the resident is not wearing them. Hot water and drying can damage them.

- Be sure that the denture container is labeled with the resident's name and room number.

- Encourage the resident to clean the dentures if possible, and check the care plan for use of assistive equipment.

Dentures are expensive to replace, and replacement may be extremely difficult or impossible for some elderly residents. Nutrition may become a major problem when dentures are broken or missing. A limited variety of foods can be eaten without teeth. Without the ability to chew food, a resident may lose much of his or her appetite. Weight

PROCEDURE

Giving Oral Care to the Comatose Resident

■ **Beginning Steps.**

Before any procedure, you always must follow the five basic steps: wash your hands, collect the equipment, identify the resident, explain the procedure and protect privacy.

Follow standard precautions.

1. Place equipment and supplies on paper towels on the overbed table.
2. Raise the bed to a comfortable working height, lock the wheels, and lower the side rail.
3. Place the resident in a side-lying position.
4. Place a bath towel under the resident's head and face and the emesis basin under the side of the chin.
5. Put on gloves.
6. Use a padded tongue depressor to separate the teeth and open the mouth (see Figure 13-4 ■).
7. Clean the mouth using Toothettes or lemon-glycerine swabs or applicators with diluted mouthwash. Clean all surfaces of the mouth (tongue, cheeks, roof, and teeth).
8. Apply petroleum jelly to the lips for lubrication.
9. Reposition the resident.
10. Raise the side rail.
11. Clean and put away equipment and discard disposables.

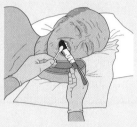

FIGURE 13-4 ■ A padded tongue blade may be used to hold the mouth open during oral hygiene of the comatose resident.

12. Wipe off the overbed table.
13. Remove your gloves and wash your hands.

■ **Ending Steps**

To complete the procedure, perform the following steps:

Make the resident comfortable, positioning in good body alignment. Make the resident safe, placing the call signal within reach, lowering the bed, and raising the side rails, if appropriate. Wash your hands. Record and report the procedure as required.

■

loss and declining health may result. Protect the resident's dentures. You may be found negligent if you fail to use precautions.

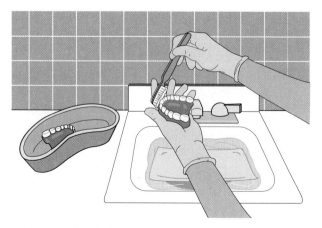

FIGURE 13-5 ■ Brushing dentures over a sinkful of water will protect them.

People who wear dentures usually prefer to clean them themselves. You may assist some residents to the bathroom to clean their own dentures, and it may be necessary for you to clean the dentures for others.

BATHING AND PERSONAL HYGIENE

Although many residents will be able to bathe themselves, others will need your assistance. A bath cleanses the skin and prevents odor. It also provides exercise for the resident.

You have an excellent opportunity to observe for skin problems while assisting with bathing. Areas that are prone to skin problems are bony prominences and skin creases and folds, such as breasts, knees, and **axillae** (underarms). Report any unusual skin problems to the nurse.

$\mathscr{P}$ROCEDURE

Care of Dentures

■ Beginning Steps

Before any procedure, you always must follow the five basic steps: wash your hands, collect the equipment, identify the resident, explain the procedure, and protect privacy.

◉ Follow Standard Precautions

1. Place the necessary equipment at the sink.
2. Take the denture cup, emesis basin, mouthwash, glass of water, and gloves to the bedside.
3. Place the towel over the resident's chest.
4. Put on the gloves.
5. Ask the resident to remove the dentures and place them in the emesis basin.
6. If the resident cannot remove the dentures, you may do so as follows:
   a. Move the upper denture up and down slightly by grasping it with your thumb and index finger at the front. This breaks the seal (see Figure 13-6A ■).
   b. When loose, remove the denture and place it into the emesis basin.
   c. Grasp the lower denture at the front with your thumb and index finger.
   d. Remove it gently, turning it if necessary to bring the end of one side out before the other (see Figure 13-6B ■). Place the lower denture in the emesis basin.
7. Take the dentures, denture cup, and emesis basin to the sink.
8. Place a paper towel in the sink or fill the sink with water to cushion the dentures in case they slip from your hands (see Figure 13-5).
9. Place toothpaste or denture cleaner on each denture in the emesis basin.
10. Holding one denture in your palm, brush all surfaces thoroughly. Return it to the emesis basin while you brush the other denture in the same manner.
11. Rinse each denture thoroughly, one at a time, under cool running water.
12. Place the dentures in the denture cup with fresh cool water.
13. Rinse the emesis basin.
14. Bring the emesis basin and dentures (in the cup) to the resident.

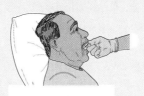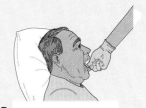

A   **B**

FIGURE 13-6 ■ Dentures are removed for denture care.

15. Dilute the mouthwash with water, and assist the resident to rinse out the mouth. You may hold the emesis basin to one side of the resident's chin for expectoration (see Figure 13-2).
16. Have the resident replace the dentures in the mouth.
17. If the resident is unable to replace the dentures, proceed as follows:
    a. With your thumb and finger at the front of the upper denture, insert it into the resident's mouth. You may lift the upper lip with your other hand.
    b. If necessary, you may turn the denture slightly to the side to insert one side, and then turn it gently against the inner cheek to insert the other side.
    c. Secure it by pressing it into place lightly.
    d. With your thumb and index finger at the front of the lower denture, insert it. You may lower the bottom lip with your free hand. You may also turn the denture as described in step 17b to insert it. Gently press downward to secure it.
18. Leave the denture cup with clean water at the resident's bedside. If dentures are not to be replaced in the resident's mouth, leave them in the labeled denture cup at the bedside.
19. Return equipment and supplies to proper storage.
20. Remove the gloves and wash your hands.

■ Ending Steps

To complete the procedure, perform the following steps:

Make the resident comfortable, positioning in good body alignment. Make the resident safe, placing the call signal within reach, lowering the bed, and raising the side rails, if appropriate. Wash your hands. Record and report the procedure as required.

Bath time observation includes the opportunity to listen to the resident and allows the nursing assistant to observe physical complaints as well as mental, emotional, and speech changes. Questions may be asked to encourage conversation. The movement that is required for bathing exercises the resident's limbs and allows you to observe any limitations of movement.

The skin and circulation are stimulated by bathing. It is a very nurturing process that often results in an improved sense of well-being.

Methods of bathing include the complete bed bath, partial bath, tub bath, shower, and specialty bath. In long-term care, showers or specialty baths are most frequently used because of their restorative value. The resident's personal preference, doctor's orders physical condition, and level of independence will determine the method of bathing required. Bath time should be chosen according to the resident's preference.

Daily partial baths usually are adequate for the elderly who receive a complete bath or shower twice a week. Bathing may tend to dry the skin. The use of soap may be limited to prevent drying and irritation. A partial bath must be provided with each episode of incontinence for the resident who experiences bowel or bladder incontinence.

GUIDELINES

BATHING

- Check the care plan or your assignment sheet to determine the type of bath required for the resident.
- Protect the resident's dignity and modesty.
- Encourage the resident to bathe as independently as possible.
- Communicate with the resident while you are providing a bath. This is a good time for conversation with the resident in addition to communicating each step before beginning it.
- Remember the importance of communicating as consistently with the comatose resident as you would with any other resident.
- Observe the resident thoroughly throughout the bath.

GUIDELINES (Continued)

- Allow the resident to use the toilet before bathing, as water stimulates the urge to void.
- Provide for privacy by pulling the privacy curtain, closing the door, and closing window coverings.
- Provide for warmth by checking room temperature, preventing drafts, and using a bath blanket.
- Protect the resident from falls. *Never* leave a resident unattended in the tub or shower.
- Check the water temperature before bathing.
- Use correct body mechanics, standing with your feet apart and your back straight.
- Raise the bed to a comfortable working height when giving a bed bath.
- Wear gloves for washing the genital area or if there will be contact with any body fluids. Gloves may be worn for the entire bath.
- Make a mitt out of the washcloth when bathing the resident (see Figure 13-7 ■).
- Change water as frequently as needed for temperature or when it becomes soapy.
- Wash from the cleanest to the dirtiest areas, beginning with the face and finishing with the genital area.
- Protect privacy and prevent chilling by uncovering, washing, rinsing, and drying only one part at a time.
- Rinse soap from the skin thoroughly.
- Apply deodorant.
- Check pockets of clothing for valuables before placing in the laundry hamper.
- If the resident is incontinent, the skin must be cleansed and linen must be changed before continuing with the bath.

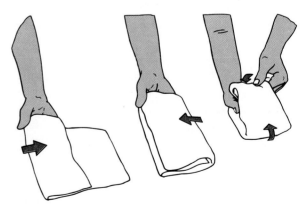

FIGURE 13-7 ■ Using the washcloth as a mitt will prevent water from dripping.

PERINEAL CARE

Perineal care (peri-care) is the cleansing of the genital and rectal areas. This procedure prevents infection and odor in areas that are susceptible to bacterial growth. You will recall that bacteria grow best in a moist, dark, warm environment. Be sure to place a clean pad under the buttocks before and after providing peri-care. Peri-care is an important part of daily care for all residents. Residents who are incontinent and those who have catheters must receive peri-care frequently. A procedure for caring for residents with catheters is located in Chapter 17. Peri-care is provided every day, usually at bath time, and as often as necessary.

The resident should be allowed to perform peri-care if able to do so. When speaking of the procedure, use words that are familiar to the resident. The resident may not understand the medical term for this procedure. The procedure for peri-care is located on this page.

Aseptic Principles

In performing peri-care, follow the principles of asepsis. The area is cleansed from the cleanest to the dirtiest. It is important to cleanse away from the urinary meatus (entrance to the urinary system). This helps to prevent urinary infections by removing germs. The rectal area contains bacteria that can cause infection in the vaginal and urinary areas. A buildup of ammonia and bacteria causes severe skin breakdown. Incontinent residents must receive peri-care immediately after urination or defecation. **Defecation** is the elimination of solid wastes from the body. Remind the resident to follow aseptic practices.

Thorough cleansing is necessary to remove urine and feces. The most common method for providing peri-care is washing with soap and water. Solutions are available for peri-care. The solution should be warmed to body temperature before

PROCEDURE

Perineal Care

■ Beginning Steps

Before any procedure, you always must follow the five basic steps: wash your hands, collect the equipment, identify the resident, explain the procedure, and protect privacy.

Follow Standard Precautions

1. Raise the head of the bed to a comfortable working height and lock the wheels.
2. Raise the side rail on the opposite side, and lower the side rail on the side nearest you.
3. Assist the resident to a supine position with legs separated and knees bent (see Figure 13-8 ■).

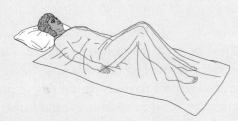

FIGURE 13-8 ■ Position the resident for peri-care.

4. Place a protective pad or towel under the buttocks.
5. Cover the resident with a bath blanket. Fold top linens to the foot of the bed. Raise the side rail when you leave the bedside.
6. Fill a wash basin with water at a comfortable temperature (approximately 105°F, or 40.5°C) and place it on paper towels on the overbed table.
7. Put on gloves.
8. Using either soap or a solution as specified in the care plan, provide peri-care for the male and female as follows:
   a. For the female (see Figure 13-9A ■): Separate the labia and wash from front to back (away from the urinary meatus) with the washcloth. Use a different area of the cloth for each stroke, beginning with the center and finishing with either side of the labia. With a clean washcloth, rinse in the same manner. Pat dry.
   b. For the male (see Figure 13-9B ■): Cleanse the head of the penis with the washcloth, using motions

(continued)

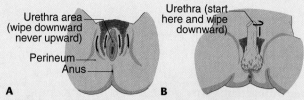

FIGURE 13-9 ■ The cleansing motion for peri-care should be away from the urinary meatus.

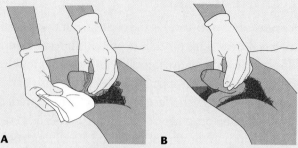

FIGURE 13-10 ■ After the foreskin is retracted for peri-care, it must be returned to its natural position.

away from the urinary meatus. Using a clean wash-cloth, rinse in the same manner. Dry thoroughly. If the male resident is uncircumcised, the foreskin must be retracted (see Figure 13-10A ■) to cleanse the head of the penis. After rinsing and patting dry, the foreskin must be returned to its natural position (see Figure 13-10B ■).

9. Turn the resident to the side facing away from you.
10. Cleanse with a wet, soapy washcloth from the vagina or scrotum to the rectal area. Use a different area of the cloth for each stroke. Rinse in the same manner. Pat dry.
11. Remove the protective pad and replace it with a clean one.
12. Raise the side rail.
13. Empty, rinse, and dry the basin.
14. Remove the gloves and wash your hands.

15. Return equipment and supplies to their proper location.
16. Lower the side rail on the side of the bed nearest you.
17. Remove the bath blanket after covering the resident with the top linen.

■ **Ending Steps**

To complete the procedure, perform the following steps:

Make the resident comfortable, positioning in good body alignment. Make the resident safe, placing the call signal within reach, lowering the bed, and raising the side rails, if appropriate. Wash your hands. Record and report the procedure as required.

spraying directly onto the genitalia. It may also be used by spraying it into a wet, warm washcloth. A kit may be used for peri-care. These kits contain antiseptic wipes or swabs and disposable gloves. Follow the policy and procedure at your facility. Although peri-care procedures vary, the principles remain the same. The procedure for perineal care starts on page 167.

𝕋HE COMPLETE BED BATH

The resident who requires a bed bath may be able to participate in bathing. If necessary, place the wet washcloth in the resident's hands and give step-by-step instructions. Encourage self-care. Give praise for the slightest effort, and prevent frustration. (See the procedure, on page 169).

𝕋HE PARTIAL BATH

Although residents may receive a shower, tub bath, or bed bath only twice a week, a partial bath is completed every day. The areas of the body that require daily hygiene include the face, hands, axilla, perineal area, all creases, and skin folds. Excessive perspiration, vomitus, and incontinence may increase the need for bathing.

Many residents may be able to take a partial bath with minimal assistance. Getting equipment and supplies together and assisting the resident to the bathroom can help promote independence. Stay nearby and be prepared to help as needed. Bathing may be done in the bed or chair or at the sink. It may be necessary for the nursing assistant to provide the partial bath for the resident. The guidelines for a complete bed bath also apply to the partial bath.

PROCEDURE

Giving a Complete Bed Bath

■ Beginning Steps

Before any procedure, you always must follow the five basic steps: wash your hands, collect the equipment, identify the resident, explain the procedure, and protect privacy.

🖑 Follow Standard Precautions

1. Raise the bed to a comfortable working height, lock the wheels, and raise the side rail on the far side of the bed.

2. Offer the bedpan to the resident. Raise the side rail nearer to you.

3. Adjust the bed in as flat a position as possible.

4. Check for drafts and proper room temperature.

5. Arrange the equipment on the overbed table. Place the bath basin on clean paper towels.

6. Be sure the resident is lying on the side of the bed near to you.

7. Remove the bedspread and blanket from the bed. Fold them over the back of the chair.

8. Place the bath blanket over the top sheet. Remove the top sheet from under the bath blanket without uncovering the resident (see Figure 13-11A ■ and 13-11B ■).

9. Remove any clothes and jewelry that the resident is wearing.

10. Fill the bath basin two-thirds full with water that is at a comfortable temperature (approximately 105°F, or 40.5°C).

11. Lower the side rail on the side of the bed near you.

12. Place the bath towel over the resident's chest.

13. Make a mitt with the washcloth (see Figure 13-7).

14. Wash the eyes from the nose (inner aspect) toward the ear, using a different corner of the wash mitt for each stroke and for each eye. Do not use soap. Wash the face, ears, and neck. Pat dry.

15. Place a towel lengthwise under the arm farther from you to protect the bed. Support the arm with your palm under the elbow while using long, firm strokes to wash the arm, axilla, and shoulder. Observe the axilla, elbow, and shoulder carefully. The hand may be soaked in the basin of water (see Figure 13-12 ■). Rinse, pat dry, and cover the arm.

16. Repeat step 15 for the arm nearer to you.

17. While the fingernails are damp, clean under them with an orange stick.

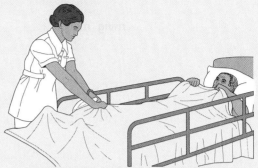

A Remove the top sheet from under the bath blanket by working from the side.

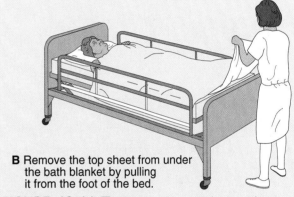

B Remove the top sheet from under the bath blanket by pulling it from the foot of the bed.

FIGURE 13-11 ■ Remove the top sheet without uncovering the resident.

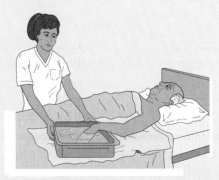

FIGURE 13-12 ■ Soaking the hands and feet may be enjoyable for the resident, and it makes the nails easier to clean and trim.

18. Place a towel across the resident's chest. Fold the bath blanket to the waist. Lifting the towel partially, wash and rinse the chest. Carefully observe the breast

(continued)

Giving a Complete Bed Bath (Continued)

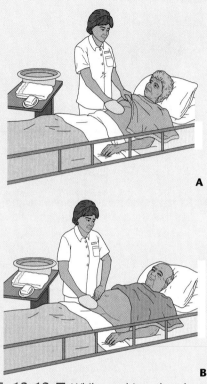

FIGURE 13-13 ■ While washing the chest and abdomen, observe skin creases.

creases for the female resident. Rinse and pat dry (see Figure 13-13A ■).

19. With the towel covering the chest, fold the bath blanket to the pubic area. Wash the abdomen and navel. Observe any abdominal folds for irritation (see Figure 13-13B ■). Rinse and pat dry. Cover the chest and abdomen with the bath blanket and remove the towel.

20. Change the water, if needed, and rinse the basin. Raise the side rail when you leave the bedside.

21. Uncover the leg farther from you and place a towel under it lengthwise. Have the resident flex the knee to support the leg. Wash the leg and foot carefully, observing for skin problems at the knee, ankle, and heel and between the toes. Wash thoroughly between the toes. The foot may be soaked in the basin of water. Pat dry, taking special care to dry thoroughly between the toes. Observe the toenails. Cover the leg and foot with the bath blanket.

22. Repeat step 21 for the leg nearer to you. Raise the side rail when you leave the bedside.

23. Change the bath water and rinse the basin.

24. Lower the side rail and assist the resident to turn onto the side facing away from you.

25. Place the towel lengthwise on the bed along the resident's back. Wash the back, the back of the neck, and the buttocks with firm, long, circular strokes. Carefully observe bony prominences of the shoulder blades, sacrum, coccyx, and hips. Pat dry and remove the towel. A backrub may be given at this time (see next procedure). Assist the resident to return to the back.

26. Perform peri-care (see the previous procedure) if the resident is unable to wash the genital area. Pat dry and observe carefully for skin problems.

27. Provide a backrub using strokes from the base of the spine and working toward the neck and shoulders. Use gentle strokes and circular motions. Remove unabsorbed lotion.

28. Assist the resident to dress and complete grooming.

29. Raise the side rail when you leave the bedside.

30. Empty, rinse, and dry the bath basin, and return equipment and supplies to their proper place. Place soiled linen in the hamper.

31. Wipe off the overbed table with a paper towel.

32. If the resident is to remain in bed, make an occupied bed. Lower the bed and make the resident comfortable. Raise the side rail if required.

33. Assist the resident out of bed, when possible, and make the bed.

34. Open the window covering if the resident desires it. Open the privacy curtain and/or door.

■ **Ending Steps**

To complete the procedure, perform the following steps:

Make the resident comfortable, positioning in good body alignment. Make the resident safe, placing the call signal within reach, lowering the bed, and raising the side rails, if appropriate. Wash your hands. Record and report the procedure as required.

GIVING A BACKRUB

The backrub is an enjoyable part of personal care. Besides producing a refreshing feeling and a sense of well-being, the backrub relaxes muscles and stimulates circulation. Backrubs are routinely given during A.M. care, during H.S. care, and every time a bedridden resident is turned and repositioned. This is a good time to observe for skin problems related to pressure and poor circulation.

The resident may be in a lateral or prone position for the backrub. Lotion should be warmed to body temperature in one of the following ways before being applied:

* Rub a small amount between your hands.
* Hold the bottle under warm running water.
* Place the bottle in warm water for a few minutes.

After warming the lotion, apply it to the resident's back. Use strokes to work from the base of the spine towards the neck and shoulders. Use gentle strokes and circular motions. Circular motions promote circulation to pressure areas over bony prominences. Massage around reddened areas. Remove unabsorbed excess lotion from the resident's back.

THE SHOWER AND TUB BATH

Showers and tub baths are additional methods of bathing. The choice is a matter of personal preference, doctor's orders, and mobility. The use of showers and tubs increases the need for safety precautions.

The Shower Chair

A shower chair (see Figure 13-15 ■) improves the safety and opportunity of showering for weak and paralyzed residents. This chair is a vinyl or metal wheeled chair with a seat similar to a toilet seat. The resident should remain seated in the shower chair throughout the shower. Because the chair is lightweight and could be upset easily, always stay with the resident who is sitting in one.

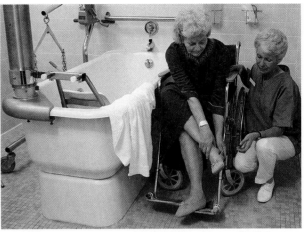

FIGURE 13-14 ■ Staff assistance prevents falls in the tub area.

GUIDELINES

ASSISTING WITH A SHOWER OR TUB BATH

* Encourage the resident to use the toilet before a shower or tub bath.
* Assist the resident into and out of the shower chair while in the shower area.
* Stay with the resident who is in the shower, tub, or shower chair (see Figure 13-14 ■).
* Use of a shower chair prevents falls. Be sure to lock the wheels.
* Prevent chilling.
* Clean the tub or shower before and after each use.
* Assist the resident to undress in the shower or tub area.
* Wear skidproof shoes in wet areas.
* Assist the resident into the tub after the water temperature is set and the tub is half full.
* Wear gloves as indicated in the procedures.
* Protect the resident's privacy. Close the door, pull the shower curtain, and keep the resident covered as much as possible.
* Take the resident to the shower or tub area fully clothed. Re-dressing should also be done in the shower or tub area.
* Assist the resident out of the tub after draining it.
* Encourage the resident to bathe as independently as possible.

PROCEDURE

Assisting the Resident to Shower

■ Beginning Steps.

Before any procedure, you always must follow five basic steps: wash your hands, collect the equipment, identify the resident, explain the procedure, and protect privacy.

🖐 Follow standard precautions.

1. Arrange supplies and equipment on a chair near the shower.
2. Assist the resident to the shower and close the door. Use a shower chair if necessary.
3. Turn the water on, and adjust the temperature and pressure.
4. Assist the resident to undress.
5. Assist the resident into the shower. If a shower chair is used, lock the wheels.
6. Provide the resident with soap and a washcloth. Encourage self-care and stand by to assist.
7. After the resident has finished bathing and rinsing, turn off the water.

8. Provide towels for drying. Assist as necessary to be sure the resident is completely dry.
9. Remove the gloves, if used. Wash your hands.
10. Assist the resident to dress and leave the shower area.
11. Apply gloves to clean the shower. Place soiled linen in the hamper.
12. Remove gloves and wash your hands.
13. Return equipment and supplies to their proper place.
14. Wash your hands.
15. Assist the resident to complete grooming.

■ Ending Steps

To complete the procedure, perform the following steps:

Make the resident comfortable, positioning in good body alignment. Make the resident safe, placing the call signal within reach, lowering the bed, and raising the side rails, if appropriate. Wash your hands. Record and report the procedure as required. ■

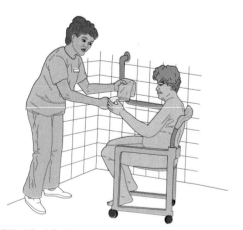

FIGURE 13-15 ■ A shower chair may be used for weak or paralyzed residents.

THE SPECIALTY BATH

There are several types of specialty tubs that are used for bathing. Many of these combine bathing with whirlpool action. Whirlpool action stimulates circulation and relaxes muscles. These tubs must be cleaned before and after use. Always check the water temperature before the resident enters the

tub. Some tubs have special transport chairs, and many use a hydraulic lift (see Figure 13-16 ■). If a seat belt is available, it always should be used.

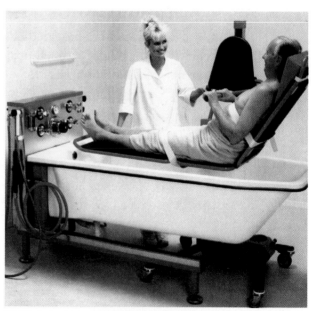

FIGURE 13-16 ■ Some specialty tubs have transport chairs and hydraulic lifts. *Ferno Inc.*

PROCEDURE

Assisting the Resident with a Tub Bath

■ Beginning Steps

Before any procedure, you always must follow the five basic steps: wash your hands, collect the equipment, identify the resident, explain the procedure, and protect privacy.

🖐 Follow Standard Precautions

1. Arrange supplies and equipment on a chair near the bathtub.
2. Assist the resident to the bathroom or tub room. Close the door.
3. Wear gloves to clean the tub according to facility policy.
4. Remove gloves and wash your hands.
5. Fill the tub half full of water at 105°F (40.5°C). Test the temperature with a bath thermometer.
6. Place a towel or bath mat on the floor beside the tub.
7. Assist the resident to undress.
8. Assist the resident into the bathtub.
9. Provide the resident with soap and a washcloth. Encourage self-care.
10. Stay with the resident and prepare to help. Wear gloves if assistance is necessary.

11. Place a towel on the chair and drain the tub. Put a towel over the resident's shoulders to prevent chilling.
12. Assist the resident out of the tub and into the chair.
13. Provide towels for drying. Assist as necessary to be sure the resident is completely dry.
14. Remove gloves and wash your hands.
15. Assist the resident to dress and leave the tub area.
16. Wear gloves to clean the tub. Place soiled linen in the hamper.
17. Remove the gloves and wash your hands.
18. Return supplies and equipment to their proper place.

■ Ending Steps

To complete the procedure, perform the following steps:

Make the resident comfortable, positioning in good body alignment. Make the resident safe, placing the call signal within reach, lowering the bed, and raising the side rails, if appropriate. Wash your hands. Record and report the procedure as required.

Because procedures may vary between types of tubs and chairs, it is your responsibility to learn the correct procedure for each tub that you use. *Never leave the resident alone in the tub.* Prevent chilling and protect privacy.

The procedure for assisting with a tub bath may be followed when using a specialty tub. The steps for assisting the resident into and out of the tub will vary according to the type of specialty tub you are using. Follow the policies and procedures of your facility.

CARE OF THE HAIR AND NAILS

Care of the hair and nails affects health, as well as appearance and self-esteem. Hair combing and brushing are done every day and more often as desired. Residents should be encouraged to comb and brush their own hair. Nursing assistants should not cut residents' hair.

Most facilities have professional beauticians with whom residents can make appointments for hair care. Appointments should not be made without the permission of the resident or legal guardian. If the resident has regularly scheduled appointments with the beautician, the hair should not be washed in the shower.

GUIDELINES

COMBING AND BRUSHING HAIR

- Place a towel over the pillow or around the shoulders.
- Remove the resident's glasses and place them in a case.
- Allow the resident to comb or brush his or her own hair.
- Part the hair in sections and comb or brush from the roots to the ends.

(continued)

GUIDELINES (Continued)

- Remove tangles by working from the ends of the hair toward the scalp.
- Arrange hair according to the resident's preference.
- Wash your hands.

Shampooing the Hair

Shampooing usually is done one to three times a week. Shampooing may be done in the bed or shower if it is not to be done by a beautician. Special equipment such as a shampoo tray and bucket make bed shampooing more manageable (see Figure 13-17 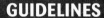). Shampoos should be done as indicated on the assignment. The hair should be dried as quickly as possible after a shampoo. Allow the resident to choose a hairstyle.

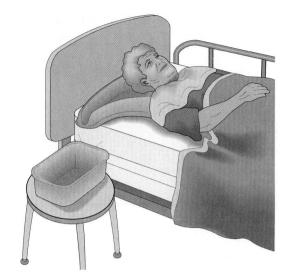

FIGURE 13-17 ■ A shampoo tray may be used to shampoo the resident's hair while she is in bed.

GUIDELINES

ASSISTING WITH A SHAMPOO

- Use a hand-held shower nozzle if available.
- Encourage the resident to perform self-care.
- Prevent shampoo from getting in the resident's eyes.
- Massage the scalp while washing the hair.
- Clean the hair thoroughly.
- Rinse shampoo out completely.
- Dry as quickly as possible.
- Style the hair according to the resident's preference.
- Wash your hands.

Nail Care

Proper care and observation of fingernails and toenails is very important. Infection or injury can cause serious problems. Fingernails must be kept clean and at a reasonable length. Nails are cleaned and trimmed easily while damp. Soak them in a basin of warm water before removing the residue under nails. Scissors are not used to cut fingernails. Usually, nursing assistants may not trim the resident's toenails and should never trim fingernails or toenails for diabetic residents. Observing the condition of nails and reporting to the nurse when care is needed is very important.

GUIDELINES

NAIL CARE

- Soak the hands or feet in warm water at 105°F (40.5°C).
- Place a paper towel under each hand.
- Use an orange stick to clean under the nails. Wipe the orange stick on the paper towel after cleaning each nail.
- Dry the hands or feet thoroughly before trimming the nails.
- Use clippers to trim the nails.
- File rough nail edges with an emery board.
- Apply lotion to the hands or feet and massage well.
- Record the procedure and report observations.

An attractive hairstyle, makeup, and manicured, polished nails can change a resident's poor self-image into a more positive one. Remember that appearance is important to both men and women.

SHAVING THE RESIDENT

Many men shave daily. This usually is done in the morning or at bath time. Residents should be encouraged to shave themselves if possible.

GUIDELINES

SHAVING THE RESIDENT

- Wear gloves and follow standard precautions.
- Place a towel across the resident's chest.
- Soften the beard with warm water and apply shaving cream before shaving.
- Dentures in the mouth make shaving easier.
- Hold the skin taut with the fingers of one hand while shaving away from your fingers in the direction the hair grows (see Figure 13-18 ■).
- Rinse the razor after each stroke.
- Dispose of razors in a puncture-proof container for sharps.

Shaving affects the self-image of many male residents in the same way that makeup improves many females' self-image. The male resident has a right to make decisions concerning shaving and to choose the shape and length of a beard, mustache, and/or sideburns. Some female residents may wish to shave their legs and underarms. Female residents also may choose to remove facial hair. Personal electric razors, brought from home, or safety razors may be used for shaving. Safety rules for electrical equipment should be followed.

Before shaving with a safety razor, the beard must be softened by applying a warm, damp washcloth for a few minutes. Soap and water or shaving cream are then applied.

DRESSING THE RESIDENT

Assisting the Resident to Dress

In the long-term care facility, many residents are able to get out of bed, so they usually dress in street clothes. Clothing is part of an individual's identity. The choice of clothing a person wears reflects and affects mood and self-esteem (see Figure 13-19 ■). Can you recall days when you chose particular colors or types of clothing because of the way you felt? A person's choice of dress is very personal and continues to be important throughout life.

Allowing and encouraging the resident to choose the clothing to be worn stimulates thinking and supports independence. Making choices returns control to the resident.

Some may choose what they would like to wear by considering the entire wardrobe. By contrast, choosing from more than one or two pieces of clothing may be overwhelming to other residents.

GUIDELINES

ASSISTING THE RESIDENT TO DRESS

- Encourage residents to choose what they would like to wear.
- Offer the resident a choice of color-coordinated, well-fitting, clean and wrinkle-free clothing that is appropriate for the weather and activities of the day.

(continued)

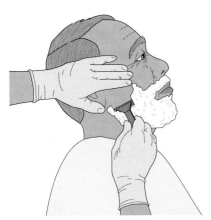

FIGURE 13-18 ■ Hold the skin taut and shave in the direction that the hair grows.

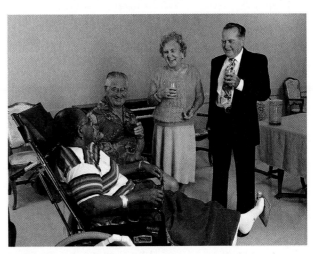

FIGURE 13-19 ■ Clothing is a personal choice that reflects a person's mood and personality.

GUIDELINES (Continued)

- Offer sweaters or jackets even when you feel warm. The elderly are more sensitive to temperature changes.

- Be sure the resident wears undergarments.

- Organize the clothing within reach in the order in which the resident will put it on (see Figure 13-20 ■).

- Check the care plan for assistive equipment and provide it.

- Allow the resident to sit to dress.

- Do not rush the resident. Be patient and assist as needed. This might be a good time to tidy the room or make the bed for the other resident in the same room.

- If you are assisting a resident who has a paralyzed arm, cast, or IV, *always dress the affected arm first and undress the affected arm last.*

- Gather up the sleeve to ease pulling it over the affected arm.

- Compliment the resident's appearance when dressing and grooming are complete.

- If you are assisting the weak resident to put on shoes, have her lie in bed to do so. Place the shoes on paper towels to protect the linen.

- Change clothing throughout the day if it becomes soiled.

GUIDELINES

FOR CHANGING THE RESIDENT'S CLOTHES

- Allow choices whenever possible.

- Provide privacy.

- Place clothing on the affected limbs first and remove it from the affected limbs last.

- Residents should wear undergarments.

- Support weak or paralyzed limbs.

- Gather up the sleeve to ease pulling it over the affected arm or leg.

- Assist the resident to turn from side to side as needed.

- Put socks and shoes on while the resident is in bed. (Protect linen from shoes with a paper towel under them.)

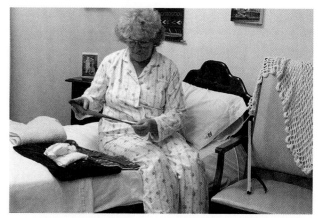

FIGURE 13-20 ■ The resident may dress herself if clothing is organized within her reach.

Praise the resident's small accomplishments as well as the major ones and emphasize how nice the resident looks.

Dressing the Resident

Some residents may be unable to dress and undress themselves. If the resident is dependent upon you, it is easier and safer to change the clothing while the resident is lying in bed (see Figure 13-21 ■).

Dressing the Resident with an IV

Some residents may be receiving fluids by the intravenous route. An **intravenous (IV)** is a needle into the vein. The presence of an IV requires special assistance in dressing and undressing. Common

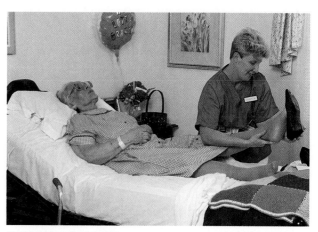

FIGURE 13-21 ■ It is easier to put the resident's shoes on while she is in bed.

locations for an IV are the arm, wrist, or hand. Care must be taken to prevent tension and pressure on the tubing or needle. Allow for slack in the tubing when moving the resident. Clothing should be loose and short-sleeved so that the IV site is visible for frequent observation. Most IVs are attached to a pump. Nursing assistants are not allowed to disconnect them. The nurse will assist you in changing the clothing unless clothes with snaps on the shoulder are used. If a pump is not in use for the IV, you may use the following guidelines to change the resident's clothes.

and personal items so that they will be within easy reach of the resident.

The nurses and occupational therapist will establish a plan of care to assist the resident with ADLs and personal care. You will need to be familiar with the plan for your resident and follow it consistently. The plan of care may include the use of assistive equipment. Some assistive devices that are designed for use in personal care can be seen in Figure 13-22. ∎

Your patience and understanding can affect the resident's success or failure. Relearning to groom, bathe, or dress oneself can be time-consuming and frustrating. Your praise and encouragement will relieve the resident's anxiety and frustration.

GUIDELINES

CHANGING THE CLOTHES OF A RESIDENT WITH AN IV

To remove clothing:

- Remove clothing first from the arm without the IV.
- Carefully slide the sleeve down the arm, over the site of the IV, and then off the arm.
- Remove the IV bag or bottle from the pole and slide it through the sleeve.
- Do not lower the bag below the IV site.
- Return the bag to the pole.

To place the clean clothing on the resident:

- Gather the sleeve to be placed on the arm with the IV.
- Remove the bag from the pole and slip it through the sleeve as if the bottle was the resident's hand.
- Slide the sleeve over the tubing, hand, arm, and IV site and onto the shoulder.
- Ask the nurse to check the IV as soon as you have finished dressing the resident.

RESTORATIVE PERSONAL CARE AND DRESSING

A restorative approach must be taken in all personal care, bathing, grooming, and dressing. Always encourage the resident to do as much as possible. Be sure that you have arranged equipment, supplies,

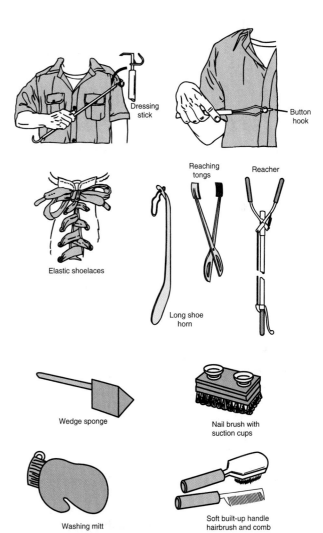

FIGURE 13-22 ∎ A variety of assistive devices are available for personal care and dressing.

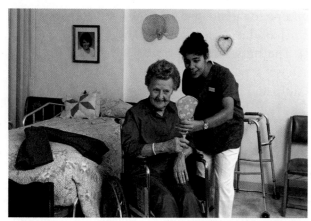

FIGURE 13-23 ■ Praise and encouragement help the resident to overcome the anxiety and frustration of relearning to bathe, groom, and dress.

Being able to bathe, groom, and dress oneself is vital to self-esteem. Each small effort that is successful increases the resident's confidence, self-image, and sense of control over his or her own body and life (see Figure 13-23 ■). Independence in personal care allows residents to protect the most personal and private part of themselves; their own bodies.

CHAPTER HIGHLIGHTS

1. Attending to personal care helps to improve self-esteem and maintain health.
2. Residents have the right to make choices about personal care.
3. H.S. care helps the resident to relax and sleep well.
4. Feeding tubes, oxygen, illness, and some medications increase the need for more frequent mouth care.
5. Steps must be taken to protect dentures from breaking.
6. Bath time is an excellent time for thorough observation of the skin; movement; and mental, emotional, and speech changes.
7. Bathing is a very nurturing process that results in an improved sense of well-being.
8. Always wash from the cleanest to the dirtiest area.
9. Perineal care should be provided immediately after urinary or fecal incontinence.
10. During the bath, carefully observe all skin creases, folds, and pressure areas.
11. Protect the resident's privacy during bathing by uncovering only the part of the body that is being bathed.
12. Backrubs stimulate circulation and relax muscles.
13. Never leave a resident unattended in the tub or shower.
14. The water temperature should be set before the resident enters the tub or shower.
15. Remove clothing from the unaffected limb first. Place it on the affected limb first.
16. Clothing is part of an individual's identity and reflects personality and self-esteem.
17. Regaining independence in personal care improves the resident's confidence, self-image, and sense of control over his or her life.

VOCABULARY REVIEW

Fill in the blanks with the vocabulary term that best completes the sentence.

1. The procedure for cleansing of the genital area and rectum is called _____ or _____.

2. To _____ is to spit.

3. A needle into the vein is a/an _____.

4. Mouth care is_____.

5. _____ is the medical term for the underarms.

6. The act of having a bowel movement is _____.

7. The inability to control urine or feces is _____.

8. A person who is unconscious or unresponsive is _____.

9. _____ are a product for oral hygiene.

10. A small, curved basin is a/an _____ _____.

CHECK YOUR UNDERSTANDING

The following questions cover the highlights of this chapter. Choose the best answer for each question.

1. Encouraging residents to make choices in personal care and dressing is helpful in which of the following ways?
   A. The resident will look better.
   B. The resident will like you.
   C. Care will be completed more quickly.
   D. A sense of control is developed in the resident.

2. What is the purpose of peri-care?
   A. To awaken the resident for breakfast
   B. To prevent skin breakdown, odor, and infection.
   C. To prevent pressure sores on the back
   D. To cleanse the resident's eyes.

3. The resident has a paralyzed right arm. What is the correct way to remove his shirt?
   A. Remove it from the left arm first.
   B. Remove it from the right arm first.
   C. Remove it over his head.
   D. Tell the resident to do it himself

4. How should you position a comatose resident for oral care?
   A. On his back with the head of the bed elevated
   B. On his back with the head of the bed flat
   C. On his side with the foot of his bed elevated
   D. On his side with a towel under his chin

5. Which of the following is the correct way to perform denture care?
   A. Clean the dentures over a sink of water.
   B. Clean the dentures in a basin at the resident's bedside.
   C. Store the dentures in hot, soapy water.
   D. Carry the dentures in your gloved hand to the bathroom.

6. When beginning a bed bath, which of the following is correct procedure?
   A. Wash the eyes first.
   B. Wash the arms first.
   C. Wash the back first.
   D. Wash the perineal area first.

7. What is the correct way to perform female peri-care?
   A. Cleanse from back to front.
   B. Cleanse from side to side.
   C. Cleanse from front to back.
   D. Cleanse away from the rectum.

8. How can you protect the resident's privacy during a bed bath?
   A. Expose one part of the body at a time.
   B. Remove the bath blanket to begin.
   C. Open the blinds to let the sunshine in.
   D. Expose one side of the body at a time.

AGE-SPECIFIC TIP

Elderly residents may be slow to respond early in the morning. Awakening the resident for hygiene and conversation before breakfast may improve morning food intake.

CULTURALLY SENSITIVE TIP

Personal care choices are affected by culture. Encourage and assist the resident in continuing his or her usual routines.

EFFECTIVE PROBLEM SOLVING

The nursing assistant is bathing Mrs. Giddens, a resident who is comatose. While giving care, the nursing assistant is silent in order to allow the resident to rest as much as possible. Was the nursing assistant's decision appropriate? If not, what would have been more appropriate?

_____
_____
_____
_____
_____
_____
_____
_____
_____
_____

INTERPERSONAL COMMUNICATION

Complete the sentence.

The resident asks you to trim her toenails. You observe that the toenails are long and yellow-colored. You should tell the resident that you will

_____
_____
_____

OBSERVING, REPORTING, AND RECORDING

List five observations during a bath that should be reported and recorded.

_____
_____
_____
_____
_____
_____
_____
_____
_____
_____
_____

EXPLORE MEDIALINK

Check out www.prenhall.com/grubbs for additional chapter-specific interactive study and review activities.

14

MEASURING VITAL SIGNS

OBJECTIVES

1. List seven factors that affect vital signs.
2. Identify the normal range of body temperature.
3. List five guidelines for reading a glass thermometer.
4. Record vital signs accurately.
5. Identify three observations to be made when counting a radial pulse.
6. List seven guidelines for counting respirations.
7. Explain the meaning of systolic and diastolic pressure.
8. List eight guidelines for measuring blood pressure.
9. Perform the procedures described in this chapter.

VOCABULARY

The following words or terms will help you to understand this chapter:

Vital signs
Body temperature
Tympanic membrane
Pulse
Radial pulse

Apical pulse
Stethoscope
Respiration
Dyspnea
Blood pressure (BP)

Hypertension
Hypotension
Systolic pressure
Diastolic pressure
Sphygmomanometer

The temperature, pulse, respirations, and blood pressure are **vital signs**. They are abbreviated TPR and BP. These are measurements of body functions (heart function, breathing, and temperature regulation) that are vital to life. Changes in any of these may indicate illness or a life-threatening condition. Since the early days of medicine, physicians have measured vital signs to evaluate a person's condition.

Vital signs are taken when a resident is admitted to a health care facility. They are measured at regular intervals (as ordered by the doctor or as required by facility policy) and anytime there is an unusual occurrence or a suspected change in the resident's condition. For example, vital signs should be taken if a resident falls or complains of chest pain. The progress of treatment may be determined by these measurements.

A person's vital signs normally may vary slightly. Factors that may affect vital signs include

- Illness
- Emotions
- Exercise and activity
- Age
- Weather
- Caffeine
- Medications

Accuracy in the measurement of vital signs is extremely important to the well-being of the resident. If you are unsure of the measurement or the measurement varies from the normal range, report it immediately to the nurse. All vital signs are recorded according to facility policy. Respond to residents' and visitors' questions about vital signs measurements according to the policy of your facility.

MEASURING BODY TEMPERATURE

A thermometer is used to measure **body temperature** (the amount of heat in the body). Body heat is produced when food is used for energy. Heat is lost from the body through breath, urine, feces, and perspiration. The same factors that affect body temperature affect all other vital signs. Body temperature normally remains fairly constant, although it is usually slightly lower in the morning and slightly higher in the evening.

The normal body temperature is determined by the site of measurement. Temperatures commonly are measured in the rectum, mouth, axilla (underarm), and ear. The mouth is used most often for measurements. The axilla is used least often because it is considered to be the least accurate.

Fahrenheit and centigrade are two types of temperature measurement systems. Celsius is the same as centigrade. Normal adult temperatures are shown in the Temperature Measurement Table (Table 14-1). Temperatures outside the normal ranges should be reported to the nurse immediately.

TABLE 14-1 TEMPERATURE MEASUREMENT TABLE			
	Axillary	Oral	Rectal
Normal temperature	97.6°F (36.5°C)	98.6°F (37°C)	99.6°F (37.5°C)
Temperature range	96.6–98.6°F (36°–37°C)	97.6°–99.6°F (36.5°–37.5°C)	98.6°–100.6°F (37°–38.1°C)
Measurement time (glass thermometer)	10 minutes	3 to 5 minutes	3 to 5 minutes
Color code (may have the words "oral" or "rectal" printed on the side)	Blue (oral)	Blue	Red
Site	Underarm	Mouth	Rectum
Recording examples	97.6°A	98.6° (no letter after oral temperature)	99.6°R

Note: An electronic thermometer measures the temperature in 2–60 seconds.

Recording Temperatures

It is important that you record temperatures accurately. Temperatures usually are recorded in decimals; for example, an oral temperature might be recorded as 98.2°, 99.4°, or 100.6°. It usually is not necessary to designate Fahrenheit or centigrade. Most facilities use only one scale. Temperatures that are measured with an electronic thermometer should be recorded exactly as read on the digital display of the thermometer. Because normal temperature ranges vary between sites, it is necessary to indicate the site when recording axillary, rectal, and tympanic temperatures. If the site is not indicated, the temperature is presumed to be oral (see Table 14-1).

TYPES OF THERMOMETERS

There are many types of thermometers available (see Figure 14-1 ■), including glass and electronic thermometers, disposable oral thermometers, and temperature-sensitive tape. Electronic thermometers include oral, rectal, and tympanic thermometers.

Oral and rectal thermometers (both glass and electronic) can be identified by color coding. Oral thermometers have a visible blue-colored area and rectal thermometers have a red area. It may be helpful to remember the letter **R**. Some glass thermometers have the words "rectal" and "oral" printed on them for identification. Oral and rectal thermometers should never be switched. Oral thermometers may be used to measure temperatures in the axilla.

Electronic Thermometers

Electronic battery-operated thermometers are more commonly used today. They are rapid and easy to use (they have a digital readout), and they don't contain mercury that would pose an environmental hazard.

Use of an Electronic Thermometer

Temperature measurement with electronic thermometers is much faster than with glass thermometers. A signal indicates when the temperature measurement is completed. The measurement usually takes less than a minute.

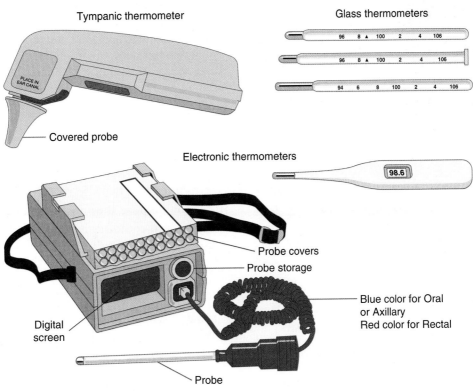

FIGURE 14-1 ■ Types of thermometers

GUIDELINES

CARE AND USE OF ELECTRONIC THERMOMETERS

- Attach the correct probe for the temperature measurement site to be used. Different colored probes are available for taking oral and rectal temperatures.
- Make sure that there is a supply of probe covers with the thermometer.
- Leave the thermometer in place until it signals.
- Discard the probe cover after every use.
- Replace the probe in the holder after discarding the cover.
- Return the thermometer to the charging unit when the procedure is complete.
- Be careful not to drop or jar the thermometer.

Glass Thermometers

The glass thermometer is a small glass tube that is marked with measurements and contains mercury in a bulb at one end. Heat expands the mercury, causing it to rise in the tube.

Reading a Glass Thermometer

Glass thermometers are calibrated (marked) with either a Fahrenheit or a Celsius scale for measurement (see Figure 14-2 ■).

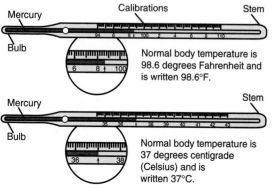

FIGURE 14-2 ■ Thermometers may be calibrated with a Fahrenheit or centigrade scale.

The Fahrenheit scale on the thermometer has long lines that represent 1 degree each. There are four short lines that divide the distance between the two long lines into four sections. These short lines divide each degree (the distance between two long lines) into sections of two-tenths each. These are read as two-tenths (.2), four-tenths (.4), six-tenths (.6), and eight-tenths (.8). Therefore, if the mercury stopped at two lines past (to the right of) the 98° line, the reading would be 98.4°F (see Figure 14-3 ■).

GUIDELINES

READING A GLASS THERMOMETER

- Hold the thermometer by the stem (the end opposite the mercury bulb) in a horizontal position at eye level.
- Light should shine on the thermometer from behind you.
- Holding the thermometer with your thumb and index finger, rotate it slowly until you can see both the numbers and lines.
- Read the temperature to the nearest degree (long line) and then to the nearest tenth of a degree (short line).
- Record the temperature and report any abnormality immediately.

Care and Use of Glass Thermometers

Because the mercury is an environmental hazard care must be taken to prevent breakage of glass thermometers. They also require cleansing and disinfecting because they are used for more than one resident and could easily transmit infection.

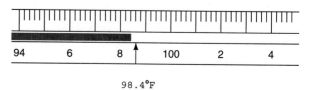

98.4°F

FIGURE 14-3 ■ If the mercury stops at two lines past the 98° line the reading would be 98.4°F.

GUIDELINES

CARE AND USE OF A GLASS THERMOMETER

- Check the glass thermometer for chips or breaks before using it.
- Firmly hold the glass thermometer stem with your index finger and thumb. Shake the mercury down to below 96° by snapping your wrist (see Figure 14-4 ■). Be sure that you do not hit furniture or fixtures that might break the thermometer.
- Before reading the temperature, remove the cover or sleeve by wiping the thermometer from stem to bulb with a tissue and discard it. Saliva and lubricant must also be wiped off with a tissue before reading the thermometer (see Fig. 14-5 ■).
- Glass thermometers usually are washed in cool soapy water before soaking them in a disinfectant solution.
- Rinse the thermometer with cool water to remove disinfectant.
- Store and disinfect oral and rectal glass thermometers in separate containers.
- Follow the facility procedures for cleaning and storing thermometers.

Taking an Oral Temperature

There are some residents for whom you may not take an oral temperature. These include residents who

- Have tubes in the nose or mouth
- Are receiving oxygen

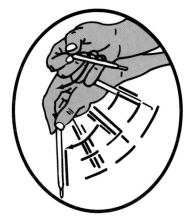

FIGURE 14-4 ■ Use a snapping action of the wrist to shake down a glass thermometer.

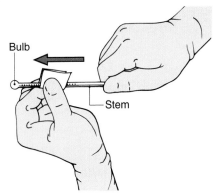

Bulb

Stem

FIGURE 14-5 ■ Clean the glass thermometer from the stem to the bulb.

- Are unconscious
- Breath through the mouth
- Have seizures
- Are confused or disoriented
- Have had recent surgery of the mouth, nose, or face

The thermometer must be placed on the unaffected side of the mouth for residents who are paralyzed on one side (hemiplegics).

The normal oral temperature is 98.6°F or 37°C. Drinking, eating, smoking, or chewing gum can change the oral temperature. It is necessary to wait 15 minutes to take the temperature after the resident has participated in any of these activities. The resident should be sitting or lying down when the temperature is being taken. Stay with the resident until the procedure is completed.

Taking a Rectal Temperature

A rectal temperature is taken when the nurse instructs you to do so. The normal rectal temperature is 99.6°F or 37.5°C. This is the most accurate method of temperature measurement. A rectal temperature cannot be taken if there has been rectal injury or surgery. Wear gloves when taking a rectal temperature.

Lubricant must be applied to the thermometer cover or probe tip before inserting it into the rectum. Lubrication promotes comfort and prevents injury. Membranes of the rectum and anus are fragile and easily injured. The tip is lubricated by dipping it into a small amount of water-soluble lubricant that has been placed on a tissue.

PROCEDURE

Taking an Oral Temperature Using a Glass Thermometer

■ **Beginning Steps**

Before any procedure, you always must follow the five basic steps: wash your hands, collect the equipment, identify the resident, explain the procedure, and protect privacy.

Follow Standard Precautions

1. After rinsing and drying the glass thermometer, check it for cracks, shake it down, and (if applicable) place a cover on it.
2. Place the bulb under the resident's tongue on one side of the mouth.
3. Ask the resident to lower the tongue and close the lips around the thermometer.
4. Leave the glass thermometer in place for 3 to 5 minutes before removing it.
5. Remove the cover from the thermometer, or wipe it from stem to bulb with a tissue, and read the thermometer.
6. Note any abnormal temperature to report immediately to the nurse.
7. Shake down and prepare the thermometer for disinfection and storage according to facility policy.

■ **Ending Steps**

To complete the procedure, perform the following steps:

Make the resident comfortable, positioning in good body alignment. Make the resident safe, placing the call signal within reach, lowering the bed, and raising the side rails, if appropriate. Wash your hands. Record and report the procedure as required.

PROCEDURE

Taking an Oral Temperature Using an Electronic Thermometer

■ **Beginning Steps**

Before any procedure, you always must follow the five basic steps: wash your hands, collect the equipment, identify the resident, explain the procedure, and protect privacy.

Follow Standard Precautions

1. Make sure the oral probe is attached to the electronic thermometer.
2. Insert the electronic probe firmly into the probe cover (see Figure 14-6A ■).
3. Place the probe under the resident's tongue on one side of the mouth.
4. Ask the resident to lower the tongue and close the lips around the thermometer.
5. Leave the probe in place until the thermometer signals.
6. Remove the probe and read the temperature on the digital display.
7. Discard the cover (see Figure 14-6B ■) and return the probe to its holder (see Figure 14-6C ■).
8. Note any abnormal temperature to report immediately to the nurse.
9. Return the electronic thermometer to the charging or storage unit.

(continued)

Taking an Oral Temperature Using an Electronic Thermometer (Continued)

■ Ending Steps

To complete the procedure, perform the following steps:

Make the resident comfortable, positioning in good body alignment. Make the resident safe, placing the call signal *within reach, lowering the bed, and raising the side rails, if appropriate. Wash your hands. Record and report the procedure as required.*

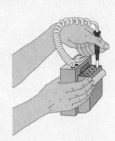
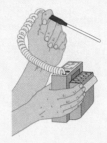
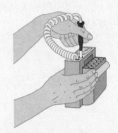

A Insert the probe into a probe cover.　　**B** After measuring the temperature, press to eject the probe cover.　　**C** Replace the probe in the holder.

FIGURE 14-6 ■ Using the electronic thermometer

*P*ROCEDURE

Taking a Rectal Temperature Using a Glass Thermometer

■ Beginning Steps

Before any procedure, you always must follow the five basic steps: wash your hands, collect the equipment, identify the resident, explain the procedure, and protect privacy.

🖐 Follow Standard Precautions

1. After rinsing and drying the glass rectal thermometer, check it for damage, shake it down, and (if applicable) place a cover on it.
2. Flatten the bed and assist the resident into a side-lying position.
3. Put on disposable gloves.
4. Lubricate the tip of the thermometer (or its cover) with a small amount of lubricant.
5. Fold the linen back to expose the rectal area.
6. Raise the upper buttock with one hand so that you can see the anus.

7. Gently insert the tip of the glass thermometer 1 inch into the rectum (see Figure 14-7 ■).

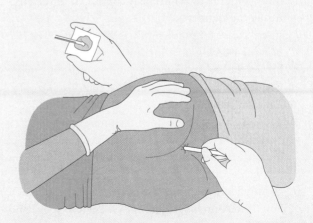

FIGURE 14-7 ■ After lubricating the tip (or cover) of the rectal thermometer, insert the tip into the rectum.

(continued)

8. Hold the glass thermometer in place for 3 to 5 minutes before removing it.

9. Remove the cover from the thermometer or wipe it from stem to bulb with a tissue and read the temperature.

10. Wipe the anal area with toilet tissue to remove excess lubricant or feces.

11. Discard the tissue in the toilet.

12. Remove the gloves and wash your hands.

13. Record a rectal temperature by recording an "R."

14. Note any abnormal temperature and report it immediately to the nurse.

15. Prepare the glass thermometer for disinfection and storage according to facility policy.

■ Ending Steps

To complete the procedure, perform the following steps:

Make the resident comfortable, positioning in good body alignment. Make the resident safe, placing the call signal within reach, lowering the bed, and raising the side rails, if appropriate. Wash your hands. Record and report the procedure as required.

ℙROCEDURE

Taking a Rectal Temperature Using an Electronic Thermometer

■ Beginning Steps

Before any procedure, you always must follow the five basic steps: wash your hands, collect the equipment, identify the resident, explain the procedure, and protect privacy.

🖐 Follow Standard Precautions

1. Make sure the rectal probe is connected to the electronic thermometer.

2. Insert the rectal probe firmly into a probe cover (see Figure 14-6A).

3. Flatten the bed and assist the resident into a side-lying position.

4. Put on disposable gloves.

5. Apply lubricant to the tip of the probe cover.

6. Fold the top linen back to expose the rectal area.

7. Raise the upper buttock with one hand so that you can see the anus.

8. Gently insert the tip of the electronic probe 0.5 inch into the rectum (see Figure 14-7). Remove your hand from the upper buttock.

9. Hold the probe in place until the thermometer signals.

10. Remove the probe from the resident's rectum and read the temperature on the digital display of the thermometer.

11. Dispose of the probe cover (see Figure 14-6B) and return the probe to its holder (see Figure 14-6C).

12. Wipe the anal area with toilet tissue to remove excess lubricant and feces.

13. Discard the tissue in the toilet.

14. Remove the gloves and wash your hands.

15. Record a rectal temperature by recording an "R."

16. Note any abnormal temperature and report it immediately to the nurse.

17. Return the electronic thermometer to the charging or storage unit.

■ Ending Steps

To complete the procedure, perform the following steps:

Make the resident comfortable, positioning in good body alignment. Make the resident safe, placing the call signal within reach, lowering the bed, and raising the side rails, if appropriate. Wash your hands. Record and report the procedure as required.

The resident must be lying down while a rectal temperature is being measured. It is very important to hold the thermometer in place until measurement is complete. This prevents the thermometer from being drawn into the rectum; it also ensures that the resident will not turn onto the thermometer. Glass thermometers are fragile, and injury could result from a broken thermometer.

Taking an Axillary Temperature

An axillary temperature is taken only when no other temperature measurement can be used. Axillary temperatures are the least accurate. The normal axillary temperature is 97.6°F or 36.5°C. The glass thermometer must be held in place for 10 minutes. The resident must be sitting or lying down during the measurement of an axillary temperature. An oral glass thermometer or oral probe for the electronic thermometer is used to measure the axillary temperature. Stay with the resident during the procedure and hold the thermometer if necessary.

Taking a Tympanic Temperature

The ear thermometer measures the temperature of blood vessels in the **tympanic membrane** (ear drum). A disposable probe is inserted gently into the ear canal, and within a few seconds the temperature is displayed in the window of the thermometer.

𝒫ROCEDURE

Taking an Axillary Temperature Using a Glass Thermometer

■ Beginning Steps.

Before any procedure, you always must follow the five basic steps: wash your hands, collect the equipment, identify the resident, explain the procedure, and protect privacy.

🖑 Follow standard precautions.

1. After rinsing and drying the oral glass thermometer, check it for cracks, shake it down, and (if applicable) place a cover on it.
2. Expose the axilla.
3. Place the bulb of the thermometer into the center of the axilla. Place the resident's arm over the chest (see Figure 14-8 ■).
4. Hold the thermometer in place for 10 minutes before removing it from the axilla.
5. Remove the cover from the thermometer, or wipe it from stem to bulb with a tissue, and read the thermometer.
6. Record an axillary temperature by recording an "A."
7. Note any abnormal temperature and report it immediately to the nurse.
8. Shake down and prepare the thermometer for disinfection and storage according to facility policy.

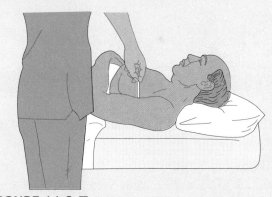

FIGURE 14-8 ■ Taking an axillary temperature

■ Ending Steps

To complete the procedure, perform the following steps:

Make the resident comfortable, positioning in good body alignment. Make the resident safe, placing the call signal within reach, lowering the bed, and raising the side rails, if appropriate. Wash your hands. Record and report the procedure as required.

PROCEDURE

Taking an Axillary Temperature Using an Electronic Thermometer

■ **Beginning Steps.**

Before any procedure, you always must follow the five basic steps: wash your hands, collect the equipment, identify the resident, explain the procedure, and protect privacy.

Follow standard precautions.

1. Attach the oral probe to the electronic thermometer.
2. Insert the electronic probe firmly into the probe cover (see Figure 14-6A).
3. Expose the axilla.
4. Place the bulb of the thermometer into the center of the axilla. Place the resident's arm over the chest.
5. Hold the resident's arm in place over the probe until the thermometer signals.
6. Remove the probe from the resident's axilla and straighten the clothing.

7. Read the temperature on the digital display.
8. Dispose of the probe cover (see Figure 14-6B) and return the probe to its holder (see Figure 14-6C).
9. Record an axillary temperature by recording an "A."
10. Note any abnormal temperature and report it immediately to the nurse.
11. Return the electronic thermometer to the changing or storage unit.

■ **Ending Steps**

To complete the procedure, perform the following steps:

Make the resident comfortable, positioning in good body alignment. Make the resident safe, placing the call signal within reach, lowering the bed, and raising the side rails, if appropriate. Wash your hands. Record and report the procedure as required. ■

PROCEDURE

Taking a Tympanic Temperature

■ **Beginning Steps.**

Before any procedure, you always must follow the five basic steps: wash your hands, collect the equipment, identify the resident, explain the procedure, and protect privacy.

Follow standard precautions.

1. Make sure the probe is connected to the unit.
2. Insert the cone-shaped end of the thermometer into a probe cover.
3. Position the resident's head so that it is directly in front of you.
4. Pull the outer ear up and back gently to open the ear canal.

5. Gently insert the probe into the ear canal (see Figure 14-9 ■). If necessary, use a slight rocking motion to insert the probe as far as possible and seal the ear canal.
6. Watch and listen for a signal such as a flashing light or beep that indicates that the measurement is complete.
7. Remove the probe from the resident's ear and read the digital display.
8. Eject the probe cover into the wastebasket.
9. Make a note of the resident's name and temperature.
10. Note any abnormal temperature to report immediately to the nurse.
11. Return the tympanic thermometer to the battery charger or base unit.

(continued)

Taking a Tympanic Temperature *(Continued)*

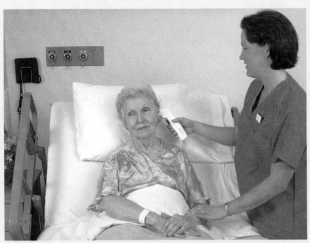

FIGURE 14-9 ■ Taking a tympanic temperature.

■ **Ending Steps**

To complete the procedure, perform the following steps:

Make the resident comfortable, positioning in good body alignment. Make the resident safe, placing the call signal within reach, lowering the bed, and raising the side rails, if appropriate. Wash your hands. Record and report the procedure as required.

Some tympanic thermometers have a built-in converter that provides equivalent oral or rectal values in either Fahrenheit or centigrade. When recording the tympanic temperature, be sure to indicate whether it is based on oral or rectal values because each would present a different normal temperature. Like other electronic thermometers, the unit works quickly and accurately.

THE PULSE

The most basic indicator of heart function is the pulse. The **pulse** is the heartbeat. Each pulse beat is a wave of blood passing through the artery. Each time the heart contracts, a wave of blood is forced into circulation. The pulse can be counted at several points on the body by pressing an artery against a bone near the surface of the skin.

The adult normal pulse range is between 60 and 100 beats per minute. Any pulse above or below the range should be reported to the nurse immediately.

When counting the pulse, you should observe and report the following:

Rate—The number of beats per minute.
Rhythm—The pattern of heartbeats, which may be regular (evenly spaced) or irregular (unevenly spaced). An irregular pulse must be counted for 1 full minute and reported to the nurse.

Force—The strength of the pulse may vary from weak to very strong or bounding.

A normal pulse is regular. Any abnormal or unusual pulse should be noted and reported immediately.

Counting the Radial Pulse

The **radial pulse** is the pulse that you usually will count. This pulse is located on the inner aspect of the wrist, at the base of the thumb (see Figure 14-10 ■). With the resident sitting or lying down, place your first three fingers against the radial artery and locate the pulse. Do not use your thumb to count the pulse or you will count your own pulse as well.

Counting the Apical Pulse

The doctor may order that pulses be taken at sites other than the radial pulse. In most long-term care

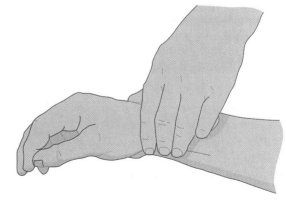

FIGURE 14-10 ■ Taking the radial pulse

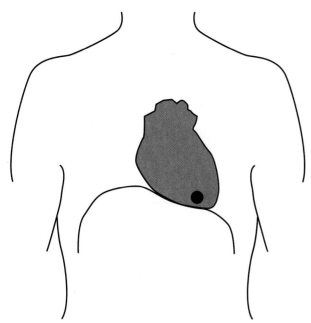

FIGURE 14-11 ■ The apical pulse site

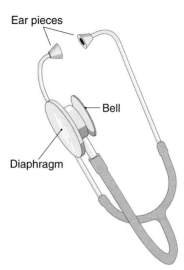

FIGURE 14-12 ■ A stethoscope

facilities, these procedures are done by a licensed nurse. The **apical pulse** is taken by listening to the heartbeat over the apex (bottom point) of the heart. This position is located 2 to 3 inches to the left of the sternum (breastbone) and slightly below the nipple.

To hear the apical pulse, **stethoscope** (an instrument used for listening to body sounds) must be used. The diaphragm (flat part) is placed against the chest over the apex of the heart (see Figures 14-11 ■ and 14-12 ■). The heartbeat will be heard as two sounds ("lub-dub"). Only one of these sounds (the "lub") is counted for each pulse beat. The apical pulse is counted for a full minute. It is recorded with an "AP" after the measurement (76 AP). "AP" indicates that the recorded pulse was an apical pulse.

PROCEDURE

Counting a Radial Pulse

■ **Beginning Steps**

Before any procedure, you always must follow the five basic steps: wash your hands, collect the equipment, identify the resident, explain the procedure, and protect privacy.

Follow Standard Precautions

1. Place the resident in a comfortable position, either lying down or sitting. The arm should be resting on a table or across the resident's chest.
2. With the first three fingers of your hand, locate the radial pulse and apply gentle pressure.
3. Using the second hand of your watch, count for 30 seconds and multiply the count by 2.
4. Note the rhythm and strength of the pulse.

5. Remove your fingers from the pulse site and make a note of the resident's name and the pulse rate.
6. Note any abnormal pulse and report it immediately to the nurse.

■ **Ending Steps**

To complete the procedure, perform the following steps:

Make the resident comfortable, positioning in goody body alignment. Make the resident safe, placing the call signal within reach, lowering the bed, and raising the side rails, if appropriate. Wash your hands. Record and report the procedure as required.

GUIDELINES

USING A STETHOSCOPE

- Clean the earpieces and diaphragm with an antiseptic wipe.
- Turn the earpieces slightly forward to fit snugly into the ears.
- If the stethoscope has both a bell and a diaphragm (see Figure 14-12), check to be sure that it is turned so that sound will travel through the diaphragm. This may be done by gently stroking your finger across the diaphragm while you have the earpieces in place.
- Place the diaphragm of the stethoscope flat against the skin.
- Apply firm, gentle pressure on the diaphragm with two fingers.

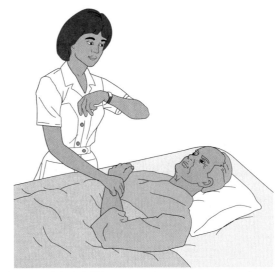

FIGURE 14-13 ■ The resident must not realize that you are counting respirations.

RESPIRATIONS

Counting **respirations** (breathing) is another routine vital sign measurement. Each respiration that is counted includes one inhalation (the chest rises) and one exhalation (the chest falls). The adult normal range is 12 to 20 respirations per minute.

When counting respirations, you should observe and report the following:

> *Rate*—The number of inhalations per minute.
> *Rhythm*—The pattern of breathing. This may be regular (evenly spaced) or irregular (unevenly spaced).
> *Quality*—The depth, shallowness, ease, or difficulty of breathing. The term for difficult or labored breathing is **dyspnea**.
> *Sounds*—These include wheezes, gurgles, rattles, and coughs.
> *Verbal complaints*—The resident may complain of pain, a tickling airway, or shortness of breath.

Normal breathing is regular, effortless, comfortable, and quiet. Abnormal respirations should be noted and reported to the nurse immediately.

Counting Respirations

The resident should not be aware that respirations are being counted (see Figure 14-13 ■) because the breathing pattern may change unintentionally. Breathing can be changed voluntarily or involuntarily by conscious thought. Does your breathing pattern change when you think about it? This is an involuntary change due to conscious awareness. To avoid the resident's awareness, you may begin counting respirations immediately after counting the pulse. Continue to hold the wrist as if continuing to count the pulse. After making a mental note of the pulse, begin to count respirations. The resident will think that you are still counting the pulse.

If you are asked about the rate of respirations by the resident or visitors, respond according to facility policy.

GUIDELINES

COUNTING RESPIRATIONS

- Watch the chest rise and fall.
- Count one each time the chest rises (each inhalation counts as one respiration).
- Count the respirations for 30 seconds, and multiply the number by 2 to determine the rate of respirations.
- The rate is the number of respirations per minute.
- If the respirations are irregular, count for 1 full minute.
- Record the respirations for each resident when you finish counting them.
- While counting, observe the rate, rhythm, quality, and sound of respirations.
- Report any abnormal or unusual findings to the nurse immediately.

BLOOD PRESSURE

Blood pressure (BP) is the force of blood against the artery walls as it is pumped by the heart. Blood pressure is affected by internal factors. These include the strength of the heart contractions, the amount of blood flowing, and the resistance or elasticity of the blood vessels. Blood pressure that is abnormally high is called **hypertension** ("hyper"—above normal or high; "tension"—pressure). **Hypotension** ("hypo"—low or below normal; "tension"—pressure) is abnormally low blood pressure.

Systolic and Diastolic Pressures

Two pressures are measured while taking the blood pressure. The higher pressure is the **systolic pressure**, which measures the pressure of the blood flowing during the heart's contraction (systole). The **diastolic pressure**, the lower measurement, is the pressure of the blood flowing during the heart's relaxation (diastole). The blood pressure is recorded as a fraction, with the systolic pressure as the top number and the diastolic as the bottom number (for example, BP 120/70). Blood pressures are measured in millimeters (mm) of mercury (Hg).

For many years the adult normal systolic pressure was determined to be 100 to 140 mm hg while the diastolic was 60 to 90 mm hg. New research suggests that the adult systolic pressure should not be higher than 120 and the diastolic pressure should not exceed 80. Follow facility policy in reporting blood pressure measurements.

Using Blood Pressure Equipment

Measuring the blood pressure requires the use of a stethoscope, a sphygmomanometer, and alcohol wipes. The stethoscope is used to listen to pulse sounds. The alcohol wipes are used to clean the earpieces and the diaphragm of the stethoscope before and after use.

The blood pressure cuff is called a **sphygmomanometer** (see Figure 14-14 ■). The four main parts of the sphygmomanometer are the cuff, bulb, valve, and measuring device (manometer or gauge). Some manometers are designed with a column of mercury that is calibrated (marked). These may be attached to a stand on wheels, folded into a case, or fastened to a wall. Another type, the aneroid manometer, uses a calibrated circular dial and a pointer. These are smaller and are transported more easily.

The cuff is wrapped around the arm and fastened. The cuff is a bladder, which is inflated with air to apply pressure on the artery. When the valve is closed (clockwise), the bulb can be pumped by hand to inflate the cuff. The valve is then turned counterclockwise to open it and deflate the cuff by allowing air to escape. The valve and bulb are connected to the bladder and cuff by a tube. A tube also connects the bladder to the manometer, which indicates the pressure.

Blood pressure cuffs are available in a variety of sizes. The cuff must fit the resident's arm snugly and must stay fastened when inflated. If the resident is very thin, so that the cuff slides, or if a larger size is needed, tell the nurse.

A sphygmomanometer is fragile, expensive equipment, so handle it with care. Do not drop it. Accuracy of this instrument is very important. If you feel that the instrument is not functioning properly, do not use it. Follow your facility policy regarding broken equipment.

Reading the Manometer (Gauge)

Manometers are calibrated with long lines, which represent 10 mm Hg (millimeters of mercury), and

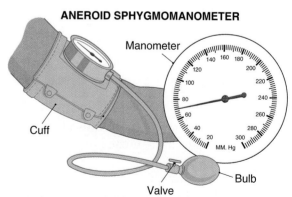

ANEROID SPHYGMOMANOMETER

FIGURE 14-14 ■ A sphygmomonometer is the blood pressure instrument. Long lines represent 10 mm Hg and short lines represent 2 mm of Hg.

Aneroid Manometer

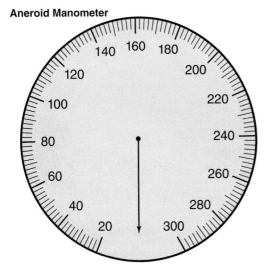

FIGURE 14-15 ■ Accuracy of measurement depends on reading the gauge correctly.

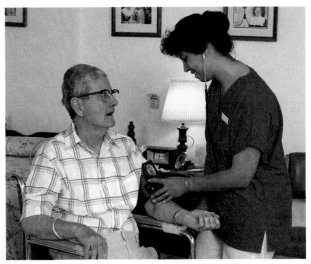

FIGURE 14-16 ■ Measuring a blood pressure

short lines, which represent 2 mm Hg (see Figure 14-15 ■). When reading the manometer, you will see that the pressure is dropping as air leaves the cuff. Read the systolic (upper) pressure first and the diastolic (lower) pressure second. Practice reading the calibrations so that you will be able to take a blood pressure accurately.

Measuring a Blood Pressure

After you have learned how to read the manometer, you will be ready to take a blood pressure (see Figure 14-16 ■). This is a complicated procedure because you must read the gauge, listen for pulse sounds, and use your hands. Be patient with yourself and practice so that you will be accurate.

Table 14-2 provides a summary of the normal TPR measurements.

TABLE 14-2	NORMAL TPR MEASUREMENTS	
Temperature	Pulse	Respirations
Axillary 97.6°F	60–90 per minute; regular rate, rhythm, and force	12–20 per minute; regular rate, rhythm, and quality
Oral 98.6°F		
Rectal 99.6°F		

GUIDELINES

MEASURING A BLOOD PRESSURE

- Do not take a blood pressure on an arm that is paralyzed or has a wound, cast, or IV.
- Place the cuff on skin, not over clothing.
- The entire surface of the stethoscope diaphragm should be held firmly and flat against the bend of the elbow, over the brachial artery (see Figure 14-17).
- Repeating the procedure will change the pressure. If you are not sure of the reading, do not re-inflate the cuff until you have completely deflated it for 1 minute.
- Deflate the cuff slowly so that you can read the pressure accurately.
- Inflate the cuff to 160 mm Hg, or inflate it to 30 mm Hg above the resident's usual systolic pressure.
- If you are not sure of a resident's pressure after two attempts, tell the nurse.
- Deflate the cuff immediately after the reading is complete. The needle will be on zero when all the air is out of the cuff.
- If you are asked about the blood pressure reading by the resident or visitors, respond according to facility policy.

PROCEDURE

Taking the Blood Pressure

■ Beginning Steps

Before any procedure, you always must follow the five basic steps: wash your hands, collect the equipment, identify the resident, explain the procedure, and protect privacy.

⟨ᵐ⟩ Follow Standard Precautions

1. Clean the stethoscope earpieces and diaphragm with alcohol wipes.
2. Have the resident sitting or lying down with the arm resting at heart level. The palm of the hand should be turned up.
3. Remove clothing over the area of the arm where the cuff will be placed.
4. With the valve open, squeeze the cuff to be sure it is completely deflated.
5. Wrap the cuff comfortably around the arm 1 inch above the elbow, with the arrow on the cuff pointing to the brachial pulse site.
6. The gauge should be clearly visible.
7. Place the stethoscope earpieces (turned slightly forward) snugly into your ears.
8. Locate the brachial pulse with your fingertips (see Figure 14-17 ■).
9. Place the diaphragm of the stethoscope flat on the pulse site, holding it firmly in place with the index and middle fingers of one hand. The stethoscope should not touch the cuff.
10. Close the valve (clockwise) until it stops. Do not tighten it.
11. Inflate the cuff to 160 mm Hg (or 30 mm Hg above the resident's usual systolic pressure). You will no longer hear a pulse.
12. With your thumb and index finger, open the valve slightly (counterclockwise). Allow the air to escape slowly as you listen for a pulse sound. (If you hear it immediately, you will have to begin again after deflating the cuff for 1 minute and reinflating it to 30 mm Hg higher than the first time.)
13. Remember the reading at which you hear the first clear pulse sound. This is the systolic pressure.
14. Continue listening for a change or muffling of the pulse sound. The reading at the point of change is the

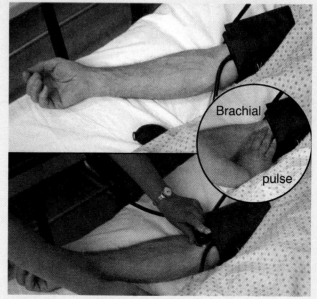

FIGURE 14-17 ■ Locate the brachial pulse with your fingertips.

diastolic pressure. (If no change of pulse sound is detectable, the point at which the sound disappears is the diastolic pressure.) Remember this reading.
15. Open the valve to deflate the cuff completely and remove it from the resident's arm.
16. Note any abnormality and report it to the nurse.
17. Wipe the stethoscope earpieces and diaphragm with alcohol.
18. Return the stethoscope and sphygmomanometer to storage.

■ Ending Steps

To complete the procedure, perform the following steps:

Make the resident comfortable, positioning in good body alignment. Make the resident safe, placing the call signal within reach, lowering the bed, and raising the side rails, if appropriate. Wash your hands. Record and report the procedure as required.

CHAPTER HIGHLIGHTS

1. The temperature, pulse, respirations, and blood pressure are measurements of body functions that are vital to life.

2. Wait 15 minutes before taking an oral temperature if the resident has been eating, drinking, smoking, or chewing gum.

3. Lubricate the rectal thermometer and hold it in place until the measurement is complete.

4. The tympanic thermometer measures the temperature of the tympanic membrane in the ear.

5. When counting the pulse, also observe its rhythm and force.

6. Do not use your thumb when taking a pulse or you will count your own pulse as well as that of the resident.

7. Observe the sounds, quality, and rhythm of breathing while counting the respiratory rate.

8. The respiratory pattern may change if the resident is aware that you are counting respirations.

9. The blood pressure cuff must fit the resident's arm snugly and stay fastened when inflated.

10. The first clear sound you hear when taking a blood pressure is the systolic pressure. The second clear sound is the diastolic pressure.

11. Deflate the cuff slowly so that you can read the gauge accurately.

12. Clean the earpieces and diaphragm of the stethoscope before and after use.

13. The resident should be sitting or lying down, with the arm resting at heart level, while a blood pressure is being taken.

14. If you are unsure of the vital signs that you have taken, notify the nurse.

15. Follow facility policy regarding information that you may give the resident or family about vital signs.

16. Report abnormalities in any of a resident's vital signs to the nurse immediately.

VOCABULARY REVIEW

Fill in the blanks with the vocabulary term that best completes the sentence.

1. The _____ is the amount of heat in the body.

2. An instrument used for listening to body sounds is a _____.

3. The _____ is the pressure of blood flowing while the heart is contracting.

4. The _____ is the pressure of blood flowing while the heart is resting.

5. The correct name for the ear drum is the _____.

6. The blood pressure cuff is called a _____.

7. The _____ is the heartbeat.

8. The temperature, pulse, respirations, and blood pressure are _____.

9. _____ is difficult or labored breathing.

10. Abnormally high blood pressure is called _____.

CHECK YOUR UNDERSTANDING

The following questions cover the highlights of this chapter. Choose the best answer for each question.

1. A normal adult oral temperature on the Fahrenheit scale is
   A. 96.6°   C. 98.6°
   B. 97.6°   D. 99.6°

2. The short line on a Fahrenheit glass thermometer represents
   A. one-tenth degree   C. one degree
   B. two-tenths degree   D. two degrees

3. How long should you leave a glass rectal thermometer in place?
   A. 1 minute   C. 3 to 5 minutes
   B. 2 minutes   D. 8 to 10 minutes

4. A tympanic thermometer measures the temperature in the
   A. mouth   C. rectum
   B. axilla   D. ear

5. Where is the radial pulse located?
   A. on the thumb side of the wrist
   B. on the side of the neck
   C. on the top of the foot
   D. behind the knee

6. An irregular pulse should be counted for
   A. 15 seconds and multiplied by 4
   B. 30 seconds and multiplied by 2
   C. 1 full minute
   D. 3 to 5 minutes

7. You have taken the resident's temperature, pulse, and respiration (TPR), and your measurements are T98.4°, P74, and R16. What action will you need to take?
   A. Chart the measurements. They are within the normal range.
   B. Report them to the nurse immediately. The pulse is too high.
   C. Retake the pulse. It is not within the normal range.
   D. Report them to the nurse immediately. All the measurements are abnormal.

8. Who should *not* have oral temperatures taken with a glass thermometer?
   A. A resident who is receiving oxygen
   B. An oriented elderly resident
   C. A resident who is lying in bed
   D. A resident who has visitors.

9. How long should the nursing assistant hold the rectal thermometer in place?
   A. Until the resident says it is all right to stop
   B. Until the resident is turned to the side
   C. Until the thermometer is inserted
   D. Throughout the procedure

AGE-SPECIFIC TIP

When taking the oral temperature of an elderly resident, you may need to remind the resident to keep his or her mouth closed around the thermometer.

CULTURALLY SENSITIVE TIP

Culture may affect whether or not the resident wants family members to stay in the room when his or her vital signs are being measured. Be aware of and honor the resident's wishes.

EFFECTIVE PROBLEM SOLVING

While measuring vital signs, the nursing assistant notes that the resident's pulse is 120. As she begins to repeat the procedure to check for accuracy, the resident anxiously asks, "Why are you taking my pulse again? Is something wrong?" The nursing assistant responds, "It's a little high, but you're probably alright." Was the nursing assistant's communication appropriate? If not, what would have been more appropriate?

_____

_____

_____

_____

_____

_____

_____

_____

INTERPERSONAL COMMUNICATION

The nursing assistant should always explain before beginning to measure the resident's vital signs. Check the example/s that are appropriate.

_____ "You don't look so good. I'd better take your vital signs."
_____ "I'm going to measure your BP now."
_____ "I'm going to count your breathing now.
_____ "I'm going to take your blood pressure."

OBSERVING, REPORTING, AND RECORDING

The resident's axillary temperature was 97.8, the pulse was 70, and the respirations were 14. The systolic blood pressure was 138 and the diastolic pressure was 78. Correctly record this information on the lines below.

_____

_____

_____

_____

_____

_____

_____

_____

_____

_____

Check out www.prenhall.com/grubbs for additional chapter-specific interactive study and review activities.

15

NUTRITION AND DINING

OBJECTIVES

1. Explain how dining can meet the needs of the whole person.
2. Explain what is meant by proper nutrition.
3. List five guidelines for using the food guide pyramid.
4. List nine factors that affect nutrition in the elderly.
5. Identify five residents' rights related to nutrition.
6. Describe assistive equipment and methods to assist the resident with dining.
7. Describe the clock method used in assisting the visually impaired resident at mealtime.
8. List ten guidelines to follow when feeding the resident who is unable to eat independently.
9. Identify five guidelines for assisting residents with swallowing problems.
10. List ten guidelines for restorative dining.

VOCABULARY

The following words or terms will help you to understand this chapter:

Nutrition	Peristalsis	Nasogastric (NG) tube
Calorie	Colon	Gastrostomy (G) tube
Nutrients	Aspirate	NPO
Metabolism	Aspiration pneumonia	PO

Nutritional needs, special diets, the digestive process, and specific needs of elderly residents are discussed in this chapter. Guidelines are provided for meeting nutritional needs of long-term care residents with nutritional problems.

THE NEED FOR FOOD

Dining can meet physical, emotional, social, and spiritual needs and can offer an opportunity to share love and compassion. Food is one of the most basic physical needs because it is used to create energy for all body functions. It also is used to build, maintain, and repair body tissues. Food helps meet emotional needs and is associated with love. A quiet meal with a special person can be emotionally uplifting (see Figure 15-1 ■). Dining meets social and spiritual needs. Many religious celebrations involve the sharing of food. Dining nourishes the whole person.

PROPER NUTRITION

Nutrition is the intake and use of food by the body. Proper nutrition means a well-balanced diet that contains all the elements necessary for physical and emotional health. Unmet nutritional needs can cause many problems such as irritability, fatigue, lack of energy, fear, and anxiety.

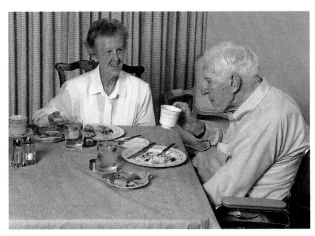

FIGURE 15-1 ■ A quiet meal with a special person can be emotionally uplifting.

Foods are measured in calories. A **calorie** is a unit of heat produced as the body burns food. Some foods produce more calories than others. The number of calories a person needs depends on many factors, such as height, body build, age, and activity.

Food contains **nutrients**, food elements that are necessary for metabolism. **Metabolism** is the combination of all body processes. The proper combination of nutrients is necessary to keep these processes in balance. Most foods contain more than one nutrient, but no one food contains all the essential nutrients. The three major nutrients are carbohydrates, fats, and protein. Consult Table 15-1 for an understanding of basic nutrients.

Water

The body needs water for proper nutrition. Water is as essential to life as food and oxygen. It is found in many foods and beverages. In fact, some fruits and vegetables are mostly water. The importance of water is discussed in detail in the next chapter.

FOOD GUIDE PYRAMID

Food Groups

Foods can be divided into basic groups: breads, cereals, rice, and pastas; vegetables and fruits; milk, cheese, and dairy products; meat, poultry, fish, dry beans, eggs, and nuts; and fats, oils, and sweets.

All foods can be classified into one or more of these groups. A well-balanced diet contains a variety of foods from each group every day.

In 1992, the U.S. Department of Agriculture developed the food guide pyramid (see Figure 15-2 ■). Following these guidelines will help you to eat a well-balanced diet daily. The food guide pyramid can easily be adapted for residents with special needs. For example, elderly residents may not be able to eat the recommended amounts of each food group. However, they can still eat more carbohydrates and fewer fats, oils, and sweets.

TABLE 15-1 BASIC NUTRIENTS

Nutrient	Body Function	Food Source
Carbohydrates	Major source of energy. Provides fiber for elimination.	Bread, cereal, grains, pasta, fruits, and vegetables.
Fats (lipids)	Provides energy, carries vitamins, protects organs from injury.	Meat, mayonnaise, butter, margarine, milk, cheese, oil, and nuts.
Protein	Builds muscle, blood, and other tissues. Used for tissue growth and maintenance.	Meat, poultry, fish, eggs, milk, cheese, nuts, peanut butter, dry beans, and whole-grain cereals.
Calcium (mineral)	Builds bones and teeth, muscles, and nerves.	Milk, cheese, yogurt, sardines, and green leafy vegetables.
Sodium (mineral)	Regulates body fluid, nerve and muscle function. Some persons must limit sodium intake.	All salty foods. Lunch meat, ham, hot dogs, catsup, mustard, pickles, and commercially prepared foods.
Potassium (mineral)	Regulates nerve, muscle, and heart function.	Bananas, oranges, cranberries, prunes, and the juices of these fruits.
Iron (mineral)	Builds hemoglobin that carries oxygen in the blood.	Meat, eggs, dry beans, whole-grain cereals, and green leafy vegetables.
Vitamin A	Contributes to healthy skin, mucous membranes, and vision. Helps fight infection.	Yellow fruits and vegetables, milk, cheese, liver, and green leafy vegetables.
Vitamin B Complex (B_1, B_2, B_6, B_{12}, Niacin)	Aids digestion, muscle tone, and growth. Maintains healthy nervous system. Builds red blood cells.	Meat, liver, fish, milk, cheese, eggs, cereal, bread, and green leafy vegetables.
Vitamin C	Builds tissue. Aids mineral absorption and healthy skin. Helps fight infection.	Citrus fruits (oranges and grapefruit), tomatoes, strawberries, cantaloupe, and many other fruits and vegetables.
Vitamin D	Builds healthy bones and teeth.	Milk, butter, cheese, eggs, liver.
Vitamin E	Helps build red blood cells and maintain muscle tone.	Eggs, liver, green leafy vegetables, and vegetable oils.
Vitamin K	Necessary for blood clotting.	Eggs, liver, and green leafy vegetables.

GUIDELINES

USING THE FOOD GUIDE PYRAMID

- Eat more foods located at the base of the pyramid (bread, cereal, rice, and pasta).
- Eat plenty of fruits and vegetables.
- Eat two or three servings daily of meat, poultry, fish, dry beans, eggs, and nuts.
- Use two or three daily servings of milk, yogurt, and cheese.
- Use fats, oils, and sweets sparingly.
- Eat a variety of foods.

TYPES OF DIETS

The doctor orders the type of diet that a resident will have. The order is given before or upon admission to the facility. Any change in the diet also requires a doctor's order. A dietician specializes in diets and directs the preparation of meals according to the doctor's orders.

Regular Diet

A regular diet is one in which a person may eat whatever he or she likes. There are no restrictions. This is sometimes called a "house diet" or "general diet."

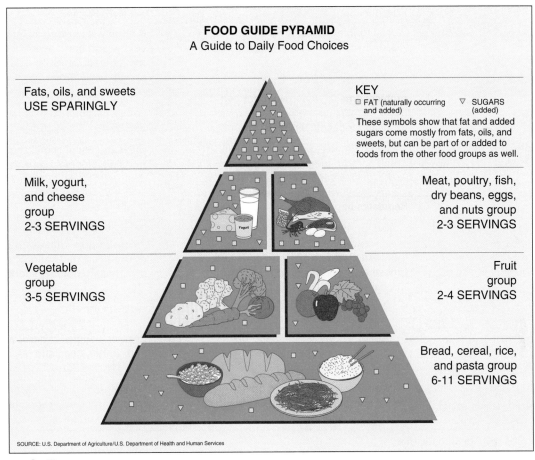

FIGURE 15-2 ■ Food guide pyramid

Therapeutic Diet

A therapeutic diet is used to treat a disease condition. It often is called a "special diet." In a therapeutic diet, the amount and type of food may be controlled. Examples of therapeutic diets are shown in Figure 15-3 ■.

The Diabetic Diet: The purpose of the diabetic diet is to maintain the correct blood sugar level and prevent complications. It is based on the resident's age, sex, height, weight, and activity level. The resident's current diet, cultural background, and food preferences are also considered. Diet is an important part of the treatment of diabetes. The following guidelines will help you assist the diabetic resident to control his or her disease.

GUIDELINES

ASSISTING A RESIDENT WITH A DIABETIC DIET

- Serve meals and snacks on time.
- Check the tray carefully to be sure that the resident is getting the correct diet.
- Encourage the resident to eat all the food on the tray.
- Remind the resident that he or she can exchange a food for one of equal value.
- Let the nurse know if the resident is not following his or her diet or does not eat everything on the tray.

Diet	Description	Foods
Diabetic	Used to treat diabetes mellitus. Carbohydrates, fat, protein, and calories are controlled.	A variety is allowed as long as the calorie and nutrient count is maintained. Candy and desserts should be avoided.
Clear Liquid	Liquids that have no residue. Used after surgery, for nausea and vomiting, and for acute illness.	Water, broth, apple juice, tea, coffee, carbonated beverages, and Jell-O.
Full Liquid	All liquid foods and solids that will melt at room temperature, may be used for residents who have problems swallowing. Next diet after clear liquids.	Clear liquids, plus milk, custard, pudding, cream soup, and ice cream.
Low-Sodium	Used for residents who have heart problems, hypertension, or kidney disease. Restricts all salty foods and those with a high sodium content. Usually, no salt is added to food. Doctor specifies amount of salt allowed.	Restricted: salt, ham, bacon, luncheon meat, hot dogs, pickles, mustard, canned soup, and vegetables that are not low-sodium.
Low-Cholesterol	Used for residents with heart disease, gallbladder problems, or a high cholesterol count.	Restricted: eggs, cheese, whole milk, butter, beef, and pork.
High-Residue/Fiber	Used for constipation and other bowel problems. Increases peristalsis and adds bulk.	Whole-grain bread and cereals, cheese, fruits and vegetables—especially green leafy vegetables.

FIGURE 15-3 ■ Therapeutic diets

Mechanical Diet

A mechanical diet is one in which the texture of the food is changed. A regular or therapeutic diet may be ordered as mechanical. This type of diet may be ordered for the person who has difficulty chewing or swallowing. The food may be chopped, pureed, or blended.

DIGESTION

Food is taken in through the mouth, where it is moistened by saliva and chewed by the teeth. The tongue pushes it to the back of the throat and it is swallowed. From there it enters the esophagus and moves by peristalsis into the stomach. **Peristalsis** is the muscular contractions that move food through the digestive system. The stomach stores and mixes the food. It secretes digestive juices that help to break down the food. The pancreas, liver, and gallbladder also contribute digestive juices. Most of digestion takes place in the small intestine, where nutrients from food are absorbed into the bloodstream through the villi. By the time food enters the **colon** (large intestine) very little is left except water and waste material called "feces." Fluid is removed from the colon and delivered to the body. Feces enters the rectum at the end of the colon and is eliminated through the anus (the opening of the rectum).

NUTRITION AND THE ELDERLY RESIDENT

Most older people require fewer calories because a decrease in metabolism and activity reduces the body's need for fuel. However, the amount of protein, minerals, and vitamins needed does not change.

Factors That Affect Nutrition

Some elderly residents have difficulty meeting their nutritional needs. Some factors that affect nutrition in the elderly are

- Physical changes of aging
- Difficulty chewing and dental problems
- Impaired mobility
- Disease or illness
- Confusion or emotional problems
- Decreased appetite
- Culture and religion
- Personal preferences
- Medication

Many people eat the same kind of cultural foods that they grew up eating. As people age, their desire for favorite foods may grow stronger. It is a real challenge for the staff in the long-term care facility to meet the residents' individual needs and preferences.

Nutritional Care Plan

A nutritional assessment of the resident is completed at admission and is revised as necessary. The care planning team attempts to create a plan that is as close as possible to the resident's usual eating habits. Check the nutritional care plan for each of your residents and follow it as closely as possible. Let the nurse know if any problems occur.

Residents' Rights as Related to Nutrition

The residents' bill of rights addresses nutrition and food. The facility and the caregivers must ensure that these rights are honored. They include the rights to

- Be served food according to ethnic, cultural, and/or religious beliefs
- Be served food according to personal preferences
- Be served attractive, tasty food at the correct temperature, in a pleasant environment, in a pleasant manner (see Figure 15-4 ■).
- Participate in traditional holiday meals
- Be offered substitutions and snacks

ASSISTING THE RESIDENT TO EAT

As a nursing assistant, you will have the opportunity to provide physical assistance and emotional

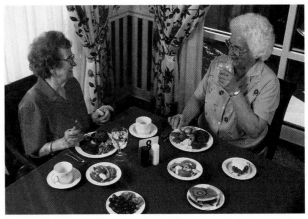

FIGURE 15-4 ■ Food should be served in an attractive manner in a pleasant environment.

support to help the resident meet nutritional needs. You may be the one who hears about food likes and dislikes. Be sure to make the nurse aware of those preferences. Observe the resident's behavior and emotional state because eating habits may change when a person is upset. Encourage the resident to share feelings, and listen attentively. Identify problems quickly, and offer help as necessary. Encourage physical activity to improve appetite and digestion.

Observe and record food and fluid intake accurately. You may need to figure the percentage or fraction of the amount consumed by the resident. An example of food intake percentages that may be used for reporting and recording is shown in Figure 15-5 ■.

Assistive Equipment

There is equipment available to assist the resident in eating. The occupational therapist will recommend and obtain assistive equipment that is specific to a resident's needs. This equipment may be useful to a resident who has weakness, paralysis, or impaired coordination. Figure 15-6 ■ shows some common assistive equipment.

Preparing the Resident for Meals

It is important to help the resident get ready for meals. Assist the resident with oral hygiene and grooming. Being well groomed is emotionally satisfying, and a clean, fresh mouth makes eating more pleasant. The guidelines will help you prepare the resident for meals.

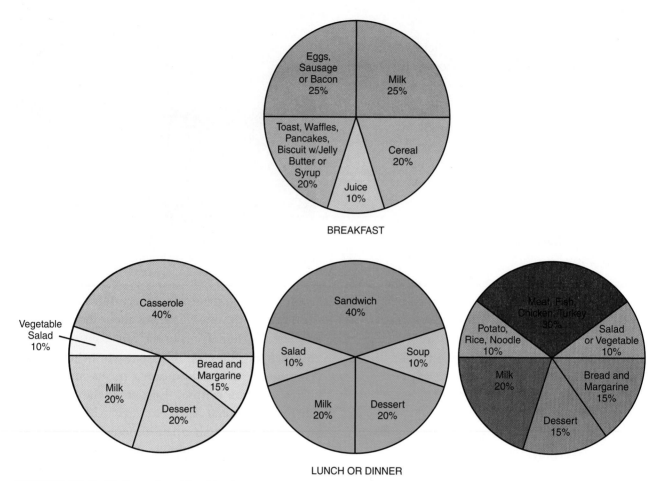

BREAKFAST

LUNCH OR DINNER

FIGURE 15-5 ■ Examples of food intake percentages

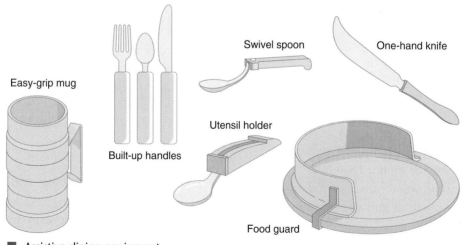

Easy-grip mug

Built-up handles

Swivel spoon

One-hand knife

Utensil holder

Food guard

FIGURE 15-6 ■ Assistive dining equipment

Serving Trays

Meal trays may be served by dietary or nursing personnel. Nursing assistants usually participate in this task. Always check the tray carefully before serving it to the resident, and follow the guidelines.

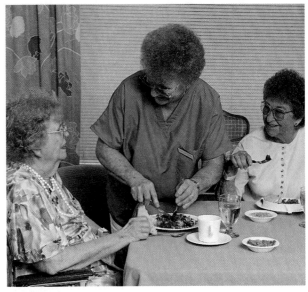

FIGURE 15-7 ■ Cutting up the resident's meat makes it easier for her to feed herself.

GUIDELINES

PREPARING RESIDENTS FOR MEALS

- Offer toileting before meals.
- Assist residents' handwashing and oral care.
- Be sure residents are clean and well groomed.
- Remind residents to wear glasses, hearing aid, and dentures if needed.
- Encourage residents to go to the dining room if possible.

GUIDELINES

SERVING FOOD TRAYS

- Wash your hands before serving meals.
- Match the name tag on the tray with the resident's ID bracelet.
- Check according to facility policy for allergies.
- Check the food on the tray with the diet that has been ordered.
- If there is food on the tray that the resident does not like, offer to get something else.
- Unwrap the silverware and napkin.
- Provide special equipment if required.
- Open cartons and remove covers.
- Offer salt, pepper, and other condiments that are allowed.
- Assist as needed by buttering bread or cutting up meat (see Figure 15-7 ■).

GUIDELINES

ASSISTING THE RESIDENT IN THE DINING ROOM

- Help the resident to be seated and positioned in correct body alignment.
- Introduce residents seated at the table if they do not know each other.
- Check the tray for the correct name and diet before bringing it to the table.
- Remove the food from the tray and arrange it in front of the resident.
- Encourage the resident to be as independent as possible.
- Stay near the table and observe for problems with chewing or swallowing.
- Observe the food that is eaten and report to the nurse if the resident is not eating well or is eating only certain foods.

Assisting the Resident in the Dining Room

Encourage the resident to eat in the dining room whenever possible because it is a familiar setting and there are more opportunities for socialization. Follow the guidelines for assisting the resident in the dining room.

Assisting Residents to Eat in Their Rooms

Some residents will need to eat their meals in their rooms. The resident should sit up as straight as possible in the bed or chair. This position improves digestion and helps to prevent choking.

GUIDELINES

ASSISTING RESIDENTS TO EAT IN THEIR ROOMS

- Assist the resident with hygiene and grooming.
- Encourage the resident to sit up in a chair if possible.
- Assist the resident who must stay in bed to sit up as straight as possible (see Figure 15-8 ■).
- Encourage independence and self-care.
- Provide a food protector for the resident's clothing if needed.
- Clean the overbed table before placing the tray on it.
- Allow the resident as much time as needed.
- Place the call signal within reach when you leave the room.

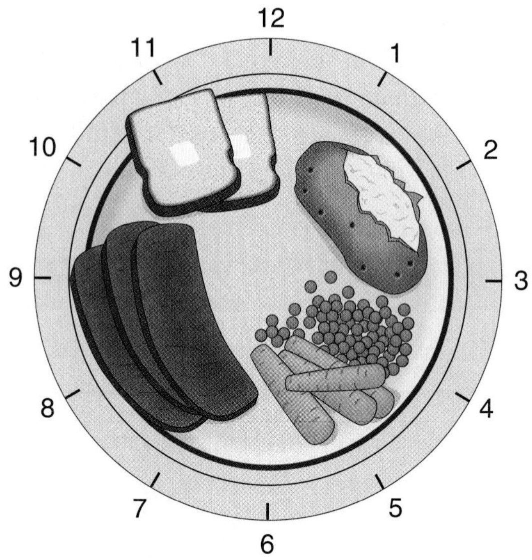

FIGURE 15-9 ■ Use the "clock method" to describe food placement to the vision-impaired resident.

Assisting the Vision-Impaired Resident with Meals

Use the "clock method" to help the blind or vision-impaired resident maintain independence. This means that you compare placement of food to the face of a clock. For example, in Figure 15-9 ■, the potato is at 2 o'clock. If the food was at 3 o'clock, it would be on the right side of the plate. Remember, the vision-impaired resident cannot see what is on the plate and has no idea what to expect.

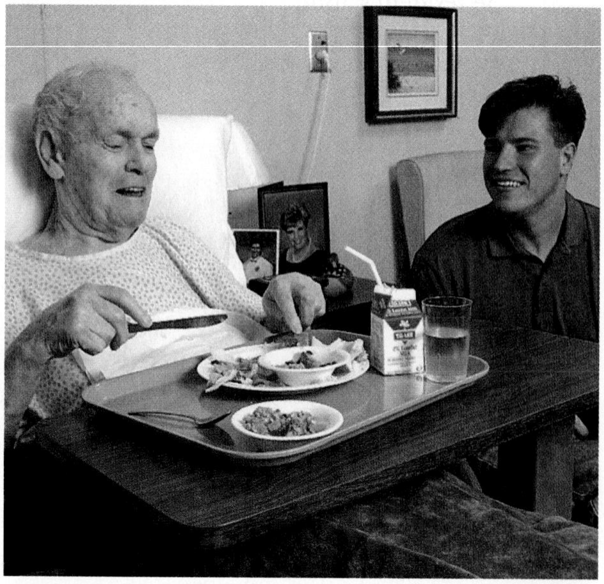

Feeding the Resident Who Cannot Eat Independently

Some residents may have physical or emotional problems that interfere with their ability to feed themselves. For example, a paralyzed resident unable to handle utensils or a confused resident with Alzheimer's disease may need to be fed. It is important to observe for any sign that the resident is improving. The resident who shows the ability or desire for self-feeding may need to be in a restorative dining program.

The helpless resident may be fed in the dining room, in the room, or in the bed. Make sure the resident is positioned correctly, sitting up as straight as possible. If a geri-chair is used, bring the recliner forward to an upright position. Do not attempt to feed the resident while the head is tilted back. Remember, when you tilt the head back and bring up the chin, you open the airway. The resident may **aspirate** (choke) if you try to offer food while the airway is open because food will enter the airway instead of the esophagus. If the resident

FIGURE 15-8 ■ The resident should sit up as straight as possible while eating in bed.

is choking, you must take action immediately. Send for the nurse and encourage the resident to cough. The Heimlich maneuver is used only if the airway is poor or completely obstructed.

GUIDELINES

FEEDING THE RESIDENT WHO CANNOT EAT INDEPENDENTLY

- Position the resident to sit up as straight as possible.
- Sit down so that you are at eye level with the resident (see Figure 15-10 ■).
- Provide a clothing protector.
- Tell the resident what is on the tray.
- Season the food as the resident desires.
- Serve the food as desired.
- Name each food as it is offered.
- Be sure that liquids are not too hot.
- Tell the resident when you are offering hot liquids or food.
- Encourage the resident to help (hold the bread or cracker).
- Alternate foods and offer fluids frequently, beginning with fluids.
- Fill the spoon no more than half full.
- Feed with the tip of the spoon.
- Feed on the unaffected side if the resident is paralyzed.
- Use a different straw for each liquid.

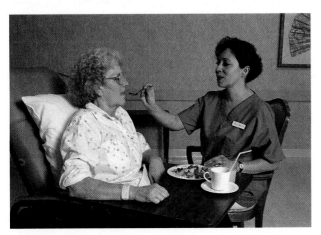

FIGURE 15-10 ■ When feeding a resident, sit down so that you are at eye level with her.

Communicate with the resident even if there is no response. Wipe the resident's mouth as needed. Make sure the resident is clean, neat, and comfortable after completing the meal. Record the amount eaten, and report to the nurse if the resident did not eat well.

ASSISTING RESIDENTS WITH SWALLOWING PROBLEMS

Many elderly residents have swallowing problems that cause them to choke easily. A major complication of choking is **aspiration pneumonia**. This kind of pneumonia results when the resident chokes and food or fluid enters the lungs and causes infection. You can help prevent complications by observing for swallowing problems. Symptoms to observe include the following:

- Poorly chewed food
- Frequent coughing or throat clearing
- Drooling
- Pocketing of food in the cheek
- Weakness of the lips or tongue
- Numerous swallows with each bite
- Excessively slow eating

If you observe any of these symptoms, inform the nurse immediately.

Residents with swallowing problems frequently are restricted to thickened liquids. Thickening increases the resident's ability to control fluid while it is in the mouth and throat. The speech therapist will indicate the necessary thickness to be used. Special products are used for thickening. If thickening is ordered, it must be used with *all* liquids. Be sure to follow the directions for each resident as ordered. You may be working directly with the speech therapist, who usually assists residents who have swallowing problems.

Lemon ice or Italian ice may be ordered with meals for residents with swallowing difficulties. Ice cream is not used for this purpose because of the sugar and fat content. Be aware that it is not provided as a dessert, but is to be used throughout the meal before every bite of food. The coldness of the ice and the tartness of the lemon stimulate muscles for swallowing and help to prevent choking. If you are assisting a resident who uses lemon

GUIDELINES

ASSISTING RESIDENTS WITH SWALLOWING PROBLEMS

- Follow the instructions of the speech therapist.
- Notify the nurse when you observe problems with swallowing.
- Position and feed the resident in an upright position.
- Allow the resident time to chew the food thoroughly.
- Make sure swallowing is completed after each bite.
- Gently stroke the resident's throat if swallowing does not occur.
- Ask the resident to swallow a second time if food appears to be stuck in the throat.
- Encourage coughing as necessary.
- Encourage the resident to sit up for at least 30 minutes after eating.

GUIDELINES

RESTORATIVE DINING

- Encourage independence.
- Maintain a quiet environment, free from distraction.
- Provide assistive equipment as needed.
- Place only one dish at a time in front of the resident who is distracted easily or who lacks confidence.
- Place food within the resident's reach.
- Use the clock method to identify food for the vision-impaired resident.
- Give directions one step at a time. For example, "Pick up your spoon. Put the spoon in your mashed potatoes. Bring the spoon to your mouth. Now swallow. That's great!"
- Help the resident maintain proper positioning while eating.
- You may need to place your hand over the resident's hand to guide it.
- Allow time for the resident to chew and swallow.
- Repeat instructions patiently, as often as necessary.
- Offer praise and encouragement frequently.
- Encourage the resident to try; don't point out mistakes.

ice, it may be necessary to remind him or her to use it before every mouthful of food.

RESTORATIVE DINING

Any assistance that is given the resident in dining should be given in a restorative manner. Encourage the resident to eat as independently as possible. Develop a positive attitude. Your belief in the success of restorative dining can contribute to the resident's success.

Restorative Dining Program

Some residents will be in a restorative dining program. They will be divided into groups according to their dining needs.

Retraining may be needed by some residents. Residents who have had strokes, for example, may need to learn how to feed themselves again. Each resident is assessed carefully for problems, strengths, weaknesses, and motivation. Both short-term and long-term goals are set. Measures are suggested to help meet those goals, and evaluations are made on a regular basis. All are part of a plan of care for meeting nutritional needs.

SUPPLEMENTAL NUTRITION

Residents who do not eat well may be offered supplemental feedings. This type of feeding also is provided for the resident who has an increased need for calories. For example, some cancer patients need to follow a diet that is nutritionally high in calories.

Between-Meal Snacks

Nutritious foods are provided for between-meal snacks. Milk shakes, ice cream, cheese, and peanut butter on crackers are examples of these snacks. It is important that you serve the snacks to the residents and encourage them to eat. Many times, however, the resident who doesn't eat well at meals will refuse nourishment that is offered between meals. In that situation, the doctor may order a liquid nutritional supplement.

Oral Supplements

Liquid supplements provide the necessary nutrients and calories in a small amount of fluid. Many products that are equal to a well-balanced meal are available. They are nutritious enough to be used as a complete diet or they may be added to a standard diet. Liquid supplements come in a variety of flavors.

Tube Feedings

The resident who is unable to take food or fluids by mouth or is unable to swallow may be fed through a tube. The two types of tubes most commonly used in a long-term care facility are nasogastric tubes and gastrostomy tubes.

A **nasogastric (NG) tube** is a tube that is placed through the nose into the stomach. A **gastrostomy (G) tube** is a tube that is placed through a surgical opening directly into the stomach. Residents with feeding tubes are often **NPO** (nothing by mouth). The abbreviation **PO** is used when the resident can have something by mouth. Check with the nurse before giving food or fluids to a resident with a feeding tube. Care of residents with feeding tubes is explained in Chapter 25.

CHAPTER HIGHLIGHTS

1. Dining can meet physical, emotional, social, and spiritual needs.
2. Food is used to create energy for all body functions.
3. Proper nutrition means a well-balanced diet that contains all the elements necessary for physical and emotional health.
4. A resident's diet is ordered by the doctor.
5. Residents' rights ensure a resident the right to be served food according to his or her individual preferences.
6. Encourage the resident to eat in the dining room, if possible.
7. Check the meal tray carefully before serving it to the resident.
8. Do not rush the resident; allow time for eating and socializing.
9. Use the clock method to describe the location of food for the vision-impaired resident.
10. Notify the nurse immediately when you observe a resident having difficulty swallowing.
11. Provide assistive equipment and help the resident maintain proper positioning while eating.
12. Check with the nurse before giving anything to eat or drink to a resident with a feeding tube.

VOCABULARY REVIEW

Fill in the blanks with the vocabulary term that best completes the sentence.

1. _____ is the combination of all body processes.

2. A tube that is placed through the nose into the stomach is a _____.

3. _____ is the intake and use of food by the body.

4. The correct name for the large intestine is the _____.

5. A/an _____ is a unit of heat produced as the body burns food.

6. The abbreviation for "nothing by mouth" is _____.

7. To _____ is to choke.

8. _____ are food elements necessary for metabolism.

9. The muscular contractions that move food through the digestive system are called _____.

10. The abbreviation for "by mouth" is _____.

CHECK YOUR UNDERSTANDING

The following questions cover the highlights of this chapter. Choose the best answer for each question.

1. Proper nutrition involves
   A. eating a 1200-calorie diet
   B. eating a high-calorie diet
   C. eating a well-balanced diet
   D. having a full liquid diet

2. Mrs. Jones, who has a feeding tube, asks you for a glass of water. What should you do?
   A. Get her a glass of water.
   B. Tell her she's not allowed to have water.
   C. Give her water through her feeding tube.
   D. Check with the nurse.

3. A mechanical diet may be ordered for residents who have problems with
   A. breathing   B. urinating
   C. walking and moving
   D. chewing and swallowing

4. According to the food guide pyramid, which type of food should provide the least part of the diet?
   A. Fruits and vegetables
   B. Meat, poultry, and fish
   C. Breads and cereals
   D. Fats, oils, and sweets

5. Who orders the diet for the resident?
   A. The nurse   C. The dietician
   B. The doctor   D. The nursing assistant

6. What type of pneumonia can result when the resident chokes and food or fluid enters the lungs?
   A. Aspiration pneumonia
   B. Chronic pneumonia
   C. Walking pneumonia
   D. Hypostatic pneumonia

7. The resident tells you that he doesn't like the fish on his food tray. What should you do?
   A. Tell him to try it and he might find he likes it.
   B. Chart that he refused to eat his fish.
   C. Tell him to eat the rest of his food and leave the fish.
   D. Ask the dietician to replace the fish.

8. The clock method of arranging food on the plate helps maintain the independence of which residents?
   A. hearing-impaired C. vision-impaired
   B. speech-impaired D. mobility-impaired

9. Mr. Chen must remain in his bed for meals. What is the best way to position him to prevent aspiration?
   A. lying flat on his back
   B. sitting up as straight as possible
   C. lying on his side
   D. leaning back as far as possible

AGE-SPECIFIC TIP

The elderly resident who is relearning to feed himself may need frequent reminders. Remind the resident to chew thoroughly and swallow completely before taking another bite.

CULTURALLY SENSITIVE TIP

Food preferences and table manners are influenced by culture. Support the resident's rights by encouraging choices.

EFFECTIVE PROBLEM SOLVING

Mrs. Chang is in a restorative dining program. She is feeding herself very slowly. The nursing assistant says, "Hurry up and eat before your food gets cold. Shall I feed you?" Was the nursing assistant's communication appropriate? If not, what would have been more appropriate?

_____
_____
_____
_____
_____
_____
_____
_____
_____
_____
_____
_____
_____

INTERPERSONAL COMMUNICATION

You are assisting a blind resident to eat independently. Check the examples that are appropriate.

_____"There is a slice of roast beef at 3 o'clock."

_____"Your cup of coffee is at 1 o'clock, and it is very hot."

_____"The roast beef is on the right side of your plate."

_____"Your plate is right in front of you."

_____"Your glass of water is at the tip of your knife."

OBSERVING, REPORTING, AND RECORDING

You are assisting residents in the dining room. List indications of swallowing problems that you would report and record.

_____
_____
_____
_____
_____
_____
_____
_____
_____
_____
_____
_____

EXPLORE MEDIALINK

Check out www.prenhall.com/grubbs for additional chapter-specific interactive study and review activities.

16

FLUID BALANCE

OBJECTIVES

1. Explain the importance of fluids.
2. Explain the meaning of fluid balance.
3. Identify four guidelines for care of the resident with edema.
4. List four reasons why the elderly do not drink enough fluids.
5. List five guidelines for preventing dehydration.
6. List three alternative methods of hydration.
7. List six guidelines for accurate intake and output.
8. Identify five guidelines for measuring fluid intake.
9. List four guidelines for measuring urinary output.
10. Calculate fluid intake and output correctly using the metric system.

VOCABULARY

The following words or terms will help you to understand this chapter:

Hydration
Edema

Dehydration
Intake and output (I&O)

Graduate
Foley catheter

This chapter describes the relationship between fluid and the human body and discusses the risk factors for proper hydration that commonly occur among elderly residents. The nursing assistant's role in maintaining fluid balance is explained, and practical approaches for maintaining hydration are provided.

THE IMPORTANCE OF FLUID

Water is essential to life. It is more important than food and necessary for all body processes. The amount of water in the body affects cell activity, and if the amount of water becomes very low, cells will die.

The Functions of Water

The body uses water in many ways. It is needed inside the cells and between the cells. Water provides fluid for the body's circulatory system. It is the major element of blood. The functions of water in the body include the following:

- Carries oxygen, nutrients, and other substances to the cells
- Carries waste products away from the cells
- Provides lubrication to body tissues
- Helps to regulate body temperature
- Helps to regulate the body's chemistry balance
- Helps to regulate fluid balance
- Satisfies thirst (see Figure 16-1 ■)

MAINTAINING FLUID BALANCE

The human body is over 60 percent water. Food and fluid provide water for the body. To achieve adequate **hydration** (amount of fluid), an adult requires 2 to 3 quarts (approximately 2,000–3,000 cc) of fluid daily. Because the body is using water continually, fluid must be replaced daily. There may be an increased need for fluids during hot weather or if a person is ill. In order to maintain fluid balance, the amount of fluid taken in must equal the amount of fluid that is eliminated.

Water is important to maintain the chemical balance of the body. Chemicals, such as sodium and potassium, are necessary for cell function. A change in the fluid balance causes a change in the chemical balance. When the chemicals in the body are not balanced, physical or mental problems may result.

EDEMA AND DEHYDRATION

Medical problems occur when the body is not in fluid balance. Either too much or not enough fluid can have serious effects on the body. Measures must be taken to restore the balance as soon as possible.

Edema

When there is too much fluid, it tends to collect in parts of the body. The accumulation of fluid that causes swelling of a body part is called **edema.** The swelling usually is noticed first in the hands and feet. Edema may be caused by poor circulation, fluid retention, or medications. It may be a complication of heart or kidney disease. Symptoms of edema include swelling, weight gain, increased blood pressure, and wet, noisy respirations.

Treatment for edema may include diet, fluid restriction, and medication. A low-sodium diet may be ordered because sodium (salt) causes the body to retain fluid. Since there is already too much fluid in the body, oral fluids may be restricted. In this case a specific amount of fluid will be ordered daily, with the amount divided between shifts. The amount of fluid taken in and eliminated must be recorded carefully. Medications (diuretics) may be ordered to reduce edema. These "water pills" cause the resident to urinate more frequently. Call signals must be answered promptly because the need to urinate may be urgent.

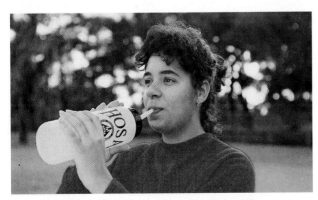

FIGURE 16-1 ■ A drink of water satisfies thirst.

GUIDELINES

CARE OF THE RESIDENT WITH EDEMA

- Elevate the swollen extremity when possible.
- Place a footstool under the feet of the resident who is sitting.
- Provide restorative skin care as explained in Chapter 12.
- Provide oral care frequently.
- Answer call signals promptly.
- Encourage the resident to follow the diet that is ordered.
- Carefully measure and record all fluids taken in and eliminated.
- Make sure that the resident and visitors are aware of the need to measure fluids.

Care of the Resident with Edema

Residents with edema need special care to prevent further complications.

Dehydration

The condition of having less than the normal amount of fluid in the body is called **dehydration**. Dehydration occurs when the resident loses too much body fluid or does not take in enough fluid. A person with low body weight can dehydrate very quickly. Infants and the elderly are especially at risk. It is important to observe early signs of dehydration before they become more serious.

The signs and symptoms of dehydration include

- Thirst
- Very dry skin that is less elastic than normal
- Pale or ashen skin color
- Sunken eyes
- Dry mouth and tongue
- Dry mucous membranes
- Weight loss
- Decreased urinary output
- Concentrated urine
- Constipation
- Rapid heart and respiratory rates
- Fever
- Irritability, confusion, and/or depression
- Weakness, twitching, or convulsions

Fluid is normally lost through urine, respirations, perspiration, and feces (bowel movement). Abnormal losses of fluid can be caused by vomiting, diarrhea, bleeding, or excessive perspiration. Dehydration may occur as a complication of an illness or as a side effect of medication.

The most common cause of dehydration in the elderly is an inadequate intake of fluid. Reasons why the elderly resident may not drink enough include

- Weakness and decreased mobility (has difficulty reaching, opening, or pouring fluid)
- Difficulty swallowing
- Confusion (fails to recognize thirst, forgets to drink, is unable to work the water fountain, or fears being poisoned)
- Lack of assistance (fluids offered infrequently or failure to assist)
- Fear of urinary incontinence (inability to control urine)
- Dislikes fluid offered (many people do not like water)

Treatment for dehydration includes increasing the amount of fluid intake. The doctor may order the staff to "encourage fluids." A specific amount of fluid will be divided between shifts. Fluid must be offered frequently, and residents must be encouraged to drink. Accurate measuring and recording of fluid intake will be necessary. Let the nurse know if you cannot get the resident to drink enough. Do not wait until the end of the shift to report this information.

Preventing Dehydration

The nursing assistant plays an important role in preventing dehydration. The following guidelines will help protect residents from becoming dehydrated.

ALTERNATIVE METHODS OF HYDRATION

Sometimes, despite all your efforts, the resident will not drink enough fluids. In that case, the doctor may order fluids by a different route. Some alternative methods for giving fluids are by nasogastric tube (NG tube), gastrostomy tube (G tube), or intravenous (IV). Caring for residents with these

GUIDELINES

PREVENTING DEHYDRATION

- Observe for signs and symptoms of dehydration.
- Be aware of the amount of fluid the resident is drinking.
- Accurately measure and record fluid intake and elimination.
- Offer fluids frequently and place them within the resident's reach.
- Open containers and assist as needed (see Figure 16-2 ■).
- Provide assistive equipment if necessary.
- Remind and encourage the resident to drink.
- Find out what fluids the resident likes and check the care plan for suggestions.
- Create an environment that will make drinking fluids a pleasant experience (see Figure 16-3 ■).

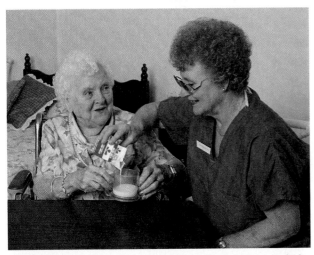

FIGURE 16-2 ■ Assist the resident with fluids as needed.

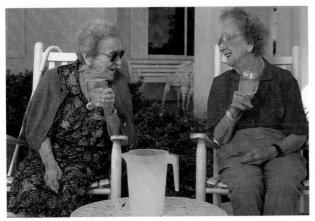

FIGURE 16-3 ■ Create an environment that will make drinking fluids a pleasant experience.

types of hydration methods are explained in Chapter 25.

MEASURING FLUID INTAKE AND OUTPUT

Intake and Output

Intake and output (I&O) includes all fluids that are taken into the body and all fluids that are eliminated. The doctor orders I&O to observe fluid balance. It is very important to measure and record all fluids accurately because this information is used in planning the resident's care and treatment. A **graduate**, a container that is used to measure fluid, will be needed (see Figure 16-4 ■). Wear gloves for measuring output.

Recording Fluid Intake and Output

An I&O recording form may be placed in the room of a resident whose fluid intake and output is being measured. The amount of intake or output is listed in the proper column, beside the correct time. At the end of each shift, the amount of fluid intake and output is totaled. The amount of fluid taken in and eliminated on all shifts is totaled every 24 hours. An example of an I&O recording form is shown in Figure 16-5 ■.

It is important to explain the need for measuring and recording I&O to the resident and visitors. They will need to tell you when the resident has had something to drink or has gone to the bathroom. You will record all the fluids taken by mouth, and the nurse will record tube feedings and IV solutions. You are

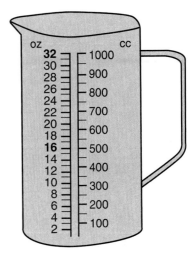

FIGURE 16-4 ■ A graduate is used to measure fluids.

also responsible for measuring and recording the amount of fluid that is eliminated. Accurate I&O depends on the cooperation of staff members, residents, and visitors. The following guidelines will help ensure accurate I&O.

Measuring Fluid Intake

Fluid intake includes water and all liquid foods that are taken into the body. Tube feedings and IV solutions are counted as fluid intake. Juice, milk, soup, coffee, and tea are examples of liquid. Solid foods that will melt at room temperature also are counted as fluid. Ice chips, popsicles, ice cream,

sherbet, pudding, jello, and custard are examples of this type of food (see Figure 16-6 ■).

The following guidelines include a formula that will help you measure and calculate fluid intake accurately.

GUIDELINES

ACCURATE I&O

- Inform the resident and visitors of the need to measure fluids.
- Place the I&O record according to facility policy.

(continued)

INTAKE AND OUTPUT SHEET

Identification # 125689400-2   Resident's Name Mary Smith Jones

Date 12-1-98   Room # 4011A

	INTAKE			OUTPUT			
				URINE		GASTRIC	
Time 11–7	BY MOUTH	TUBE	PARENTERAL	VOIDED	CATHETER	EMESIS	SUCTION
7:30a	120 cc			250 cc			
9:45	240 cc						
10:30	60 cc						
11:00				350 cc			
11:20						200 cc	
12:Noon	NPO						
TOTAL	420 cc	—	—	600 cc	—	200 cc	—
Time 7–3	NPO						
2:50p				450 cc			
3:00			1,000 cc	200 cc			300 cc
TOTAL	—	—	1,000 cc	650 cc	—	—	300 cc
Time 3–11	NPO						
5:00p				200 cc			
11:00			1,000 cc	480 cc			250 cc
TOTAL	—	—	1,000 cc	680 cc	—	—	250 cc
24-HOUR TOTAL	420 cc	—	2,000 cc	1,930 cc	—	200 cc	550 cc

24-Hour Grand Total•Intake 2420 cc   24-Hour Grand Total•Output 2680 cc

FIGURE 16-5 ■ I&O sheet

GUIDELINES (Continued)

- Answer call signals promptly.
- Measure and record fluid intake immediately.
- Measure and record fluid output immediately.
- Use a graduate to measure urinary output.
- Measure fluids accurately and figure the amounts correctly.
- Record fluid amounts in cubic centimeters on the I&O record.

GUIDELINES

MEASURING FLUID INTAKE

- Identify the foods or fluids to be measured.
- Use the following formula to calculate the amount of fluid consumed by the resident:

  1. Determine the amount of fluid originally in the container.
  2. Estimate, in a fraction, the amount of fluid taken (⅓ or ½, for example).
  3. Divide the bottom number of the fraction into the amount originally in the container.
  4. Multiply the answer in Step 3 by the top number of the fraction. This gives the amount of fluid consumed from that container.

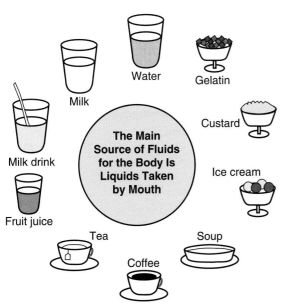

FIGURE 16-6 ■ Examples of fluid intake

GUIDELINES (Continued)

- Repeat the process for each fluid taken by the resident.
- Add the amounts of fluid taken and record the total on the I&O form.
- Record fluids as soon as the resident finishes eating or drinking.
- Mark the I&O form before the tray is removed at mealtime.

Measuring Urinary Output

Urinary output is measured after each voiding. A specimen pan can be placed under the seat of the toilet or bedside commode to collect and measure the urine (see Figure 16-7 ■). The resident who is not able to get out of bed may use a bedpan or a urinal.

The following guidelines will help you measure and record fluid that is eliminated from the body.

GUIDELINES

MEASURING URINARY OUTPUT

- Wear gloves and follow standard precautions.
- Assist the resident with a bedpan, urinal, bedside commode, or into the bathroom.
- Place a specimen container under the seat of the bedside commode or toilet to collect the urine (see Figure 16-7).
- Ask the resident not to put toilet paper into the bedpan, urinal, or specimen pan.
- Instruct the resident to signal when he or she is through so that you can measure and discard the urine.
- Pour the urine or other fluid into a graduate.
- Set the graduate on a flat surface and read the amount at eye level.
- Record the amount on the I&O form.
- Measure and record emesis if vomiting occurs.
- Discard your gloves and wash your hands when through.
- Assist the resident to wash his or her hands.
- Report bleeding, drainage, diarrhea, and excessive perspiration to the nurse, who will measure or estimate these fluids.

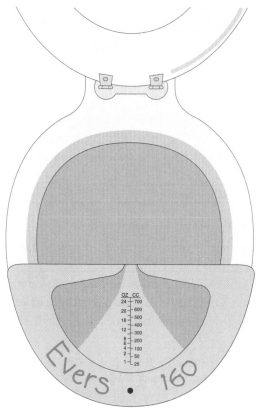

FIGURE 16-7 ■ A specimen pan may be placed under the toilet seat to collect the urine for measuring.

I&O usually is ordered for a resident with a Foley catheter. A catheter is a tube that is inserted into the bladder to drain urine. A **Foley catheter** is a urinary catheter that is left in place. It is attached to a urinary drainage bag.

The urinary drainage bag is emptied at the end of every shift and recorded on the I&O form. If the bag fills before the end of your shift, empty it and record the amount. Let the nurse know if this happens. Guidelines for emptying a urinary drainage bag are located in Chapter 17 on page 235.

SYSTEMS OF MEASUREMENT

Metric System

The metric system is an international system of weights and measures that commonly is used in health care. The units used most often are cubic centimeter (cc) and milliliter (ml). These two units are equal (1 cc = 1 ml).

Code of Measurement

The system includes many other measurements, some of which you will learn in other chapters. This chapter deals with those that are used in measuring fluids. Because you frequently will need to convert ounces to cubic centimeters, it is important to remember that 30 cc = 1 oz. The chart in Figure 16-8 ■ shows equivalent (approximately equal) measurements to be learned.

To total I&O, it will be necessary to know how much fluid various containers hold. This information usually can be found on the I&O sheet and may be posted in the nourishment room or the utility room. It is your responsibility to know the code of measurements in your facility. They are not necessarily the same in all facilities. An example of a measurement chart can be seen in Figure 16-9 ■.

Using Math Skills

A graduate may be marked in cubic centimeters (cc), milliliters (ml), ounces (oz), or a combination. Look at Figure 16-4 again. The graduate is marked in cubic centimeters and ounces. That works well in measuring output, but to measure

---

EQUIVALENT MEASUREMENTS

1 cc = 1 ml
30 cc = 1 oz
240 cc = 8 oz or 1 cup

FIGURE 16-8 ■ It is helpful to know equivalent measurements for the metric system.

CAPACITIES OF SERVING CONTAINERS

4-oz juice glass	120 cc
6-oz cup	180 cc
8-oz cup	240 cc
12-oz cup	360 cc
1-cup milk carton	240 cc
4-oz ice cream cup	120 cc
6-oz Jell-O cup	180 cc
6-oz coffee cup	180 cc
1-qt water pitcher	1,000 cc

FIGURE 16-9 ■ Sample code of measurements from a long-term health care facility.

intake, you will need to use your math skills. The math used in figuring I&O is very simple when you work the problems one step at a time. Let's look at some examples. You will need to refer to Figures 16-8 and 16-9.

Example 1: If you know how many cubic centimeters the container holds, all you need to do is add the amounts the resident drank.

> **Problem:** The resident drank 150 cc of coffee, 120 cc of milk, and 90 cc of juice. What is the total amount of intake?

$$
\begin{array}{r}
150 \text{ cc coffee} \\
120 \text{ cc milk} \\
\underline{90 \text{ cc juice}} \\
360 \text{ cc}
\end{array}
$$

The correct answer is 360 cc.

Example 2: You might use multiplication to figure the amount of intake.

> **Problem:** The resident drank three cans of a feeding supplement. Each can contains 240 cc. What is the total intake?

$$
\begin{array}{r}
240 \text{ cc} \\
\underline{\times\ 3} \\
720 \text{ cc}
\end{array}
$$

The correct answer is 720 cc.

Example 3: Sometimes you will know how many ounces are in a container, and you will need to figure the total in cubic centimeters. In this situation, you will multiply the number of ounces by 30. (Remember, there are 30 cc in 1 oz.)

> **Problem:** The resident drank one 3-oz glass of juice. What is the intake in cubic centimeters?

$$
\begin{array}{r}
30 \text{ cc} \\
\underline{\times\ 3} \\
90 \text{ cc}
\end{array}
$$

The correct answer is 90 cc.

Example 4: Probably the most difficult math will involve fractions. A fraction is a part of something. The fractions you usually will work with are quarters, halves, and thirds (see Figure 16-10 ■).

> **Problem:** The resident drank three-fourths of a glass of water that contained 240 cc. How

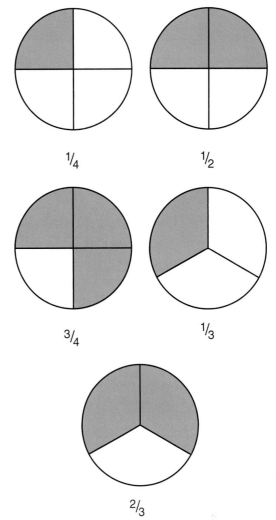

FIGURE 16-10 ■ A fraction is a part of something. The dark sections represent the fractions.

much water did he drink? Carefully follow these two steps to figure fractions.

Step 1. Divide the bottom number of the fraction into the total amount in the glass.

$$
\begin{array}{c}
3/4 \text{ of } 240 \text{ cc} \\
4 \text{ into } 240 = 60 \text{ cc}
\end{array}
$$

Step 2. Multiply the answer to step 1 by the top number of the fraction.

$$
60 \times 3 = 180 \text{ cc}
$$

The correct answer is 180 cc.

Example 5: Most of the time, you will use a combination of methods when figuring the total intake for the day. The following example shows the intake for one meal, using the code of measurements in Figure 16-9. Use the math techniques given earlier.

> ***Problem:*** At breakfast, Mrs. Ryan had one egg, one-half carton of milk, two pieces of toast, one-half of a banana, two-thirds glass of orange juice, and two cups of coffee. What is her fluid intake for this meal?

Step 1. List the fluids:
(a) 1/2 carton milk,
(b) 2/3 glass juice,
(c) 2 cups coffee.

Step 2. Figure the number of cubic centimeters in each item.
(a) 1/2 carton milk; 1 carton = 240 cc
        1/2 of 240 = 120 cc

(b) 2/3 glass juice; 1 juice glass = 120 cc
        2/3 of 120m = 80 cc
(c) 2 cups coffee; 1 coffee cup = 180 cc
        2 × 180 = 360 cc

Step 3. Add the answers to a, b, and c.

$$\begin{array}{r} 120 \text{ cc} \\ 80 \text{ cc} \\ + 360 \text{ cc} \\ \hline 560 \text{ cc} \end{array}$$

The correct answer is 560 cc. This is the total amount of fluid that Mrs. Ryan took in at breakfast.

You can substitute milliliters for cubic centimeters in any of these problems. Remember, cubic centimeters and milliliters are equal (1 cc = 1 ml)

Chapter Highlights

1. Water is necessary for all body processes.
2. Edema or dehydration can occur when there is a fluid imbalance in the body.
3. An extremity that is swollen with edema should be elevated when possible.
4. The most common cause of dehydration in the elderly resident is not drinking enough fluid.
5. Remind and encourage residents to drink fluids.
6. A resident who is not drinking enough may receive fluids through an NG tube, a G tube, or an IV.
7. Use a graduate to measure fluids accurately.
8. I&O must be recorded accurately.
9. Encourage the resident and visitors to help with I&O.
10. Solid foods that melt at room temperature are counted as fluid intake.
11. Urinary output is measured after each voiding.
12. A urinary drainage bag is emptied, measured, and recorded at the end of every shift.
13. 30 cc fluid = 1 oz

VOCABULARY REVIEW

Fill in the blanks with the vocabulary term that best completes the sentence.

1. The condition of having less than the normal amount of fluid in the body is called _____.

2. A/An _____ is a catheter that is left in place to drain urine from the body.

3. The accumulation of fluid that causes swelling is called _____.

4. A/An _____ is a container used to measure fluids.

5. _____ is a measurement of all fluids that are taken into the body and all fluids that are eliminated.

6. The amount of fluid in the body is called _____.

7. _____ are food elements that are necessary for metabolism.

8. The ability to move is called _____.

9. A/An _____ is a tube inserted through a surgical opening into the stomach.

10. The _____ is a system of weights and measurements, used in health care, that includes cubic centimeters and milliliters.

CHECK YOUR UNDERSTANDING

The following questions cover the highlights of this chapter. Choose the best answer for each question.

1. The resident's feet are swollen. Which of the following measures would be helpful when the resident is sitting in a chair?
   A. Elevate the feet.
   B. Remove the shoes.
   C. Apply ankle splints.
   D. Remove the footrest.

2. Dry skin, fever, and decreased urinary output are symptoms of
   A. dehydration
   B. edema
   C. aspiration
   D. expectoration

3. Which of the following is *not* an alternative method of hydration?
   A. an NG tube
   B. a G tube
   C. an IV infusion
   D. a Foley catheter

4. Mrs. Iona is on I&O. When should you measure and record fluid intake?
   A. at the end of each shift
   B. whenever you have time
   C. whenever she eats or drinks
   D. every 4 hours

5. A resident drank three 8-oz cans of feeding supplement. What was her total intake in cubic centimeters?
   A. 240 cc   C. 720 cc
   B. 480 cc   D. 960 cc

6. Which of the following foods would be considered fluid and would need to be counted for I&O?
   A. Jello   C. Potato
   B. Bread   D. Cake

7. Fluids located on Mr. Jones's meal tray included 240 cc of milk, 180 cc of coffee, and 90 cc of juice. Mr. Jones drank all the fluids except the juice. What was his total fluid intake?
   A. 410 cc   C. 480 cc
   B. 420 cc   D. 510 cc

8. Two ounces equals how many cubic centimeters (cc)?
   A. 30 cc   B. 50 cc
   B. 40 cc   D. 60 cc

AGE-SPECIFIC TIP

Elderly residents may not drink enough fluids. Remind them frequently and assist as needed.

CULTURALLY SENSITIVE TIP

Ethnic background may influence the resident's preference of beverages. Always ask what the resident would prefer to drink.

EFFECTIVE PROBLEM SOLVING

A resident with edema had an order for "restrict fluids." She became very upset when the nursing assistant brought her a glass with only 60 cc of water in it. She complained of being thirsty and uncomfortable and blamed it on the nursing assistant. The nursing assistant responded, "It's not my fault! I am only trying to help. You'll get sicker if you drink a lot of fluid."

Was the nursing assistant's communication appropriate? If not, what would have been more appropriate?

_____
_____
_____
_____
_____
_____
_____
_____
_____
_____
_____

INTERPERSONAL COMMUNICATION

The nursing assistant is talking to the resident about fluid intake. Check the examples that are appropriate.

_____ "You've only had 300 ccs to drink today."

_____ "Your doctor wants you to be NPO. That means you can't eat or drink anything until 6 P.M."

_____ "You haven't had enough to drink and your doctor told us to force fluids."

_____ "I'm going to empty your water pitcher now. Your doctor wants you to be NPO."

OBSERVING, REPORTING, AND RECORDING

The nursing assistant plays a major role in preventing dehydration. List six signs and symptoms of dehydration that should be observed, reported, and recorded.

_____
_____
_____
_____
_____
_____
_____
_____
_____
_____
_____

EXPLORE MEDIALINK

Check out www.prenhall.com/grubbs for additional chapter-specific interactive study and review activities.

17

ELIMINATION

OBJECTIVES

1. Explain the importance of privacy and positioning when assisting with elimination.

2. Identify infection-control measures to follow when assisting with elimination.

3. List eight guidelines for assisting with elimination.

4. List five guidelines each for assisting the resident to use a bedside commode, a bedpan, and a urinal.

5. List four signs and symptoms of a UTI.

6. Describe the physical and emotional affects of incontinence.

7. List eight guidelines for care of residents with urinary catheters.

8. Identify five guidelines for restorative bladder retraining.

9. List six restorative methods of preventing constipation.

10. List eight guidelines for giving a commercially prepared enema.

11. List six guidelines for providing colostomy care.

12. Perform the procedures described in this chapter.

VOCABULARY

The following words or terms will help you to understand this chapter:

Void	Fracture pan	Fecal impaction
Feces	Foley catheter	Diarrhea
Defecation	Peristalsis	Enema
Incontinence	Colon	Ostomy
Urinal	Flatus	Stoma
Urinary meatus	Constipation	Colostomy
Bedside commode		

Some waste that is produced during body functions is eliminated through the lungs and the skin. However, most waste material is eliminated by the urinary system and the digestive system. Liquid waste, in the form of urine, is eliminated by the urinary system. To eliminate urine is to urinate or **void**. The digestive system eliminates solid waste called **feces**. Other terms for feces include stool, bowel movement, and B.M. The elimination of solid waste is called **defecation**. The lack of control of urine or feces is **incontinence**.

*A*SSISTING THE RESIDENT WITH ELIMINATION

Important restorative measures during resident elimination include privacy, positioning, infection control, and safety. Correct body position allows the organs to be in natural alignment and provides for more efficient elimination. The use of gloves and their proper disposal, and handwashing, are important when assisting residents with elimination. Perform and assist with perineal care as needed. Safety bars and emergency call signals are available in the bathrooms for safety (see Figure 17-1 ■). Raised toilet seats (see Figure 17-2 ■) are restorative devices that may be installed to promote independence by assisting residents who have difficulty rising from chairs. Some residents will need assistance with getting to the bathroom to use the toilet or with other methods of elimination. This information will be included in the

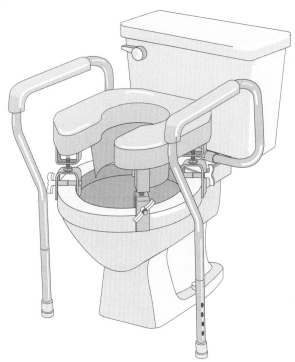

FIGURE 17-2 ■ A raised toilet seat

care plan. Confused residents may need to be reminded to use the bathroom. Confused residents may recognize the need for elimination when they actually see the bathroom. While many people have difficulty urinating or having a bowel movement when another person is present, some residents should not be left alone in the bathroom. In this case you can stand just outside the door. Guidelines for assisting the resident with elimination follow.

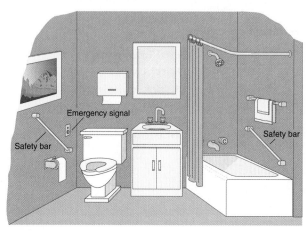

FIGURE 17-1 ■ Safety bars and an emergency signal make the environment safer.

GUIDELINES

ASSISTING WITH ELIMINATION

- Check the resident's care plan for information regarding the method of elimination and assistance that is needed.

- Encourage the resident to use the bathroom rather than the bedpan or bedside commode whenever possible.

- Protect the resident's privacy by asking visitors to leave, closing the door, pulling the curtain, and preventing unnecessary exposure of the body.

- Knock and wait for a response before entering the room or bathroom.

GUIDELINES (Continued)

- Be sure the resident is sitting as upright as possible for urination and bowel movements. Encourage male residents to stand to urinate if possible.

- Wear gloves and dispose of them properly. Wash your hands after removing gloves and follow standard precautions when assisting with elimination.

- Provide toilet paper.

- Remind the resident to use the safety bars and emergency call signal. Indicate their locations and give instructions for their use if necessary.

- Always remain with or near a resident who is on the toilet or bedside commode.

- Ask the resident to signal when finished. Watch for the call signal and answer promptly. Check back frequently.

- Cover bedpans and urinals when carrying them. A **urinal** is a portable container that a male uses when urinating.

- Observe the contents of elimination for abnormalities and report them.

- Empty the contents of elimination into the toilet.

- Wash, rinse, and dry bedpans and store them properly.

- Bedpans and urinals should never be placed on the overbed table.

- Perform or assist with perineal care as needed.

- Always cleanse or wipe with toilet paper away from the **urinary meatus** (the opening of the urinary system).

- Remind or assist the resident to wash his or her hands when elimination is complete.

- Remove gloves, dispose of them properly, and wash your hands.

- Open the privacy curtain and door and invite visitors to return.

- Be sure to record all elimination on the resident's chart.

Using a Bedside Commode

A **bedside commode** is a portable chair with a toilet seat that fits over a container or regular toilet (see Figure 17-3 ■). Sitting on a bedside commode positions the resident correctly for elimination. It may be used for the resident who can get out of bed but is unable to go into the bathroom. Because

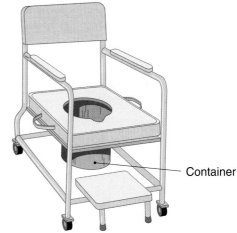

Container

FIGURE 17-3 ■ A bedside commode

the toilet may feel unsafe to the resident who is weak or poorly balanced, the bedside commode may be positioned over the toilet. This promotes the resident's independence.

GUIDELINES

ASSISTING THE RESIDENT TO USE A BEDSIDE COMMODE

- Follow the steps of the procedure for assisting the resident from the bed to a chair.

- Follow guidelines for assisting the resident with elimination.

- If the bedside commode has wheels, lock them before transferring or assisting the resident to transfer to the commode. Leave them locked while the resident remains on the commode.

- Encourage the weak or dizzy resident to hold on to the arms of the bedside commode or to lean against the back of the commode to gain a sense of security.

- Provide toilet paper. Place the call signal in reach and tell the resident to signal when finished.

- If the resident is weak or confused, stay nearby while the commode is used. Provide as much privacy as is possible and safe.

- Watch for the call signal and answer promptly. Check back frequently.

- Wear gloves while assisting with elimination.

(continued)

GUIDELINES (Continued)

- Observe the contents for abnormal findings and report them when finished.
- Empty the bedside commode container into the toilet; cleanse, dry, and return it.
- Keep the bedside commode covered when not in use.
- Bedside commodes may not be taken from resident to resident or from room to room.
- Remove gloves, dispose of them properly, wash your hands, and follow standard precautions.
- Wash the resident's hands when finished. Open the privacy curtain and door and invite visitors to return.
- Record the elimination on the resident's medical record.

Using the Bedpan

A bedpan is a container that the resident who is in bed uses for elimination. The most commonly used are the fracture pan and the regular bedpan (see Figure 17-4 ■). A **fracture pan** is a bedpan with a flat end which is placed under the resident. It is usually more comfortable and has less effect

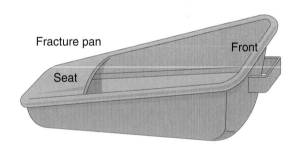

Fracture pan — Front — Seat

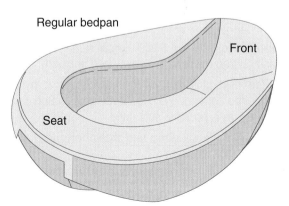

Regular bedpan — Front — Seat

FIGURE 17-4 ■ A fracture pan and a regular bedpan

on body alignment but it holds less urine and can spill easily.

Remember that it is always best to use a restorative approach in all care, including assisting with elimination. Use of the bathroom toilet is normal and should always be encouraged if the resident is able to do so. Having the resident help you to place the bedpan by raising the hips when possible will provide exercise.

GUIDELINES

ASSISTING THE RESIDENT TO USE A BEDPAN

- Follow guidelines for assisting the resident with elimination.
- Provide privacy by asking visitors to leave, closing the door, and pulling the privacy curtain.
- Prevent unnecessary exposure of the resident's body.
- Wear gloves, dispose of them properly, wash your hands, and follow standard precautions.
- While the resident's hips are raised, slide the bedpan under the buttocks (see Figure 17-5A ■). The resident can help by bending her knees and pushing up with her feet.
- If the resident is unable to raise her hips, assist her to turn onto the side while you place the bedpan against the buttocks. Then turn the resident back onto the bedpan (see Figure 17-5B ■).
- Position the bedpan correctly. Placing it too high or too low will create discomfort for the resident.
- After positioning the bedpan, adjust the head of the bed to place the resident in as upright a position as possible (see Figure 17-5C ■).
- Place toilet paper and the call signal within the resident's reach and tell the resident to signal when finished.
- Raise the side rails before leaving.
- Remove your gloves, wash your hands, and leave the room if the resident can be left alone on the bedpan.
- Watch for the signal and answer promptly. Check back frequently.
- Avoid leaving the resident on the pan for a prolonged period to prevent discomfort and skin breakdown.

(continued)

GUIDELINES (Continued)

- Assist the resident to raise her hips, or turn her to the side to remove the bedpan.
- Hold the pan to prevent spilling when turning the resident. A fracture pan will spill easily.
- Cover the pan as soon as you remove it.
- As necessary, assist the resident or wipe the perineal area away from the urinary meatus.
- Observe the contents of the bedpan to report any unusual findings.
- Measure and record the amount of urine if output is being measured.
- Empty the bedpan into the toilet.
- Cleanse, dry, and store the pan. Bedpans should never be placed on the overbed table.
- Assist the resident to wash his hands.
- Remove your gloves, dispose of them properly, and wash your hands.
- Return the bed to a comfortable position, open the privacy curtain and the door, and invite visitors to return.
- Report and record as indicated.

Using the Urinal

A urinal is a container that the male resident uses when urinating. It usually has a handle and is marked with measurements (see Figure 17-6 ■). The resident may stand to use the urinal or he may use it while in bed. Many male residents like to keep the urinal within reach when they are in bed. This allows them to remain independent.

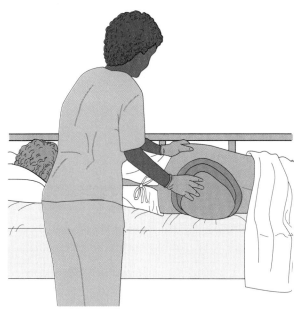

B Place the bedpan against the resident's buttocks and turn her back onto the bedpan.

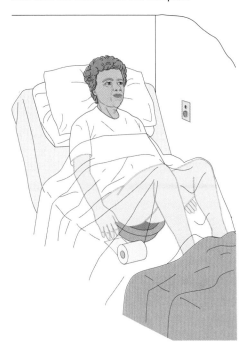

C Adjust the head of the bed so that the resident is in a sitting position.

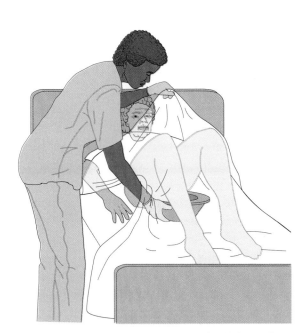

A Slide the bedpan under the resident's buttocks.

FIGURE 17-5 ■ Assisting the resident onto the bedpan

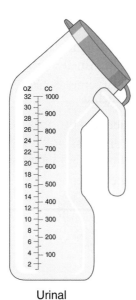

Urinal

FIGURE 17-6 ■ A urinal

- Wear gloves to remove the urinal.
- Observe the contents of the urinal to report abnormal findings.
- Measure and record the amount of urine if the resident is to have output measurements.
- Cover the urinal and empty it in the toilet.
- Cleanse, dry, and store the urinal. Urinals should never be placed on the overbed table.
- Remove your gloves, dispose of them properly, and wash your hands.
- Assist the resident to wash his hands.
- Assist the resident to return to a comfortable and safe position.
- Open the privacy curtain and invite visitors to return.

GUIDELINES

ASSISTING THE RESIDENT TO USE A URINAL

- Follow guidelines for assisting the resident with elimination.
- Provide privacy by asking visitors to leave, closing the door, and pulling the privacy curtain.
- If the resident can stand at the bedside, it is best to use the urinal while standing.
- The resident who cannot stand may use the urinal in the bed or a chair.
- Wear gloves and discard them properly, wash your hands, and follow standard precautions while assisting the resident to use the urinal.
- Assist the resident to an upright position. If the urinal is being used in bed, raise the head of the bed to a sitting position if possible and maintain privacy with the covers.
- Assist the resident to place the urinal if he is unable to do so.
- Provide toilet paper.
- Place the call signal within reach and ask the resident to signal when finished.
- Remove gloves, discard them properly, and wash your hands before leaving the room.
- Watch for the call signal and answer promptly when signaled. Check back frequently.

*U*RINARY ELIMINATION

The major organs of the urinary system are the kidneys, ureters, bladder, and urethra (see Figure 17-7 ■). The kidneys filter waste material from the blood and produce urine. Urine is normally pale yellow or straw-colored and clear, and has a distinct odor. The urine flows from the kidneys, through the ureters, to the bladder, where it is stored until it is eliminated. The average adult bladder can hold about 1,000 cc of urine. When it contains about 350 cc, the brain sends a signal that causes the urge to void (urinate). Urine flows from the bladder, through the urethra, to the outside of the body. The outer opening of the urethra is called the urinary meatus.

Most people are able to control urinary elimination. When they feel the urge to urinate, they can wait until they get to a bathroom. However, if the urge is ignored or delayed too long, the bladder will empty and release the urine.

Common Urinary Problems

A change in urine clarity, color, or odor occurs in many disease conditions. Notify the nurse if you observe any of the following in urinary drainage:

- Blood or mucus
- Stones, gravel, or sediment

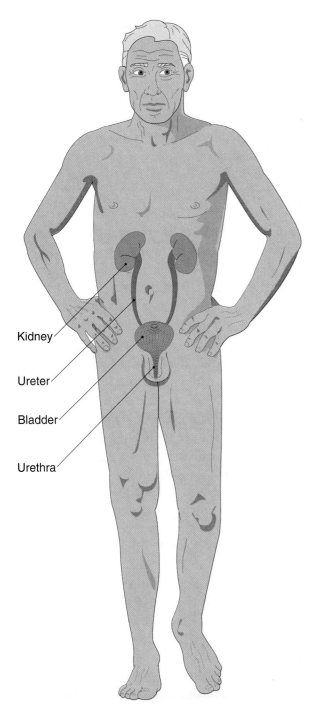

Kidney

Ureter

Bladder

Urethra

FIGURE 17-7 ■ The urinary system

- Dark color or concentration
- Unusual odor

Report residents' complaints of pain, burning, or itching in the perineal area. These symptoms, as well as frequency and urgency, may indicate a urinary tract infection (UTI). Careful observation helps to prevent infection and other urinary problems.

Some of the urinary problems that occur in residents are also a result of aging. Muscles weaken and control of urinary elimination decreases, resulting in urinary incontinence. This may result in other problems, such as

- Urinary frequency—the urge to urinate often while passing only a small amount of urine each time
- Urinary urgency—the sudden, strong urge to urinate
- Difficulty starting to urinate
- Nocturia—the urge to urinate frequently during the night

Although frequency and urgency can occur in any elderly person, they are more common in women. Many elderly men have problems with the prostate gland, which tends to enlarge and cause constriction of the urethra. Nocturia can interfere with rest and sleep and may result in incontinence.

Nursing Measures to Stimulate Urination

Sometimes, a resident may have difficulty urinating. Water can be an effective tool to use in solving this problem. Measures used to stimulate urination include turning on the faucet, placing the resident's fingers in warm water, or pouring warm water over the genitals. Offering a drink of water also may help. Male residents may be able to urinate more easily when they are standing.

The Effects of Urinary Incontinence

Although elderly residents may be incontinent, it is not a normal change of aging. The changes of aging do, however, contribute to urinary incontinence because they make it more difficult to control elimination. Other causes of incontinence include

- Disease
- Confusion
- Medications
- Failure to toilet frequently

Although incontinence affects everyone who is involved, the impact on the resident can be devastating. It can have physical, emotional, and social effects. Incontinence is a major cause of skin breakdown because urine provides a warm, moist environment for pathogens, which may attack the skin or lead to a UTI. It is difficult to maintain healthy skin when a person frequently is wet with urine.

Emotional effects of incontinence include feelings of embarrassment, shame, anger, and frustration. The loss of urinary control can damage self-esteem. Depression is not uncommon. The resident may withdraw and avoid social activities for fear of "having an accident."

Urinary incontinence presents a challenge to infection control. Follow standard precautions and wear gloves when handling soiled linen. Immediate attention should be given to urine spills. Constant effort is necessary to prevent odors and maintain a clean, pleasant environment.

Many times, incontinence can be prevented. Offering toileting at regular intervals helps to establish a routine. Explain to the resident and encourage cooperation. Answer call signals promptly because the elderly resident may not be able to wait. Check residents frequently to see whether they need to go to the bathroom.

Confused residents present a challenge. They may not be able to tell you when they need to urinate or have a bowel movement. If they are ambulatory, they may not be able to locate the bathroom. Remember, it is easier to toilet the resident than to change linen and clothing. Observe carefully for signs that the resident might need to go to the bathroom. These signs may include

- Restlessness
- Fidgeting
- Pulling at clothes or undressing
- Holding or pointing at the genitals
- Crying

If incontinence is a temporary result of an illness or medication, the problem may be relieved by treating the illness or changing the medication. Long-term urinary incontinence may be managed by restorative bladder retraining. That program is explained later in this chapter. Measures to use in treating incontinence are included in the resident's care plan.

The resident who is incontinent must be changed immediately and perineal care must be provided. If the bed is wet, the linen will need to be removed. Place a clean absorbent pad under the resident while you are cleaning the perineal area. Wear gloves and use aseptic technique with soap and water to clean the wet area of the skin. Rinse and dry well. Wiping the urine with a dry towel without washing the skin well leaves microorganisms and chemicals on the skin.

Urinary Tract Infection

A UTI results when pathogens enter the urinary system. A UTI is more common in women because the opening of the urinary system is closer to the opening of the rectum. The female bladder also is closer to the outside of the body.

A UTI may occur because of improper cleansing of the perineal area. Always cleanse from the urinary meatus to the anus when performing perineal care. The procedure for perineal care can be found in Chapter 13. If this procedure is not done correctly, pathogens from the rectal area may be brought forward to the urinary tract.

Most UTIs can be prevented by practicing aseptic technique at all times and by cleaning and changing the incontinent resident immediately.

𝒰RINARY CATHETERS

A urinary catheter is a tube that is inserted through the urethra into the bladder to drain urine. A catheter may be inserted temporarily and then removed after the bladder is drained. Another type of catheter is left in place to drain urine continuously. A urinary catheter that is left in place is called a **Foley catheter** or an indwelling catheter. The nurse inflates a balloon on one end of the catheter (see Figure 17-8 ■) with sterile water. The balloon is inside the bladder and keeps the catheter in place. The other end of the catheter is attached to a drainage tube and bag.

Nursing Care

Urinary catheterization is a procedure that is performed by a nurse or doctor and requires a doctor's order. Nursing assistants do not insert catheters. Special precautions are necessary when caring for a resident with a Foley catheter.

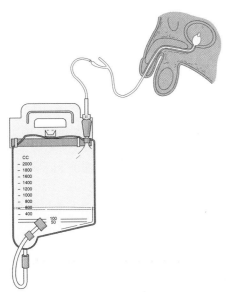

FIGURE 17-8 ■ A balloon is inflated to hold the urinary catheter in place.

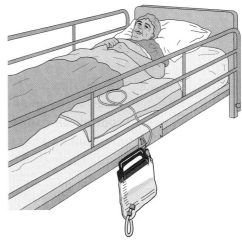

FIGURE 17-9 ■ The drainage bag should be attached to the bedframe.

GUIDELINES

CARE OF RESIDENTS WITH URINARY CATHETERS

- Keep the drainage tube below the level of the bladder. Urine drains from the bladder by gravity.

- Keep the catheter and drainage tubing free of kinks and pressure.

- When assisting a resident to move, be careful that you do not pull on the catheter.

- Keep the urinary drainage system closed and connected as much as possible to prevent infection.

- Report any leaks in the drainage system. If urine can get out, germs can enter through the same opening.

- Attach the drainage bag to the bed frame when the resident is in bed (see Figure 17-9 ■).

- Never attach the bag to the side rail or any other moving part of the bed.

- Do not allow the bag or tubing to touch the floor. Extra tubing can be looped on the bed.

- Attach the drainage bag to a wheelchair below the level of the bladder.

- Use a drainage bag cover, if available.

- Do not disconnect the drainage bag for ambulation.

- If the drainage system must be disconnected from the catheter, protect the open end of the catheter

GUIDELINES (Continued)

and the end of the drainage tube from contamination. Catheter plugs are available for this purpose.

- Use a graduate instead of the markings on the drainage bag to measure urinary output.

Urinary Leg Bags

Some residents may feel more comfortable with a leg bag (see Figure 17-10 ■). This is a small drainage bag that is worn on the upper leg. It may be held in place by a Velcro® band. If the resident is to wear a leg bag, it will be indicated in the care plan.

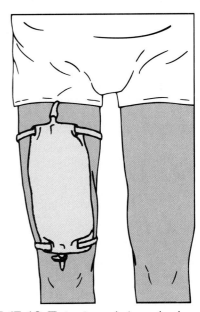

FIGURE 17-10 ■ A urinary drainage leg bag

The risk of infection is increased when a leg bag is used. It holds a smaller amount of urine and must be emptied more often. Each time it is emptied, the urinary tract is exposed to infection. Care must be taken to prevent contamination of the catheter and urinary drainage tubing. Follow facility policy and procedure in changing to and from the use of a leg bag.

Providing Catheter Care

A tube placed into the body creates an entry for germs. Using aseptic technique helps to prevent infection. The resident with a Foley catheter needs special cleansing of the perineal area. This procedure is called catheter care. The catheter care procedure begins with peri-care. Before you cleanse the catheter, the perineal area needs to be clean.

A catheter care kit may be used to perform catheter care. These kits may contain antiseptic, swabs, cotton balls, and disposable gloves. The most common method is washing with soap and water. Follow the policy of your facility.

𝒫ROCEDURE

Providing Catheter Care

■ Beginning Steps

Before any procedure, you always must follow the five basic steps: wash your hands, collect the equipment, identify the resident, explain the procedure, and protect privacy.

👐 Follow Standard Precautions

1. Raise the bed to a correct working height and lock the brakes.
2. Raise the side rail on the opposite side, and lower the rail on the side near you.
3. Assist the resident to a supine position with the legs separated and the knees bent, if possible.
4. Put on disposable gloves.
5. Place a clean protective pad or towel under the resident's buttocks, and drape as you would for perineal care.
6. Perform perineal care, following the procedure found in Chapter 13.
7. Check carefully for dried secretions.
8. Using a clean washcloth, wash the catheter for 3 or 4 inches, beginning at the urinary meatus and washing away from it (see Figure 17-11 ■).
9. Rinse and dry the catheter thoroughly.
10. Replace the protective pad with a clean, dry pad.
11. Make sure there are no kinks in the tubing.
12. Raise the side rail.
13. Empty, rinse, and dry the basin.
14. Remove the gloves and wash your hands.
15. Return equipment and supplies to the proper location.
16. After covering the resident with the top linen, remove the drape covering the resident.

■ Ending Steps

To complete the procedure, perform the following steps:

Make the resident comfortable, positioning in good body alignment. Make the resident safe, placing the call signal within reach, lowering the bed, and raising the side rails, if appropriate. Wash your hands. Record and report the procedure as required.

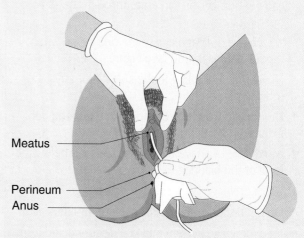

Meatus

Perineum

Anus

FIGURE 17-11 ■ Wash the catheter for 3 or 4 inches, beginning at the urinary meatus.

External Catheter

The doctor may order an external catheter for the incontinent male resident. An external catheter is a soft latex sheath that is applied over the penis. A tube leading from the sheath connects to a urinary drainage bag. The external catheter may have adhesive tape attached to it. There is less chance of infection with this device, and it is more comfortable.

However, the external catheter can present problems. It can irritate the skin or interfere with circulation if not applied correctly. An inch of space must be left between the end of the catheter and the tip of the penis. When tape is used, it is applied spirally and must not completely encircle the penis (see Figure 17-12 ■). Care must be taken not to interfere with circulation or urinary output. There are many different types of external catheters that are kept in place by various methods. Follow the procedural steps used in your facility.

The external catheter should be changed daily and as often as needed. To change the catheter, remove the tape and roll the sheath off the penis. Observe for skin irritation.

Emptying the Urinary Drainage Bag

A resident's urinary drainage bag is emptied at the end of every shift, and the amount of urine measured is recorded on the I&O record.

GUIDELINES

ASSISTING THE RESIDENT WITH AN EXTERNAL CATHETER

- Follow standard precautions and wear disposable gloves.
- Provide perineal care.
- Roll the catheter onto the penis, leaving an inch of space at the end of the penis.
- Apply tape spirally and do not completely encircle the penis with tape.
- Attach the catheter to drainage tubing and bag.

GUIDELINES

EMPTYING A URINARY DRAINAGE BAG

- Follow standard precautions and wear disposable gloves.
- Empty the drainage bag into a graduate (see Figure 17-13 ■).
- Do not use the measurements on the side of the drainage bag, as they may be inaccurate.
- Do not allow the drain to touch the inside of the graduate.
- Do not allow the drainage bag to touch the floor.
- Replace the clamped outlet in the holder.
- Record output immediately.

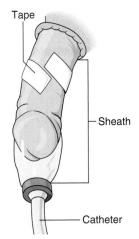

FIGURE 17-12 ■ The external urinary catheter must be applied and taped correctly.

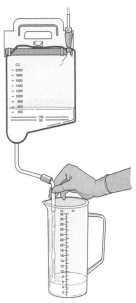

FIGURE 17-13 ■ Empty the urine directly into a graduate.

*R*ESTORATIVE BLADDER RETRAINING

Restorative bladder retraining is a program that is used to prevent incontinence and to restore urinary elimination to as near normal as possible. It involves establishing a routine of emptying the bladder at regular intervals. An individual plan of retraining is developed for each resident in the program. The need to empty the bladder varies from person to person.

GUIDELINES

ASSISTING WITH RESTORATIVE BLADDER RETRAINING

- Help residents to understand what is expected.

- Maintain a positive attitude so that you can influence the residents' attitude in a positive way.

- Build trusting relationships with residents so they will know they can depend on you. This will help them to cooperate.

- To begin retraining, a resident's normal routine of voiding is observed and recorded at 2-hour intervals of scheduled toileting.

- After observing and recording the resident's normal pattern, establish a toileting routine based on that pattern.

- The voiding schedule may be changed as often as necessary as indicated by the resident's needs and episodes of incontinence.

- Offer fluids frequently and encourage residents to drink. The voiding schedule may be changed as indicated by episodes of incontinence and by the resident's needs.

- Answer call signals promptly.

- Toilet residents at regular intervals and as soon as they ask.

- Use methods to stimulate urination.

- Be consistent.

- Record accurately.

- Progress is evaluated after 6 to 8 weeks and periodically thereafter.

- Retraining may be temporarily discontinued after approximately 2 months if the effort is not successful.

Bladder retraining is basically a four-step program of determining normal voiding habits, establishing a regular routine, evaluating results, and adjusting the routine as necessary.

The nursing assistant plays an important role in restorative bladder retraining. Often, it is your attitude that influences the resident's attitude. When you are assigned a resident who is on bladder retraining, his or her schedule must be a priority as you organize your work.

*B*OWEL ELIMINATION

The digestive system breaks down the food into a form that the body can use. It also provides for the elimination of wastes by peristalsis. **Peristalsis** is the muscular contractions that push food through the digestive system. Most of the food is digested in the small intestine, where nutrients are absorbed through the villi into the bloodstream. The nutrients are delivered by the bloodstream to all the cells. Waste material, fluid, and undigested food continue through the digestive system for elimination.

When waste material reaches the **colon** (large intestine) (see Figure 17-14 ■), it is mostly liquid. The purpose of the colon is to remove water

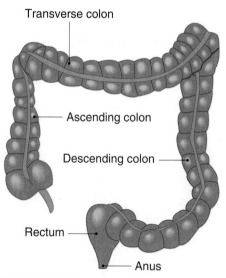

Transverse colon

Ascending colon

Descending colon

Rectum

Anus

FIGURE 17-14 ■ The colon (large intestine)

from the feces for the body's use. Feces is stored in the rectum until nerve receptors signal the urge for defecation. Feces is eliminated from the body through the anus (the outer opening of the rectum). Normally, defecation takes place once every day or two. Feces should be soft-formed and brown-colored. Let the nurse know when a resident's stool is too soft or too hard or has an unusual color. Always report the presence of blood in the stool. Bowel elimination is affected by diet, fluid intake, exercise, and medication. Some foods, such as beans or cabbage, produce **flatus** (gas or air expelled from the digestive system).

COMMON PROBLEMS OF BOWEL ELIMINATION

Constipation

The most common problem of bowel elimination is constipation. **Constipation** is the passage of hard, dry stool. Hard, dry stool collects in the rectum because it cannot pass easily through the anus. To have a bowel movement, a person who is constipated has to strain, which may cause pain or bleeding from the rectum.

Constipation can be caused by any of the following:

- Low fluid intake
- Lack of exercise
- Eating the wrong foods
- Ignoring the urge to defecate
- Medication
- Disease

Many elderly people suffer from constipation. It can be caused by any of the situations listed above or may be related to some of the changes of aging. Peristalsis slows, allowing the colon to absorb more water from the stool. The result is hard, dry feces.

Constipation may be treated with laxatives, suppositories, or enemas. However, the best plan is to prevent constipation. Restorative methods to prevent constipation include the following:

- Increase fluid intake.
- Increase activity and exercise.
- Offer foods, such as whole-grain cereals, that stimulate peristalsis.
- Answer call signals promptly, and assist the resident as needed.
- Observe and record bowel movements, noting the color, amount, and consistency (hard or soft).
- Remind the resident to toilet as needed.

The methods used to prevent constipation will be included on the resident's care plan.

Constipation that is not relieved can result in an impaction. A **fecal impaction** is a large amount of hard, dry waste material. It often is too large to be expelled from the rectum. The resident with a fecal impaction may complain of pain or nausea. The abdomen may appear swollen and hard. Smears of stool may be noticed on clothing or linen. Dark liquid feces may leak from the anus. Don't assume that this is a symptom of diarrhea, because it may be liquid stool going around the large mass of solid stool. An impaction may affect urinary elimination because of pressure exerted on the bladder by the mass of stool. Always report these signs and symptoms to the nurse. Impaction is a serious complication that may lead to bowel obstruction and prevent elimination of wastes. Enemas may be given for a fecal impaction, or it may have to be removed manually by the nurse.

Diarrhea

Diarrhea is loose, watery stool. It occurs when peristalsis pushes food too rapidly through the intestines. This results in insufficient time for the colon to absorb water, so the feces remains very liquid. Diarrhea can be caused by food, medication, infection, or other diseases. It can be very serious for the frail, elderly resident because loss of water can result in dehydration. Diarrhea requires immediate medical attention to find the cause and to treat the condition.

The resident with diarrhea will need to defecate frequently and urgently. Bowel incontinence may occur. Answer call signals promptly, and provide toileting when needed. Thorough cleansing of the rectal and perineal areas is important to prevent skin damage. Empty bedpans immediately to reduce odor and prevent the spread of infection. Wear gloves whenever there is a possibility of contact with feces, and use aseptic technique at all times. Report each occurrence of diarrhea to the nurse. Record the time, amount, and frequency of the diarrhea.

Fecal Incontinence

Fecal incontinence is the inability to control bowel movements. It can be caused by poor muscle tone, a change in peristalsis, or nervous system damage. Confusion is frequently the cause of incontinence in the elderly resident. Confused residents may not be able to understand and respond correctly to the urge to defecate. They may not be aware that the need to empty the rectum has been signaled.

An illness, such as infectious diarrhea, may cause temporary incontinence. Usually, the incontinence stops when the illness is brought under control. Long-term fecal incontinence is best treated by restorative bowel retraining.

RESTORATIVE BOWEL RETRAINING

The goal of restorative bowel retraining is to prevent fecal incontinence, constipation, and other bowel problems. The retraining program usually includes increased activity, adequate fluid intake, and a high-fiber diet. The bowel may be stimulated by using a combination of stool softeners, laxatives, suppositories, or enemas. Although the nurse is responsible for carrying out the treatment, you may be asked to assist. Bowel retraining may take several weeks to accomplish.

GUIDELINES

ASSISTING WITH RESTORATIVE BOWEL RETRAINING

- The bowel retraining program is individualized to meet the needs of each participating resident.
- Offer fluids frequently and encourage the resident to drink.
- Encourage the resident to eat high-fiber foods that are served.
- Assist the resident with toileting at regular intervals and encourage use of the bathroom for defecation.

GUIDELINES (Continued)

- Ensure an upright position for defecation. This position assists the emptying of the bowel.
- Bowel function is evaluated.
- Stool consistency should be normalized. Observe and report abnormal consistency.
- Observe to determine the resident's normal pattern of defecation.
- Establish a schedule for defecation.
- The bowel is stimulated to empty on schedule.
- Encourage ambulation and other physical activity. Perform ROM exercises if ordered.
- Be alert for signs that indicate a need to defecate. These may include complaints of fullness, abdominal cramps, goose bumps, holding the abdomen, frowning, crying, and restlessness.
- Answer call signals promptly and offer toileting immediately if the resident asks or if signs indicate the need.
- Record accurately.

The nursing assistant can help to make restorative bowel retraining successful. Develop a positive attitude, and let the resident know that you believe it will work. Remember, your expectation of success will help the resident to feel more confident.

ENEMAS

An **enema** is the introduction of fluid into the rectum and colon. Enemas are used to remove feces and empty the lower bowel. Some X-ray tests require the bowel to be empty. The doctor may order an enema to relieve constipation or an impaction. The two basic types of enemas are cleansing enemas and commercially prepared enemas.

Cleansing Enemas

A cleansing enema must be prepared before it is given. The doctor orders the type of solution to use. The solution may be plain tap water (1,000 cc), soap suds (1,000 cc water and 5 cc liquid soap), or saline (1,000 cc water and 2 teaspoons salt). The water temperature for the enema solution should be 105°F (40.5°C).

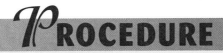

Giving a Cleansing Enema

■ The Beginning Steps

Before any procedure you must always follow the five basic steps: wash your hands, collect the equipment, identify the resident, explain the procedure, and provide privacy.

🖐 Follow Standard Precautions

1. Raise the bed to a comfortable working height and lock the wheels.
2. Raise the side rail on the opposite side, and lower the rail on the side nearest you.
3. Assist the resident into the left-sided Sims' position (see Figure 17-15A ■), and cover with a bath blanket.
4. Place an IV pole beside the bed, and raise the side rail.
5. Clamp the enema tube, and prepare the solution that is ordered, usually to 105°F (40.5°C).
6. Allow a small amount of solution to run through the tubing. Clamp the tubing.
7. Hang the enema bag on the IV pole with the tubing at the bottom. Make sure that the enema bag is no more than 12 inches above the anus (see Figure 17-15B ■).
8. Wash your hands and put on disposable gloves.
9. Lower the side rail, and uncover the resident enough to expose the anus.
10. Place the disposable bed protector under the resident's buttocks. Place the bedpan close to the resident.
11. Lubricate 4 inches of the tip of the enema tubing.
12. Ask the resident to breathe deeply during the procedure to help relieve cramps.
13. With one hand, lift the upper buttock to expose the anus. With the other hand, insert the tip of the tubing into the rectum (see Figure 17-15C ■).
14. Rotate the tubing 2 to 4 inches into the rectum. Stop if you feel resistance or the resident complains of pain. If this happens, clamp the tubing and call the nurse.
15. Allow the solution to flow slowly into the rectum. If the resident complains of cramping, clamp the tubing

and stop for a minute or so. Encourage the resident to take as much of the solution as possible.

16. When the solution is almost gone, clamp the tubing and remove the tip from the rectum. Place the tip of the tubing into the empty enema bag. Do not let it contaminate you or the linens.
17. Ask the resident to hold the solution as long as possible.
18. Assist the resident onto the bedpan or bedside commode or into the bathroom.
19. Place toilet paper and the call signal within reach. Ask the resident not to flush the toilet when finished.
20. Discard the disposable equipment and clean the area.
21. Remove your gloves and wash your hands.
22. If the resident can be left alone, leave the room for a few minutes. Remind the resident to use the call signal. Check back frequently.
23. When the resident is through, put on gloves and assist the resident to clean the perineal area and remove the bed protector. Assist the resident from the pan.
24. Empty the bedpan and observe the enema results for amount, color, and consistency. Clean the bedpan and put it away. Check the contents of the toilet if the resident was in the bathroom.
25. Remove your gloves and wash your hands.
26. Assist the resident with handwashing.
27. Remove the bath blanket, and open the window covering if the resident desires.
28. Return equipment to its proper place.

■ Ending Steps

To complete the procedure, perform the following steps:

Make the resident comfortable, positioning in good body alignment. Make the resident safe, placing the call signal within reach, lowering the bed, and raising the side rails, if appropriate. Wash your hands. Record and report the procedure as required.

(continued)

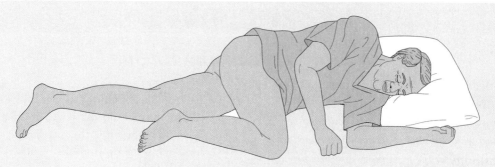

A Assist the resident into a left Sim's position.

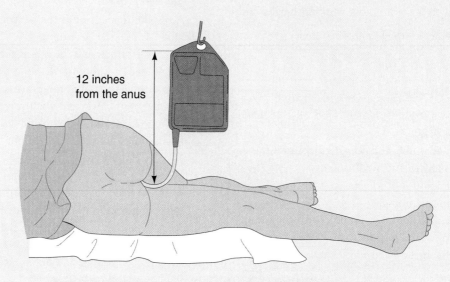

12 inches
from the anus

B The enema bag should be no more than 12 inches from the anus.

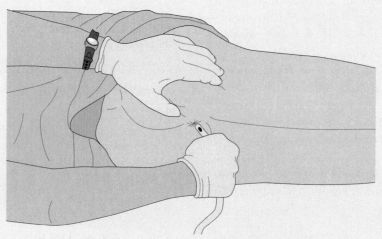

C Insert the tip of the tubing into the rectum.

FIGURE 17-15 ■ Giving a cleansing enema.

Most facilities have disposable enema kits. The kit usually contains an enema bag, tubing with a clamp, and a bed protector. Some kits may contain a package of liquid soap or salt. If the tubing is not already lubricated, a lubricant will be necessary. A bedpan and toilet paper will be needed.

Many long-term care facilities do not allow nursing assistants to give cleansing enemas. It is your responsibility to know the policy of the facility where you work.

Commercially Prepared Enemas

The commercially prepared enema (see Figure 17-16A ■) comes prepackaged and ready to use. The most common type is a disposable plastic bottle filled with solution. The tip of the bottle is lubricated and inserted into the rectum. The bottle is squeezed and rolled from the bottom until all the solution has been given. The directions for giving the enema usually are found on the container. Some facilities do not allow nursing assistants to give commercially prepared enemas. It is your responsibility to know the policy of the facility where you work.

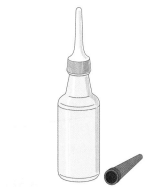

A A commercially prepared enema.

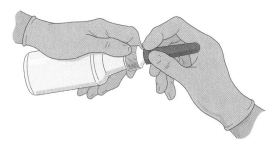

B Remove the cover from the tip of the bottle.

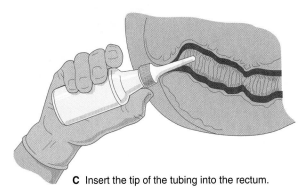

C Insert the tip of the tubing into the rectum.

FIGURE 17-16 ■ Using a commercially prepared enema.

> ## GUIDELINES
>
> ### GIVING A COMMERCIALLY PREPARED ENEMA
>
> - Collect your equipment before you begin.
> - Follow standard precautions and wear disposable gloves.
> - Position the resident on the left side.
> - Remove the protective cover from the tip of the squeeze bottle (see Figure 17-16B ■).
> - Gently insert the lubricated tip two inches into the rectum (see Figure 17-16C ■).
> - Squeeze and roll the bottle from the bottom until all the solution is used.
> - Place the squeeze bottle, tip first, into its original container and discard.
> - Encourage the resident to hold the solution as long as possible.
> - Record the procedure and report your observations.

Giving a commercially prepared enema is similar to the procedure for giving a cleansing enema. The steps for maintaining privacy, protecting bed linens, positioning, and asepsis are the same.

The oil-retention enema also may be commercially prepared. The primary purpose of this type of enema is to soften and lubricate stool. This makes defecation easier and helps relieve constipation. The oil retention enema is given like any other commercially prepared enema. The solution should be retained long enough for the oil to soften the stool. Even though you may not give the enema, you will care for the resident after the procedure. Encourage the resident to lie quietly and hold the solution as long as possible.

OSTOMIES

An **ostomy** is a surgical opening into the body. Some ostomies involve a surgical opening through the abdominal wall into the intestines or urinary tract. The mouth or opening of the ostomy is called a **stoma**. An ostomy is necessary when disease or injury prevents normal elimination. An ostomy may be permanent or temporary, and an appliance may be worn to collect the waste material. This may include a bag that fits over the stoma and supplies to keep the bag in place. There are many types of ostomy appliances (see Figure 17-17 ■). The type used depends on the size and location of the stoma as well as the resident's personal preference. This information

is a part of the resident's plan of care. Some ostomies do not require an appliance. A gauze or large Band-Aid® may be placed over the stoma.

Psychosocial Considerations

The resident with an ostomy may have feelings of anxiety, and embarrassment. Having an artificial opening in the body affects the self-image. The change in body image can lead to depression and social withdrawal. These reactions will affect independence and self-esteem. This is especially true when the ostomy surgery was fairly recent. As time passes, most people adjust to the ostomy both physically and emotionally. They usually learn to care for their own ostomy and continue to live normal lives.

As a nursing assistant, you can help the resident adjust to the ostomy. Be familiar with the problems listed in the care plan. Encourage the resident to express feelings, and listen attentively. Refer questions that you cannot answer to the nurse. Allow the resident to do as much of the ostomy care as possible. This helps build confidence and promote independence.

Colostomy

A **colostomy** is a surgical opening into the colon. A section of the colon is brought to the surface of the abdomen for defecation. Feces and flatus are eliminated from the body through the stoma.

The consistency of feces from the colostomy depends on its location in the colon (see Figure 17-18 ■). Water is removed from the feces as it moves through the colon. If the colostomy is near the beginning of the colon, the feces will be watery. The nearer the colostomy is to the rectum, the more normal the feces will appear.

The colostomy appliance may develop an odor. Proper hygiene and asepsis help to eliminate unpleasant odors. Wear gloves and follow standard precautions when caring for the ostomy. The bag should be emptied every time soiling occurs. It should be cleaned or replaced immediately.

Be aware of your feelings while providing care for the resident with an ostomy. The resident will be aware of your reactions. If you care for the ostomy in a comfortable manner, you will help the resident to feel more relaxed.

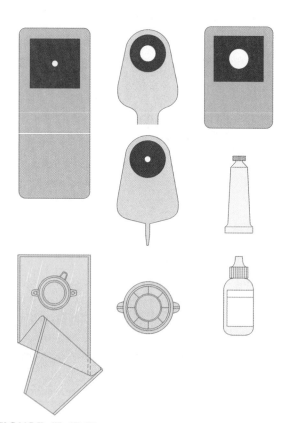

FIGURE 17-17 ■ Ostomy appliances

Sigmoid colostomy	Descending colostomy	Transverse (single barrel)	Transverse (double barrel)	Transverse-loop colostomy

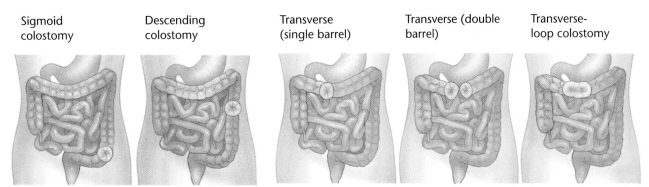

FIGURE 17-18 ■ Examples of colostomy stoma locations

Providing Colostomy Care

Colostomy care should be provided every time the resident has a bowel movement. The care might involve emptying and cleaning the bag or changing the entire appliance. Check with the nurse or the care plan to determine what care is necessary for each resident with a colostomy.

Providing skin care is very important for the resident with an ostomy. The skin around the stoma may become irritated, especially if bowel contents contact the abdominal skin. Many ostomy appliances use adhesive to secure the appliance and prevent leaking, yet the adhesive can irritate the skin. Proper cleaning and emptying of the ostomy appliance help to prevent complications. Always observe the skin around the stoma and report any signs of irritation to the nurse.

The procedure for providing colostomy care depends upon the type of appliance that is used. A belt with an attached bag that fits over the stoma may be worn. Sometimes, an adhesive wafer is applied to the skin around the stoma. The bag is attached to the wafer. Some bags are emptied and discarded after each bowel movement. Others are emptied and cleaned each time. The type of appliance required will be noted in the care plan.

Bowel and bladder elimination are private and personal body functions. Privacy, infection control, and careful observation are very important restorative measures in urinary and bowel care. Sensitivity to the resident's emotional needs must be combined with thorough and consistent physical care to maintain healthy elimination for the elderly resident.

GUIDELINES

PROVIDING COLOSTOMY CARE

- Follow standard precautions and wear gloves.
- Carefully and gently remove appliances that are applied to the skin.
- Empty and clean a reusable bag after each bowel movement.
- Observe the skin around the stoma for redness and irritation and report these to the nurse.
- Use lubricant, skin protector, or skin cream around the stoma, as ordered.
- Attach appliances securely to prevent leaking.
- Clean the reusable bag with soap and water.
- Fasten the clamp securely when you are finished.
- Observe the contents of the bag. Record and report as necessary.
- Wipe around the stoma with toilet tissue to remove feces. Use soap and water to clean around the stoma, unless otherwise ordered.
- Use the following steps to apply an adhesive wafer around the stoma.

  Step 1. Cut the hole in the center of the wafer 1/8 inch larger than the stoma (see Figure 17-19A ■).

  Step 2. Apply adhesive stoma paste around the stoma, as ordered.

  Step 3. Peel the backing from the wafer (see Figure 17-19B ■).

  Step 4. Place wafer, adhesive side down, over the stoma.

  Step 5. Attach a clean bag to the wafer (see Figure 17-19C ■).

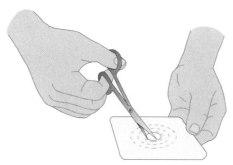

A Cut the hole in the center of the wafer 1/8 inch larger than the stoma.

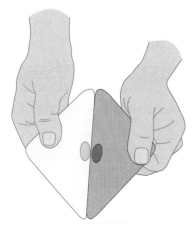

B Peel the backing from the wafer.

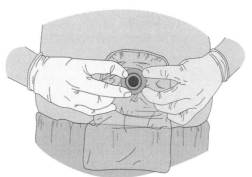

C Place the wafer over the stoma and attach a clean bag.

FIGURE 17-19 ■ Applying an adhesive wafer around a colostomy stoma.

CHAPTER HIGHLIGHTS

1. Whenever possible, the resident should go to the bathroom for elimination.
2. Do not leave a weak or confused resident alone on the toilet or bedside commode.
3. Empty and clean the bedpan and the urinal promptly after every use.
4. Urinary urgency and frequency may occur in elderly residents.
5. Incontinence affects the resident physically and emotionally.
6. The resident who is incontinent must be changed immediately.
7. Follow standard precautions and wear gloves when appropriate.
8. Always clean from the urinary meatus to the rectum.
9. Always keep the urinary drainage bag below the level of the bladder.
10. Urinary drainage systems should be left closed and connected as much as possible to prevent contamination.
11. Careful observation helps to prevent infection and other urinary problems.
12. Restorative bladder retraining involves establishing a routine of emptying the bladder at regular intervals.
13. Bowel and bladder retraining must be consistent.
14. Constipation often can be prevented by increasing fluids and exercise.
15. Recording information accurately and completely is necessary to evaluate bowel and bladder retraining.
16. Encourage the resident who has had an enema to hold the solution as long as possible.
17. The resident may feel embarrassed or depressed about having an ostomy.
18. Ostomy care should be provided every time the resident has a bowel movement.

VOCABULARY REVIEW

Fill in the blanks with the vocabulary that best completes the sentence.

1. The lack of control of urine or feces is _____.

2. Gas or air expelled from the digestive system is _____.

3. _____ is the elimination of solid waste.

4. A/an _____ is the introduction of fluid into the rectum or colon.

5. A/an _____ is a surgical opening into the body.

6. A surgical opening into the colon is called a/an _____.

7. A/an _____ is a bedpan with a flat end that is placed under the resident.

8. A portable chair with a toilet seat that fits over a container or regular toilet is a/an _____ _____.

9. _____ is the passage of hard, dry stool.

10. _____ is loose, watery stool.

CHECK YOUR UNDERSTANDING

The following questions cover the highlights of this chapter. Choose the best answer for each question.

1. Which of the following is the *most* restorative measure for assisting an ambulatory resident with elimination?
   A. Assist him to a bedside commode.
   B. Assist him into the bathroom.
   C. Place him on a bedpan.
   D. Place an incontinence pad on the bed.

2. Which of the following actions is safest for a resident using a bedside commode?
   A. Stay near the resident.
   B. Restrain the resident to the commode.
   C. Leave the resident alone.
   D. Ask the resident's family to stay.

3. You are told to place a resident on the bedpan, but she is unable to raise her hips. What will you do?
   A. Place an incontinence pad under her.
   B. Get her out of bed to a bedside commode.
   C. Tell the nurse she can't get on the bedpan.
   D. Assist her to turn onto her side, and position the bedpan.

4. What procedure should be done when you begin catheter care?
   A. Vital signs
   B. An enema
   C. Perineal care
   D. Colostomy care

5. The most important component of a successful bowel or bladder training program is
   A. Use of the bedpan
   B. Cooperation and effort of the staff
   C. Use of a catheter
   D. Making the resident hold the urine or feces

6. The urge to urinate frequently during the night is called
   A. hesitancy
   B. constipation
   C. nocturia
   D. peristalsis

7. You changed the incontinent resident 30 minutes ago, and he is wet again. What should you do?
   A. Tell him he'll have to wait awhile.
   B. Remind him that you just finished changing him.
   C. Change him immediately.
   D. Pretend not to notice.

COMMUNICATION CENTRAL

AGE-SPECIFIC TIP

Changes of aging in the digestive system may cause the elderly resident to experience discomfort. Be aware of signs and symptoms of digestive problems and ask the resident specific questions.

CULTURALLY SENSITIVE TIP

Residents of any culture may feel embarrassed by colostomy care. Be aware of your comments and facial expressions when providing colostomy care.

EFFECTIVE PROBLEM SOLVING

Mrs. Bowen has visitors in her room. The nursing assistant is completing her assignment sheet and says to Mrs. Bowen in front of her visitors, "Have you had a good bowel movement today?" Was the nursing assistant's communication appropriate? If not, what would have been more appropriate?

_____

_____

_____

_____

_____

_____

_____

_____

_____

_____

INTERPERSONAL COMMUNICATION

Fill in the blanks.

The resident who is unable to speak may indicate the need to go to the bathroom by _____, _____, or _____.

OBSERVING, REPORTING, AND RECORDING

The resident has a Foley catheter. You observe that the urine level in the drainage bag has not increased in 3 hours. What should you do?

_____

_____

_____

_____

_____

_____

_____

_____

_____

_____

_____

_____

_____

EXPLORE MEDIALINK

Check out www.prenhall.com/grubbs for additional chapter-specific interactive study and review activities.

18

ADDITIONAL CARE AND PROCEDURES

OBJECTIVES

1. List 10 guidelines for care of the resident receiving oxygen.
2. Identify eight guidelines for cast care.
3. List four guidelines for accurate weight measurement.
4. Explain how to measure the height of a resident who cannot stand.
5. List four guidelines for straining urine.
6. Identify six general guidelines for collecting specimens.
7. List five guidelines for collecting a stool specimen.
8. List two purposes of a vaginal irrigation.
9. Identify the purpose of elastic support hose and bandages.
10. Identify 10 general guidelines for heat and cold applications.
11. Perform the procedures described in this chapter.

VOCABULARY

The following words or terms will help you to understand this chapter:

Oxygen
Oxygen concentrator
Dyspnea

Sputum
Fracture
Specimen

Stool
Expectorate

This chapter contains additional procedures that are not done as part of routine care. In some facilities, they may be performed by nurses. It is your responsibility to know your facility's policy in regard to these procedures.

CARE OF THE RESIDENT RECEIVING OXYGEN

One of the main purposes of respirations is to obtain **oxygen** (a gas) from the air. An illness or injury may interfere with the respiratory process and decrease the amount of oxygen in the body. The doctor may order additional oxygen for a resident who needs it. The method, rate, and length of oxygen administration are indicated in the doctor's order.

Many methods of oxygen administration are available. These include the mask, cannula (prongs), nasal catheter, and tent (see Figure 18-1 ■). The type of device is ordered by the doctor. Nursing assistants may not begin, discontinue, or adjust the flow rate of oxygen. However, you need to understand how it is administered because you will care for residents receiving oxygen. In many facilities, nursing assistants are responsible for the care of oxygen equipment. Follow the policy of the facility where you work.

Oxygen may be administered from piped-in wall outlets, tanks, and concentrators. Oxygen from tanks or wall outlets is regulated by a flow gauge. Although it may not be your responsibility to adjust the flow, your observation, awareness, and reporting of changes in the flow gauge are important

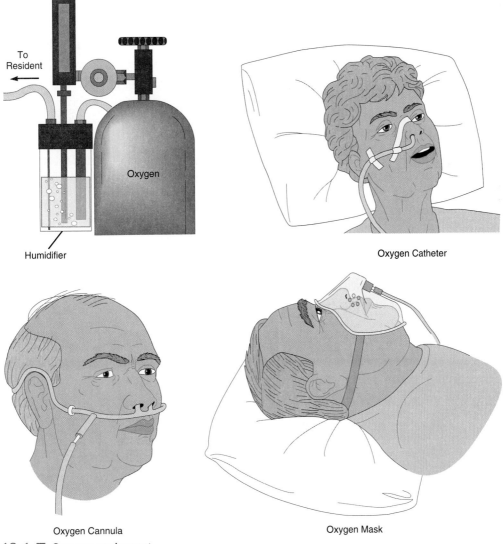

To Resident

Oxygen

Humidifier

Oxygen Catheter

Oxygen Cannula

Oxygen Mask

FIGURE 18-1 ■ Oxygen equipment

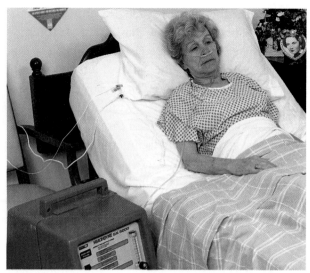

FIGURE 18-2 ■ Oxygen may be supplied to the resident through an oxygen concentrator.

to the resident's well-being. If a tank is used, be observant of the pressure gauge. This gauge indicates the amount of oxygen that remains in the tank so that staff members will know when a new supply tank is needed. Many long-term care facilities use concentrators to supply oxygen. An **oxygen concentrator** is a portable machine that pulls oxygen from the air and supplies it to the resident in a concentrated form (see Figure 18-2 ■).

Because oxygen is drying, it may be passed through moisture before reaching the resident. The device that provides moisture is a humidifier, in which oxygen bubbles through water. It may be your responsibility to keep water in the humidifier at the proper level.

Oxygen supports fire. An "oxygen in use" sign is placed in the resident's room. Check with the nurse before using any electrical equipment in the room. The resident and visitors must be advised of the safety precautions.

The resident who requires oxygen administration has increased needs. **Dyspnea** (difficult or labored breathing) is tiring and uncomfortable. The resident may perspire heavily and may become too warm or too cool. Finding a comfortable position that eases breathing can be difficult. Dizziness may occur and interfere with safety.

Coughing may produce mucous or **sputum** (mucus from the lungs). Because this material may be infectious, care must be taken to prevent contamination. Provide a convenient container for the

resident to dispose of used tissues, avoid handling contaminated tissues without gloves, and follow standard precautions.

Experiencing dyspnea is frightening. Even though the administration of oxygen is helpful, it can increase fear and cause discomfort. Maintaining the resident's independence, function, and comfort requires time, effort, and empathy. You must remain very observant, aware of, and sensitive to the resident's physical and emotional needs.

GUIDELINES

ASSISTING THE RESIDENT WHO IS RECEIVING OXYGEN

- Follow rules of safety when oxygen is in use.
- Recognize the resident's fear and suffering. Provide emotional support and reassurance as needed.
- Check on the resident frequently.
- Recognize the resident's limitations of physical and emotional energy and strength.
- Activity may require frequent periods of rest.
- Use standard precautions when in contact with mucus, sputum, and other body fluids.
- Do not handle contaminated tissues without gloves.
- Provide the resident with a bag or container for disposal of tissues.
- Frequent mouth care and lubrication are necessary. Oxygen dries the nose and mouth.
- Observe and relieve pressure on the skin or discomfort caused by oxygen devices.
- Frequent bathing, skin care, and clothing changes may be necessary due to perspiration.
- Adjust the room temperature and clothing as needed for the resident's comfort.
- An upright position often makes breathing easier (see Figure 18-3 ■).
- Allow the resident to sit on the side of the bed before standing to prevent dizziness.
- Observe for dizziness and weakness, and stay with resident as necessary.
- Observe and report changes in gauges and water level.
- Observe and report changes in the resident's condition.

Fowler's position

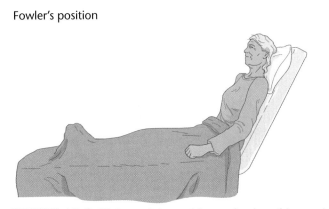

Orthopneic position

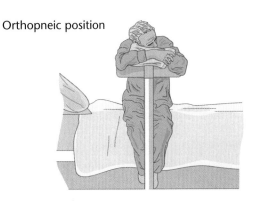

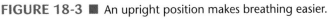

FIGURE 18-3 ■ An upright position makes breathing easier.

CARE OF THE RESIDENT WITH A FRACTURE

A **fracture** is a broken bone. Residents who have a fracture may be treated with a cast, splint, or traction. These treatments are used to immobilize (prevent movement of) the bone to promote proper healing. Restorative care is especially challenging because residents who are immobilized are more dependent on others to meet their needs. Encourage the resident to be as active as possible.

The probability of pressure sores increases when the resident has a fracture. Nutrition, elimination, and exercise may cause additional concern. It may be difficult to provide comfort. Always check with the nurse and obtain specific directions before caring for a resident who has been immobilized. Check the care plan daily.

Residents who have hip fractures or hip surgery must not rotate the affected leg outward. The knee must be kept below the hip, and the resident is not allowed to bend more than 90° from the waist. A special pillow or cushion is used between the resident's legs to support the leg in an abducted position (away from the midline of the body). Measures and precautions for caring for residents with hip fractures or hip surgery are provided in Figure 18-4 ■. Always check with the nurse regarding movement and positioning of the resident with a hip fracture.

Casts, Splints, and Traction

All casts, splints, and traction (see Figure 18-5 ■) require special care for positioning. Skin must be observed carefully for pressure from the appliance or from immobilization. Nursing assistants are not allowed to adjust traction equipment. Do not move, add, or replace any piece of the equipment. Notify the nurse if you observe anything unusual. Observation of equipment, body alignment, and skin problems is the responsibility of the nursing assistant. A new cast requires additional observation and care. Close observation may prevent complications and promote a smoother return to normal function.

GUIDELINES

CAST CARE

- Elevate and support a casted extremity with pillows.
- Observe fingers and toes for color, swelling, or temperature changes that may indicate impaired circulation.
- If the resident complains of numbness, pain, or tingling, report this immediately to the nurse.
- Observe stains or color changes in the cast material. This may indicate bleeding or drainage inside the cast. Report these changes to the nurse.
- Wear gloves and follow standard precautions any time there is a possibility of contact with blood or drainage.
- Report a foul odor to the nurse.
- Taping or padding rough edges of the cast may be necessary. Report any problems to the nurse.
- Keep the cast dry.
- Remind the resident to avoid scratching under the cast.

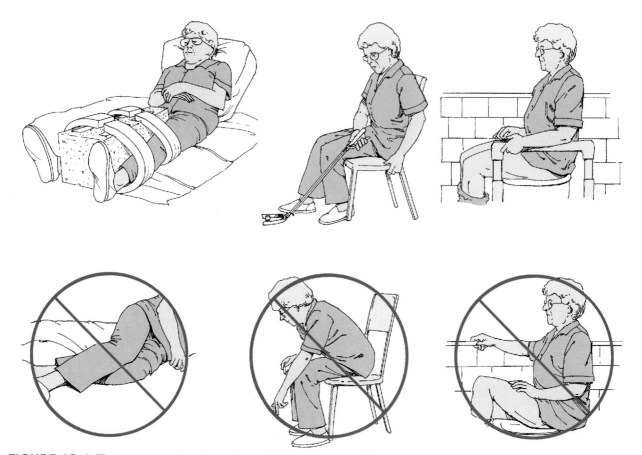

FIGURE 18-4 ■ *Some precautions for patients with hip fractures include:*

- Use an abduction device to keep the fracture in the proper position. Do not allow the patient to lie on his or her side with the legs together. Do not rotate or turn the operated leg outward.
- Have the patient use a device for reaching objects on the floor or shelves. Do not allow the patient to bend forward from the waist more than 90 degrees—to pull up blankets or socks, for example, or to tie shoes. Provide adaptive devices for these purposes.
- Have the patient sit in a high chair. Do not allow the patient to cross his or her legs or raise the knee on the affected side higher than the hip.

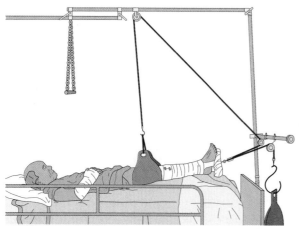

FIGURE 18-5 ■ Residents with casts, splints, and traction require special care.

MEASURING THE RESIDENT'S WEIGHT

Residents usually are weighed on admission to a facility and regularly thereafter. Monthly weighs are routine. Accuracy of measurement is important because weight changes may indicate progress or decline in the resident's condition. Treatments and dietary changes may be ordered as a result of weight measurements.

Types of Scales

Residents may be weighed on the standing balance scale or a bathroom scale. There are many other types of scales available (see Figure 18-6 ■). It is important to protect the resident's safety while

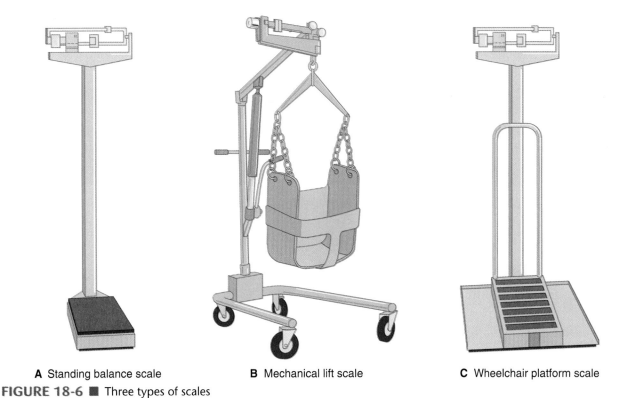

A Standing balance scale   **B** Mechanical lift scale   **C** Wheelchair platform scale

FIGURE 18-6 ■ Three types of scales

obtaining weight measurements. Never leave a resident alone on any type of scale. Always use aseptic practices to prevent the spread of infection. For example, clean linen may be used between the resident's body and the platform of a bed scale and paper towels between the resident's feet and the platform of a standing balance scale. Table 18-1 describes the types of scales commonly used in long-term care. Procedures vary, so check the procedure book for directions on using a specific scale.

TABLE 18-1 TYPES OF SCALES USED IN LONG-TERM CARE FACILITIES		
Type	Description	Use
Bed Scale	A padded platform on wheels that can be adjusted to bed height.	For residents who are unable to get out of bed
Mechanical lift scale	Similar to the mechanical lift used to transfer residents and described in Chapter 11.	For residents who must be lifted to transfer
Chair scale	An armed chair with a footrest that is balanced on a weight mechanism.	For residents too weak to stand
Wheelchair platform scale	A platform on a weight mechanism. Allows the resident to be wheeled onto the scale without getting out of the wheelchair. (The weight of the chair must be subtracted from the total for correct measurement.)	For residents who cannot stand
Standing balance scale	A small platform scale with a balance bar for weight measurement. Often has a height measurement rod as well. The procedure for weighing a resident on a standing balance scale is located on page 254.	For residents who can stand

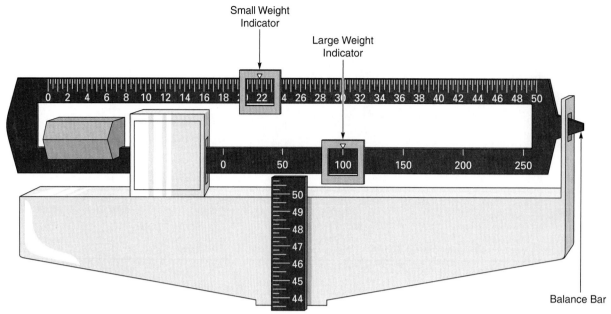

FIGURE 18-7 ■ The scale must be balanced when weighing the resident.

When using a standing balance scale, you must learn how to use the balance bar. Before the resident steps on the scale, set both weight indicators at zero. If the balance bar pointer is not in the middle of the designated area, the balance adjustment must be set. Some scales have a level bar with a bubble that must be floating in the center when balance is obtained. The scale must be balanced for accurate weight measurement (see Figure 18-7 ■).

PROCEDURE

Using a Standing Balance Scale

■ Beginning Steps

Before any procedure, you always must follow the five basic steps: wash your hands, collect the equipment, identify the resident, explain the procedure, and protect privacy.

Follow Standard Precautions

1. Assist the resident to the scale.
2. Balance the scale so that the balance bar is level.
3. Place clean paper towels on the platform.
4. Assist the resident to step out of shoes and onto the center of the scale platform.
5. Adjust the weight indicators until the scale is balanced (see Figure 18-8 ■).
6. Note the resident's weight.
7. Assist the resident off the scale and into shoes.

(continued)

8. Ensure the resident's comfort and safety.
9. Dispose of paper towels and wash your hands.

■ Ending Steps

To complete the procedure, perform the following steps:

Make the resident comfortable, positioning in good body alignment. Make the resident safe, placing the call signal within reach, lowering the bed, and raising the side rails, if appropriate. Wash your hands. Record and report the procedure as required.

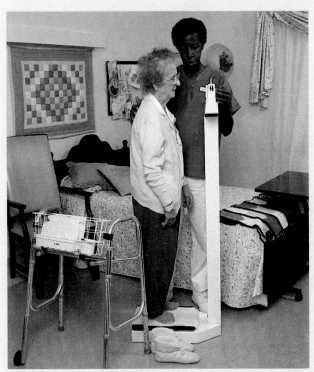

FIGURE 18-8 ■ Weighing the resident on the standing balance scale

𝓜EASURING THE RESIDENT'S HEIGHT

The height of the resident usually is measured on admission. If the resident is able to stand, you may use the height measurement rod that is attached to the standing balance scale. The rod measures the height in inches and fractions of inches. It is calibrated (marked) in 1/4-inch segments (see Figure 18-9 ■). You may be required to record the height in feet and inches. To convert a total number of inches to feet and inches, divide 12 into the total number of inches measured. (There are 12 inches in a foot.) The answer will be the number of feet, and the remainder will be the number of inches in the resident's height. A resident's height may be measured in bed with a tape measure if standing is not possible.

Guidelines are provided to help you correctly measure the height of a resident under varying conditions.

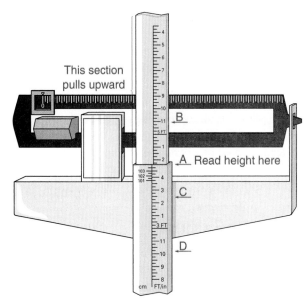

FIGURE 18-9 ■ Reading the height rod

GUIDELINES

MEASURING THE RESIDENT'S HEIGHT ON A STANDING BALANCE SCALE

- Raise the height measurement rod to a level above the resident's head.
- Assist the resident to step up on the scale and stand as straight as possible.
- Lower the height measurement device until it rests flat on the top of the resident's head.
- Note the height and record it after the resident is comfortable and safe.
- Convert the measurement to feet and inches by dividing 12 into the total number of inches indicated on the measurement rod.

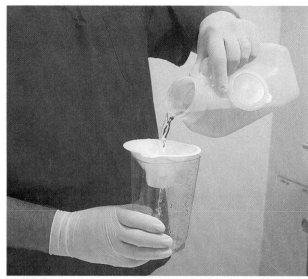

FIGURE 18-10 ■ Pour the urine through a strainer into a graduate.

GUIDELINES

MEASURING THE HEIGHT OF A RESIDENT WHO CANNOT STAND

- Bring a tape measure to the resident's bedside.
- Flatten the bed and place the resident in a supine position (on the back).
- Place a mark on the sheet at the top of the resident's head and another at the bottom of the feet.
- Measure the distance between the marks. This is the resident's height.
- Note the resident's height and record it as soon as possible.
- If the resident has contractures or is unable to lie in a straight position, begin measuring with the tape measure at the top of the head. Continue measuring to the base of the heel, following the curves of the spine and legs.
- Convert the measurement to feet and inches as explained in the previous guideline.

GUIDELINES

STRAINING URINE

- Follow standard precautions and wear gloves.
- Collect all urinary output in a urinal, bedpan, or specimen pan.
- Instruct the resident not to have a bowel movement or to put toilet paper in the urine container.
- Pour the urine through a disposable paper strainer into a graduate (see Figure 18-10 ■).
- If any particles are seen, place the paper strainer in a plastic bag or specimen container.
- Label the specimen and record the date and time of collection.
- Measure and record the urine for I&O if necessary.
- Discard the urine.
- Wash your hands.
- Record the procedure and report your observation. Report to the nurse when the specimen is collected.

STRAINING URINE

It may be necessary to strain the urine for stones, crystals, or other particles. Paper strainers usually are provided for this procedure. Ask the resident to save all urine.

COLLECTING SPECIMENS

A **specimen** is a sample of material from the resident's body. Nursing assistants collect specimens of urine, feces, and sputum. The purpose of collecting specimens is to identify and treat disease. Although collection procedures vary, certain guidelines apply to collecting any specimen.

In the hospital, most specimens are taken directly to the laboratory. However, in the long-term care facility, the specimens usually are taken to the nurses' station. Notify the nurse as soon as you collect the specimen, and take it to the designated area. Follow facility policy for packaging, storing, and labeling specimens.

GUIDELINES

COLLECTING SPECIMENS

- Wear gloves and follow standard precautions (see Figure 18-11A ■).
- Identify and label the specimen container accurately before collecting (see Figure 18-11B ■).

GUIDELINES (Continued)

- Use the correct specimen container.
- Follow the correct procedure for collecting each type of specimen.
- Take the labeled specimen to the designated area as soon as you have collected it.
- Record the procedure and report observations.

Collecting a Urine Specimen

Urine specimens are studied to determine kidney function, infection, and other disease conditions. Urine also may be tested to determine treatment.

ASEPTIC PRACTICES

- Use standard precautions.
- Wash your hands.
- Don't touch the inside of the container.
- Place the lid upside down on a clean surface.
- Clean and dry the bedpan or urinal before collecting the specimen.

A Follow aseptic practices when collecting specimens.

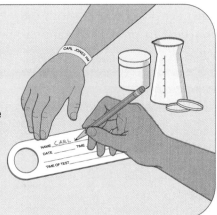

BE ACCURATE...

- Check the resident's identification bracelet.
- Copy the resident's name from the bracelet.
- Print clearly so the label can be read easily.

B Accuracy is necessary in collecting specimens.

FIGURE 18-11 ■ Aseptic practices and accuracy are important when collecting specimens.

PROCEDURE

Collecting a Routine Urine Specimen

■ Beginning Steps

Before any procedure you must always follow the five basic steps: wash your hands, collect the equipment, identify the resident, explain the procedure, and provide privacy.

👋 Follow Standard Precautions

1. Select and label the specimen container.
2. Put on disposable gloves and follow aseptic practices.
3. Ask the resident to urinate into a clean bedpan or urinal. Assist as necessary.
4. Pour the urine from the bedpan or urinal into a clean graduate.
5. Measure the urine if the resident is on I&O.
6. Pour the urine from the graduate into the specimen container. Fill the container three-fourths full, if possible (see Figure 18-12 ■).
7. Place the lid on the container, being careful not to touch the inside.
8. Clean and replace the equipment.
9. Remove the gloves and wash your hands.
10. Assist the resident with handwashing.
11. Ensure the resident's comfort and safety.
12. Take the labeled container to the designated area.

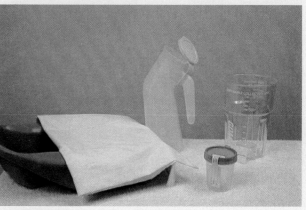

FIGURE 18-12 ■ Pour the urine from the graduate into the specimen container.

■ Ending Steps

To complete the procedure, perform the following steps:

Make the resident comfortable, positioning in good body alignment. Make the resident safe, placing the call signal within reach, lowering the bed, and raising the side rails, if appropriate. Wash your hands. Record and report the procedure as required.

Collecting Urine Specimens

Wash and dry the urinal or bedpan before collecting any urine specimen. Ask the resident not to have a bowel movement or place toilet tissue in the pan. These measures help to prevent contamination of the specimen.

GUIDELINES

COLLECTING A CLEAN-CATCH URINE SPECIMEN

- Wear gloves and follow the guidelines for collecting urine specimens.
- Perform perineal care before collecting the specimen.

GUIDELINES (Continued)

- Ask the resident to begin voiding and then to stop.
- Position the container and ask the resident to begin voiding again.
- Ask the resident to stop voiding, and remove the container when it is three-fourths full.
- Allow the resident to finish voiding.
- Wash your hands.
- Record the procedure and report observations.

Table 18-2 describes the urine specimens most commonly collected in long-term care facilities. Guidelines and procedures are also provided.

TABLE 18-2 TYPES OF URINE SPECIMENS

Name	Purpose	Special Instructions
Routine urine specimen	Routine lab tests. Often done on admission.	Whenever the doctor orders it. No special instructions.
Clean-catch urine specimen (midstream)	Free from contamination. As clean as possible.	Provide perineal care before beginning. Interrupt the flow of urine. Collected between the time the resident begins voiding and the time he stops.
Fresh-fractional urine specimen (double-voided)	Obtain "fresh" urine that has not been stored in the bladder for a long time. Used in diabetic testing.	Voids twice. Use test results from the second voiding. Only a fractional amount needed.
24-Hour urine specimen	Test results on all the urine produced by the body during a 24-hour period.	Timed collection. Save all urine produced after the test begins until it ends 24 hours later. May need to be kept on ice.

GUIDELINES

COLLECTING A FRESH-FRACTIONAL URINE SPECIMEN

- Wear gloves and follow the guidelines for collecting a urine specimen.
- Ask the resident to void at the specified time.
- Save this specimen in case the resident is unable to void again in 30 minutes.
- Return in 30 minutes and ask the resident to void again.
- Explain that you only need a small (fractional) amount of urine.
- If you are performing a diabetic urine test, use the second voiding. It will be more accurate. Use the first voiding only if you were unable to get a second one.
- Let the nurse know if you were unable to get a second voiding.

GUIDELINES (Continued)

- Ask the resident to void at the start time.
- Discard the first voiding because the urine has been in the bladder prior to the beginning of the test.
- Begin the collection after the first voiding.
- Save all the urine for the next 24 hours.
- Save the last voiding when the 24-hour collection ends.
- Pour the urine as soon as it is collected into a large container provided for the test (see Figure 18-13 ■).
- Keep the container chilled, usually in a bucket of ice.
- Refill the ice bucket as necessary.
- Let the nurse know immediately if incontinence, spilling, or accidental disposal of urine has occurred.
- Be aware that if any urine is lost during the 24-hour urine period, the test will be discontinued and restarted.

GUIDELINES

COLLECTING A 24-HOUR URINE SPECIMEN

- Explain to the resident and family that a 24-hour urine test is in progress. Be sure they are aware that all urinary output must be saved.
- A sign may be posted to remind the resident, family, and staff that a test is in progress.
- Note the start and stop times of the collection.

Collecting a Stool Specimen

Stool (feces, bowel movement, BM) is solid waste material from the digestive system. Stool specimens are collected to test for blood, fat, microorganisms, parasites (worms), or other abnormal conditions. When collecting a stool specimen, instruct the resident not to urinate or place toilet tissue in the bedpan. This will contaminate the specimen. Some tests require a warm stool specimen. In

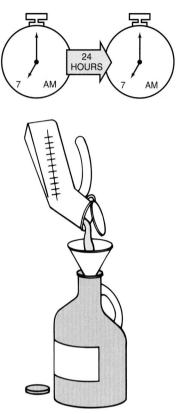

FIGURE 18-13 ■ Collecting a 24-hour urine specimen

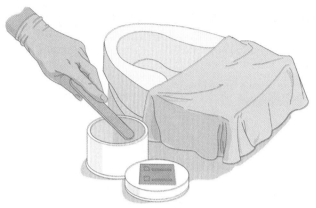

FIGURE 18-14 ■ Use a tongue blade to transfer a stool specimen from a bedpan to the specimen container.

that case, the specimen must go to the laboratory promptly.

Sometimes, stool specimens are ordered to be collected three times. The specimen container is labeled with the appropriate number. Be sure to number the specimen correctly and let the nurse know that it has been collected.

Collecting a Sputum Specimen

Some disease processes cause the respiratory system to produce mucus. Mucus from the lungs or deep in the respiratory system is called "sputum." Sputum is a thick, sticky substance that differs from saliva.

Coughing and bringing up sputum can be difficult and painful for the resident. The resident is asked to cough and **expectorate** (spit) directly into the specimen container. Nursing assistants usually are not asked to collect sputum specimens.

GUIDELINES

COLLECTING A STOOL SPECIMEN

- Wear gloves and follow standard precautions.
- Follow the guidelines for collecting specimens.
- Use a tongue blade to transfer 1 or 2 tablespoons of stool from the bedpan to the specimen container (see Figure 18-14 ■).
- Place the lid on the container without contaminating it.
- Wrap the tongue blade in a paper towel and discard it in the biohazardous waste container.
- Remove gloves and wash your hands.
- Record the procedure and report observations.

GUIDELINES

COLLECTING A SPUTUM SPECIMEN

- Wear gloves and follow standard precautions. Sputum is considered infectious.
- Sputum specimens are easier to collect in the early morning.
- The mouth should be rinsed with plain water before collecting the specimen. Do not use mouthwash.
- Instruct the resident to take three deep breaths and cough.
- The resident should expectorate directly into the container (see Figure 18-15 ■).
- Do not contaminate the container.
- Cover the container immediately.
- Remove gloves and wash your hands.
- Record the procedure and report observations.

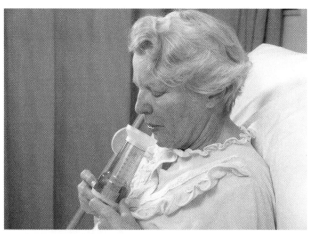

FIGURE 18-15 ■ The resident should expectorate directly into the sputum specimen container.

$\mathcal{D}$IABETIC TESTING FOR SUGAR AND ACETONE

An S&A test is a urine test for sugar and acetone for diabetics. A fresh-fractional urine specimen is needed for an S&A test. It is important that the test be done on fresh urine to obtain results that are as accurate as possible. There are many types of urine tests for diabetes.

The procedure is different for performing each of these tests. Directions for testing the urine and reading the results are on each container. Follow the directions carefully to ensure accuracy.

The reagent on the tablets and strips is poisonous and is affected by light or air. Handle tablets and strips carefully and avoid touching the reagent. When taking a reagent tablet from a bottle, pour the tablet into the lid. Then pour the tablet from the lid into a test tube or place it on a clean paper towel. Container lids should be closed tightly and the containers stored away from direct light.

Today, most facilities test the blood for sugar. In many facilities, urine testing no longer is done. Follow the policy and procedures of the facility where you work.

$\mathcal{V}$AGINAL IRRIGATIONS

The physician may order a vaginal irrigation (douche) to cleanse the vagina or relieve inflammation. A vaginal irrigation is given by allowing a solution to flow into the vagina, after which it returns by the force of gravity. Usually, a douche is used to apply heat or cold or to medicate the vaginal tissues. If the douche contains medication, it must be administered by the nurse. Frequent douches destroy the normal flora of the vagina. These normal flora are microorganisms that exist in the vaginal area and provide protection from other invading microorganisms.

Follow standard precautions and wear gloves when administering a vaginal irrigation.

$\mathcal{P}$ROCEDURE

Administering a Vaginal Irrigation

■ **Beginning Steps**

Before any procedure, you always must follow the five basic steps: wash your hands, gather the equipment, identify the resident, explain the procedure, and provide privacy.

Follow Standard Precautions

1. Ask the resident to urinate.
2. Raise the bed to a comfortable working height, lock the wheels, and lower the side rails on the side nearest you.

3. Cover the resident with a bath blanket and fold the top linen to the foot of the bed.
4. Place a protective pad under the resident's buttocks.
5. Put on gloves, and place the bedpan under the resident.
6. Provide peri-care (see the procedure for giving perineal care). Raise the side rail.
7. Clamp the tubing of the douche kit before pouring solution into the container.
8. Fill the douche container with warm solution, usually at 105°F (40.5°C). Lower the side rail.

(continued)

9. Expel air from the tubing by releasing the clamp and allowing the solution to flow through the nozzle and over the genitalia without allowing the nozzle to touch the vulva.

10. While the solution flows, insert the nozzle 2 to 3 inches into the vagina in an upward and then downward and backward motion (see Figure 18-16 ■).

11. Hold the solution container 12 inches above the vagina while the solution flows.

12. Gently rotate the nozzle.

13. Remove the nozzle after clamping the tubing, and place the nozzle inside the solution container.

14. Ask the resident to sit upright on the bedpan to allow the solution to drain from the vagina.

15. Assist the resident to dry the perineal area.

16. Empty the bedpan and observe the solution. Rinse the pan and put it away.

17. Remove the protective pad and dispose of it.

18. Remove the gloves and wash your hands.

19. Cover the resident with the top linen and raise the side rail.

■ **Ending Steps**

To complete the procedure, perform the following steps:

Make the residents comfortable, positioning in good body alignment. Make the resident safe, placing the call signal

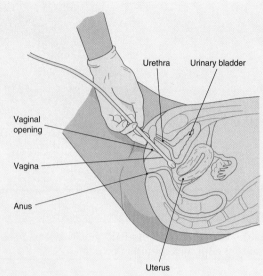

FIGURE 18-16 ■ Insert the douche nozzle 2 to 3 inches into the vagina in an upward and then downward and backward motion.

within reach, lowering the bed, and raising the side rails, if appropriate. Wash your hands. Record and report the procedure as required.

*E*LASTIC SUPPORT HOSE AND BANDAGES

Elastic support hose and bandages often are ordered for residents with heart disease and other circulatory problems or for those with limited mobility. The purpose of support hose and bandages is to

- Improve circulation by exerting pressure on the veins, which promotes blood return to the heart.
- Prevent and treat blood clots.
- Provide comfort and support.

Elastic Support Hose

Elastic support hose also are called "antiembolism stockings" or "T.E.D.® hose." They may be knee-high or full-length (see Figure 18-17 ■), and a variety of sizes are available.

Be sure to use the right size hose for the resident and apply them before the resident gets out of bed.

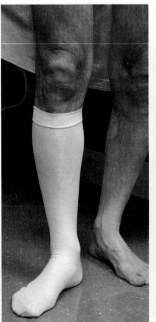
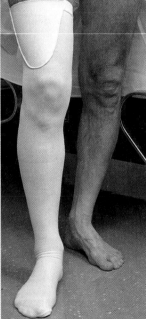

FIGURE 18-17 ■ Elastic support hose

PROCEDURE

Applying Elastic Support Hose

■ Beginning Steps

Before any procedure, you always must follow the five basic steps: wash your hands, collect the equipment, identify the resident, explain the procedure, and protect privacy.

Follow Standard Precautions

1. With side rails up and brakes locked, raise the bed to a comfortable working height.
2. Lower the side rail near you and assist the resident to a supine position.
3. Gather the stocking in your hands as you turn it inside out to the toe.
4. With the foot resting on the bed, insert the resident's toes into the stocking.
5. Support the resident's foot at the heel and handle the leg gently.
6. Slip the front of the stocking over the foot and heel (see Figure 18-18 ■).
7. Pull the stocking snugly and evenly up over the leg. Make sure the stocking is not twisted or wrinkled.
8. Instruct the resident not to roll the stocking partially down.
9. Raise the side rail, lower the bed, and adjust the side rails according to the resident's care plan.
10. Assist the resident out of bed or to a comfortable position in bed.

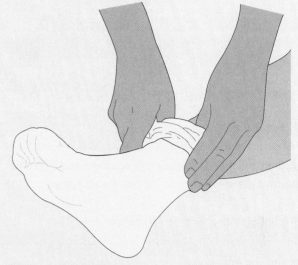

FIGURE 18-18 ■ Slip the front of the stocking over the toes, foot, and heel.

■ Ending Steps

To complete the procedure, perform the following steps:

Make the resident comfortable, positioning in good body alignment. Make the resident safe, placing the call signal within reach, lowering the bed, and raising the side rails, if appropriate. Wash your hands. Record and report the procedure as required. ■

The hose should fit snugly. After the hose are applied, check frequently to see that they are not twisted or wrinkled. Remove the hose at least twice a day and report any discoloration or signs of edema.

Elastic Bandages

Elastic bandages often are called "ACE® bandages." They are strips of elasticized material of varying lengths and widths. Elastic bandages sometimes are used to reduce swelling from a musculoskeletal injury.

The nurse will tell you what area should be bandaged. Begin applying the bandage at the smallest part of the extremity, leaving the fingers or toes exposed. Use as many bandages as you need to cover the area. Check frequently for edema, skin discoloration, or changes in the skin temperature of residents wearing elastic bandages. Reapply bandages if they become loose or wrinkled.

HEAT AND COLD APPLICATIONS

Treatment with heat and cold may be ordered by the physician to reduce swelling, relieve pain, stimulate circulation, and promote healing (see Figure 18-20 ■). Because heat and cold can cause injury, great care and constant attention are necessary in this type of application. Elderly residents may have decreased awareness or sensation of temperature changes and pain. Their skin is fragile and may be injured easily. They are at increased risk of burns. In many facilities, nursing assistants are not responsible for applying heat and cold because of the risk involved. Be sure that you are familiar with the policies of your facility.

Heat and cold applications may be dry or moist. In a dry application, moisture is not in contact with the skin. Dry applications include ice bags, collars or packs, water bottles, heat lamps, and electric, fluid-filled warming pads (often called

PROCEDURE

Applying Elastic Bandages

■ Beginning Steps

Before any procedure, you always must follow the five basic steps: wash your hands, collect the equipment, identify the resident, explain the procedure, and protect privacy.

🖐 Follow Standard Precautions

1. Hold the bandage with the loose end at the bottom of the roll.
2. To anchor the bandage, make two circular turns around the smallest part of the extremity (see Figure 18-19A ■).
3. Make overlapping spiral wraps in an upward direction. Each wrap should overlap about half the width of the bandage (see Figure 18-19B ■).
4. Apply the bandage smoothly and firmly, being careful not to wrap it too tightly. Make sure that no skin is exposed.
5. Fasten the bandage with clips to hold it in place (see Figure 18-19C ■).

■ Ending Steps

To complete the procedure, perform the following steps:

Make the resident comfortable, positioning in good body alignment. Make the resident safe, placing the call signal within reach, lowering the bed, and raising the side rails, if appropriate. Wash your hands. Record and report the procedure as required.

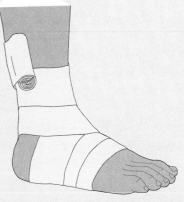

B With each spiral wrap, overlap about one-half of the width of the bandage.

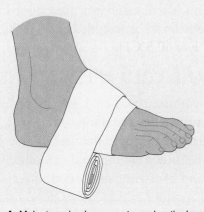

A Make two circular wraps to anchor the bandage.

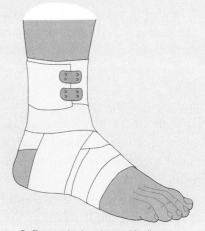

C Fasten the bandage with clips.

FIGURE 18-19 ■ Applying an elastic bandage

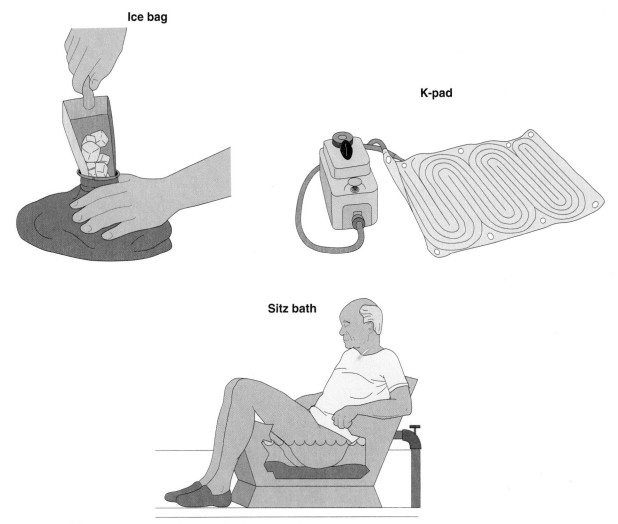

FIGURE 18-20 ■ Three types of heat and cold applications

"K-Pads®"). These devices should be covered before application to protect the skin.

Moist applications include soaks, compresses, wet packs, cooling sponge baths, and sitz baths. Moisture is in contact with the skin for these applications. Soaks, compresses, and wet compresses can be warm or cold. A wet cloth is wrung out and placed upon the skin for a wet compress. A device filled with ice or warm water may be applied to the moist compress to maintain the temperature. Soaks involve placing the resident (or a part of the resident's body) into warm water or solution.

A Cooling Sponge Bath

A cooling sponge bath may be ordered by the doctor to reduce a resident's fever. Evaporation of moisture from the skin has a cooling effect. Alcohol evaporates very quickly and may cool more effectively than water. Alcohol or cool water is sponged onto the resident's skin and is left to evaporate. The application is repeated as needed. Do not apply alcohol near the face. Check with your nurse to determine what areas should be sponged, and follow facility policy.

The Sitz Bath

To take a sitz bath, the resident must sit in warm water (105°F or 40.5°C) for 20 minutes. This procedure relieves pain, improves circulation, and cleanses wounds. It also may be used to stimulate urination.

Special equipment for a sitz bath might include a disposable plastic model that fits into the toilet, a portable sitz bath, or a built-in model. A regular bathtub may be used for a sitz bath by filling it with warm water to a level that covers the pelvis.

You must ensure the resident's safety by assisting the resident into and out of the tub. The resident may experience fatigue or weakness or feel faint. Stay with the resident and observe for these conditions.

GUIDELINES

HEAT AND COLD APPLICATIONS

- Proper temperature of heat applications must be maintained between 100° and 115°F (37.8° and 46.5°C).
- The temperature of solutions should be checked with a bath thermometer according to facility policy.
- Stop treatment, cover the resident, and notify the nurse if shivering occurs.
- Add ice to cold applications as necessary to maintain constant temperature.
- Do not fill ice bags or water bottles to the top.
- Check for leaks in ice bags, collars, or packs and water bottles.

GUIDELINES (Continued)

- Always be sure ice bags are dry before applying them.
- Always cover ice bags, hot water bottles, or vinyl containers with cloth before applying them to the skin.
- Be sure that caps or firm parts of bags are away from the skin.
- Remember, ice will burn.
- Check skin frequently, and report abnormalities or resident complaints to the nurse immediately.
- Remove the heat or cold applications immediately if you suspect burns. Report the situation immediately to the nurse.
- Be familiar with and follow the polices of your facility.

CHAPTER HIGHLIGHTS

1. Positioning, skin care, and mouth care help provide comfort for the resident who is receiving oxygen.
2. The resident who is having difficulty breathing may need extra reassurance and emotional support.
3. Residents who are immobile are more dependent on others to meet their needs.
4. Check with the nurse regarding movement and positioning of the resident with a hip fracture.
5. Observe fingers or toes for circulation when the resident has a cast.
6. Make sure that the standing balance scale is properly balanced before weighing the resident.
7. Use a tape measure to measure the height of a bedridden resident.
8. It may be necessary to strain urine for stones, crystals, or other particles.
9. Wear gloves and follow aseptic practices when collecting a specimen.
10. The purpose of a clean-catch urine specimen is to obtain a specimen as free from contamination as possible.
11. The purpose of a fresh-fractional urine test is to obtain urine that has not been in the bladder for long.
12. A 24-hour urine specimen must be kept chilled during the collection period.
13. When collecting a stool specimen, instruct the resident not to urinate or place toilet tissue in the pan.
14. Most diabetic testing for S&A is done on blood samples.
15. Frequent douches wash away the protective normal flora of the vagina.
16. Elastic support hose and bandages improve circulation by exerting pressure on the veins.
17. Because heat and cold can cause injury, use caution in this type of application.

VOCABULARY REVIEW

Fill in the blanks with the vocabulary term that best completes the sentence.

1. To _____ is to spit.

2. A gas found naturally in the air and necessary for breathing is called _____.

3. _____ is another term for solid body waste, feces, bowel movement, or BM.

4. A broken bone is called a/an _____.

5. A/An _____ is a portable machine that pulls oxygen from the air and supplies it to the resident in a concentrated form.

6. Mucus from the lungs is called _____.

7. _____ is difficult or labored breathing.

8. A/An _____ is a sample of material from the resident's body.

9. The device that provides moisture for oxygen administration is called a/an _____.

10. A/An _____ is another name for a vaginal irrigation.

CHECK YOUR UNDERSTANDING

The following questions cover the highlights of this chapter. Choose the best answer for each question.

1. Which of the following tasks is the responsibility of the nursing assistant?
   A. Discontinue the oxygen when appropriate.
   B. Change the flow rate of the oxygen as needed.
   C. Provide frequent mouth care as needed.
   D. Turn the oxygen on when appropriate.

2. Which of the following is correct cast care?
   A. Wash the cast with soap and water.
   B. Check the color of the resident's fingers or toes.
   C. Remove the cast when the resident bathes.
   D. Dry the cast with a heating pad.

3. Where do you set the weights before weighing a resident on a standing balance scale?
   A. Set both weights at 0.
   B. Set both weights in the middle.
   C. Set one weight at 0 and the other at 50.
   D. It doesn't matter where you set the weights.

4. You have measured a resident's height at 74 1/2 inches. How tall is he in feet and inches?
   A. 5 feet, 2 1/2 inches   C. 6 feet, 1 1/2 inches
   B. 5 feet, 8 1/2 inches   D. 6 feet, 2 1/2 inches

5. While straining the resident's urine, you find two tiny stones. What should you do?
   A. Throw the stones in the trash.
   B. Place the stones in a plastic bag and discard them.
   C. Save the stones and show them to the nurse.
   D. Flush the stones down the toilet.

6. The primary purpose of a clean-catch urine specimen is to
   A. obtain a specimen as free from contamination as possible
   B. obtain a specimen as fresh as possible
   C. obtain all the urine for a 24-hour period
   D. obtain a sterile urine specimen

7. Which of the following is the correct procedure when caring for a resident with a hip fracture?
   A. Position the resident on the side with the legs together.
   B. Ask the resident to sit with the legs crossed.
   C. Use an abductive device between the legs to keep the fracture in position.
   D. Rotate the resident's affected leg outward.

8. The purpose of a fresh-fractional urine specimen is to
   A. Obtain a specimen as free from contamination as possible.
   B. Obtain a specimen as fresh as possible.
   C. Obtain all the urine for a 24-hour period.
   D. Obtain a sterile urine specimen.

9. Which of the following is a purpose of elastic support hose?
   A. Improve circulation.
   B. Prevent blood clots.
   C. Provide comfort and support.
   D. All of the above.

AGE-SPECIFIC TIP

Observe carefully, and do not depend on the resident to tell you if an application is too hot or too cold. Elderly residents may have decreased awareness of temperature changes.

CULTURALLY SENSITIVE TIP

Residents with respiratory problems who cannot understand your language may be comforted by your immediate response to the call signal, your presence, and your touch. Use these forms of communication to provide support and reassurance.

EFFECTIVE PROBLEM SOLVING

Mr. Pippin is receiving oxygen because of respiratory problems. He becomes anxious and begins to cry. To calm him, the nursing assistant says, "Cheer up, Mr. Pippin, it'll be okay. I'll be right next door if you need me."

Was the nursing assistant's communication appropriate? If not, what would have been more appropriate?

_____

_____

_____

_____

_____

_____

_____

_____

_____

INTERPERSONAL COMMUNICATION

The nursing assistant is giving instructions to Mr. Jones, who is taking a sitz bath in the bathtub. Check the instructions that are appropriate.

_____"I'll be back in a minute. Don't get up."

_____"Pull the call signal if you need me."

_____"I'll be right here with you until you are finished."

_____"If the water gets cool, just run some more hot water in the tub."

OBSERVING, REPORTING, AND RECORDING

A resident has a cast on his leg. List four observations that should be recorded and reported immediately.

_____

_____

_____

_____

_____

_____

_____

_____

_____

_____

_____

_____

EXPLORE MEDIALINK

Check out www.prenhall.com/grubbs for additional chapter-specific interactive study and review activities.

19

USING COMMUNICATION SKILLS

OBJECTIVES

1. Explain the importance of communication in the long-term care facility.
2. List three effects of communication as a restorative measure.
3. List five guidelines for each verbal and non-verbal communication.
4. Demonstrate listening skills.
5. List 11 barriers to communication.
6. List three guidelines for communicating with nonambulatory vision-, hearing-, and speech-impaired residents.
7. List nine guidelines for assisting the resident with a hearing aid.
8. Describe the nursing assistant's role in communicating with the resident's family and friends.

VOCABULARY

The following words or terms will help you to understand this chapter:

Communication
Reality orientation
Verbal communication

Nonverbal communication
Listening
Communication barriers

Communication impairment
Aphasia

This chapter explains the communication process and provides guidelines for communicating with various residents for whom communication can be challenging and problematic.

THE IMPORTANCE OF COMMUNICATION

Communication is the sharing of information (a message). The receiver of the information must understand what the speaker (or sender) means (see Figure 19-1 ■). Communication is a lifelong process. The newborn baby enters this world communicating with a cry and a dying person continues to hear until death occurs (see Figure 19-2 ■).

In the health care facility, staff members must communicate to provide resident care that is efficient and helpful. For example, if a resident is having chest pain, failure to communicate could be life-threatening.

Communication ensures that the residents receive the care that is needed. The dietary department must know about diet changes, and the laundry must know when the nursing unit needs additional linen. When an employee is too ill to come to work, the supervisor is notified so that arrangements can be made for another employee to work. If the doctor has ordered "Nothing by mouth after midnight," the staff must have this information. Failure to communicate information successfully could cause significant problems.

The accurate and effective delivery of medical information uses only a small part of the communication skills that are necessary in the long-term care setting. Communication can be used to instruct, problem-solve, comfort, encourage, and convey respect, as well as to report information. This is accomplished by consciously choosing not only the words you use, but the way you use the words. Your attitude, physical distance, voice tones, inflection, facial expression, eye contact, posture, and use of touch all affect the way your message impacts the person with whom you are communicating. As well as choosing your role in a communication, you must be sensitive to the other person's needs. Your message can create reactions in another person that are influenced by that individual's age, emotional state, cultural background, familiarity with the language, and physical impairments.

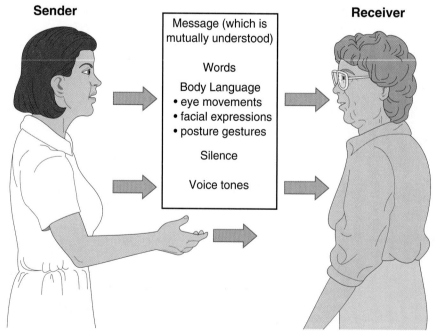

Sender   Message (which is mutually understood)   **Receiver**

Words

Body Language
• eye movements
• facial expressions
• posture gestures

Silence

Voice tones

FIGURE 19-1 ■ The communication process

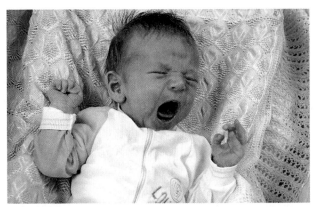

FIGURE 19-2 ■ Communication begins at birth and continues through death.

COMMUNICATION AS A RESTORATIVE MEASURE

Communication is an important part of providing restorative care. Everyone, even a person who likes being alone, needs contact with others. This is impossible without communication. Have you ever been in a room full of people and felt alone? Communication was the missing "bridge" between you and the crowd. Residents need this communication bridge to others. It is necessary for physical and emotional health. Some residents have no family or visitors and must depend upon the staff and volunteers for much of their communication (see Figure 19-3 ■).

You will find many opportunities to talk with the residents while you are providing care. Ask them questions about their interests, families, and

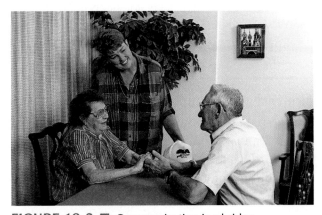

FIGURE 19-3 ■ Communication is a bridge.

histories. Because many elderly residents are no longer able to function as totally independent individuals, their self-image, and sense of individuality may be threatened. Talking about themselves, and about topics that are important to them, helps residents feel valuable and worthy and restores self-esteem. Always speak in a way that encourages independence. Avoid phrases such as "I'll have to help you." It would be better to ask if the resident would like to help with self-care. Comments such as "You're too slow" are insulting and will lessen the resident's sense of independence.

Communication also helps the confused resident to stay in touch with reality. During your conversations with residents, it is helpful to mention dates, times, places, and the names of individuals frequently. It is also important to call the resident by name. This helps to keep the resident in touch with reality (**reality orientation**).

Many residents must remain seated or stay in bed. Having to communicate with others who stand can affect the self-image and comfort level of the chair- or bedridden resident. Being "talked down to" can be demeaning to nonambulatory residents.

GUIDELINES

AGE-SPECIFIC COMMUNICATION WITH THE ELDERLY

- Address residents by titles or names that they prefer.
- Be aware of sensory impairments.
- Ask questions about the resident's interests and family.
- Encourage residents to talk about themselves.
- Avoid the use of slang or medical terms.
- Use the resident's name frequently.
- Be aware of and respect generational differences.
- Stay aware of your attitude toward the elderly.
- Speak to the elderly resident as an adult, regardless of behavior or confusion.
- Encourage and assist with the use of hearing aids, glasses, and dentures to facilitate communication.

FORMS OF EFFECTIVE COMMUNICATION

Verbal Communication

Verbal communication is the use of words to share information. This form of communication includes spoken words, written words, and sign language. Proper choice of words is important to effective communication.

GUIDELINES

COMMUNICATING WITH NONAMBULATORY RESIDENTS

- Position yourself at eye level with the resident (see Figure 19-4 ■).
- Avoid talking "over" the resident.
- Include the resident in your conversation.
- Avoid talking about residents as if they are not present.
- Avoid blocking the view of a resident in a wheelchair or bed.
- Honor and provide the space required to maneuver a wheelchair.
- Remember that many nonambulatory residents are able to communicate normally.
- Assure eye contact with the resident while communicating.

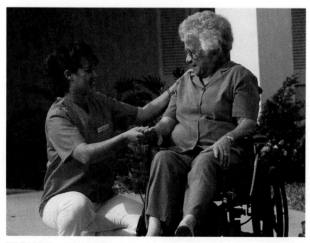

FIGURE 19-4 ■ When communicating with the resident, position yourself at eye level.

GUIDELINES

VERBAL COMMUNICATION

- Think before you speak in order to avoid offending another person.
- Use feedback by repeating what you think was said to ensure correct understanding of the message.
- Do not use medical terminology to communicate with residents and family members.
- Be aware that there are language differences that may interfere with understanding.
- Listen and have empathy when a concern is being communicated. Avoid "pat" answers such as "Everything will look better tomorrow" or "Cheer up."
- Speak frequently, always giving explanations to the unconscious resident.
- Consider possible speech, hearing, and vision impairments and use appropriate guidelines listed in this chapter for communicating with residents with each type of impairment.
- Speak slowly and clearly, with short sentences, and repeat as many times as needed for the confused resident to understand you.
- When using written communicaton with the resident who cannot hear, write clearly and follow guidelines for communicating with hearing-impaired residents.
- When recording in medical records, follow guidelines for recording information about the resident. These guidelines are located in Chapter 10.
- Sign language or written notes may be necessary when communicating with residents with hearing impairments.
- Ask questions that encourage residents to talk about themselves and what is important to them. This promotes self-esteem and helps them to feel valuable and worthy (see Figure 19-5 ■).
- Speak in a way that encourages resident independence.

Nonverbal Communication

Nonverbal communication is the sharing of information without the use of words (see Figure 19-6 ■). This form of communication often is the best indicator of a person's true feelings. Although loudness and tone of voice affect the verbal message, they are not verbal communication. For example, a pleasant or angry tone of voice adds information to

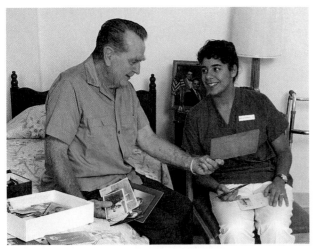

FIGURE 19-5 ■ Encouraging the resident to talk about himself promotes self-esteem.

the message. Voice tone may change the meaning of the message and may affect the receiver's perception of what is meant.

GUIDELINES

NONVERBAL COMMUNICATION

- Be sure that nonverbal communication matches verbal communication.
- Be aware that you are constantly communicating nonverbally.
- Avoid negative body language such as crossing your arms or placing your hands on your hips.
- Develop effective listening skills.
- Use touch appropriately.
- Observe the nonverbal communication of others.
- Be aware of cultural differences in the use of touch and gestures.
- Honor the other person's need for personal space.
- Avoid hurried body movements.

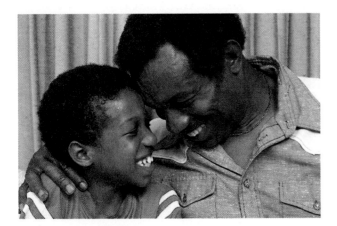

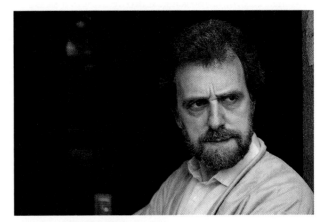

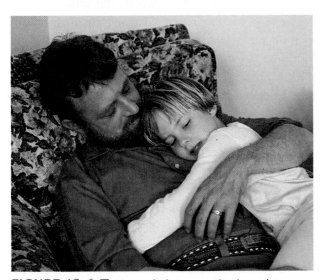

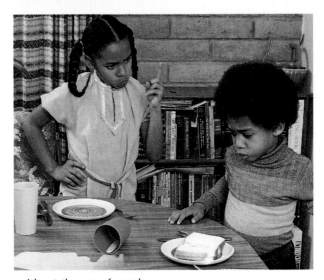

FIGURE 19-6 ■ Nonverbal communication relates a message without the use of words.

Look at the following list of nonverbal communications and recall the last time you were given a message with one of them.

- Body language—includes facial expressions (smiles, frowns, and eye movements), posture, body position, gestures, and other body movements
- Touch (patting, hugging)
- Silence
- Listening
- Personal space
- Voice tones
- Inflection

Touch is a very personal method of communication. Because you provide most of the "hands-on" care for residents, it is important that you remain aware of the significance of the touch that you provide. Remember that when you touch the resident, you are sending a message. Culture affects a person's response to touch. It should be used in a manner that is acceptable to the resident. Touch should be gentle, deliberate, kind, and calm. Hurried movements can be upsetting to the resident and may convey a lack of concern. Hurrying may be perceived as roughness when that is not your true intention. Roughness is a form of abuse.

Listening

One form of nonverbal communication is listening. **Listening** is giving your attention to what you are hearing (see Figure 19-7 ■). The quality of care that is given can be affected by your ability to listen. The health and safety of the resident depend upon your ability to understand orders and directions.

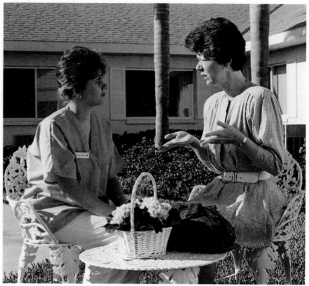

FIGURE 19-7 ■ Listening is giving attention to what you are hearing.

GUIDELINES

LISTENING

- Use eye contact to convey interest.
- Stop other activities.
- Wait quietly for the speaker to compose his or her thoughts.
- Ask questions.
- Be sincere. Don't just pretend to listen.

GUIDELINES (Continued)

- Use body language that shows interest.
- Avoid becoming defensive if the speaker is angry.
- Allow the speaker to talk without intervening.
- Don't interrupt thoughts that are being expressed.

It is important to listen to pleasant conversation as well as to the resident's verbal complaints. It reassures the resident to know that you care enough to take the time to listen. Your listening helps maintain the resident's sense of worth and value.

Have you ever recognized that someone was not truly listening, although he or she appeared to be doing so? If you have ever been ignored, think about the feelings and thoughts that you experienced at the time.

Verbal and nonverbal communication may be used together or separately. The nonverbal message may disagree with the words that are spoken. People often think about their verbal communication. Nonverbal communication usually is not planned and is more difficult to control. For better understanding, it is important to be aware of nonverbal communication. Your words, body language, and voice tones should agree so that you don't send confusing messages.

COMMUNICATING WITH CULTURALLY DIVERSE RESIDENTS

Culture affects a person's use of and response to communication. Touch, personal space, and eye contact are used and interpreted differently among cultures.

GUIDELINES

COMMUNICATING WITH CULTURALLY DIVERSE RESIDENTS

- Seek understanding in communication with residents who speak a language that is different from your own.
- Learn about the cultures of your residents.
- Be aware of cultural differences such as personal space requirements, privacy issues, and levels of formality.
- Understand and accept that family interactions may differ.
- Realize that hand gestures may have different meanings.

GUIDELINES (Continued)

- Avoid being judgmental.
- Be aware of your own feelings and discomfort.
- Show respect for individual customs and beliefs.

COMMUNICATION BARRIERS

The quality of relationships between people depends upon the quality of the communication between them. Communication does not occur if the message is misunderstood. Problems that interfere with communication are called **communication barriers** (see Figure 19-8 ■).

There are many barriers to communication, some of which are listed here:

- Different language levels (using medical terms with the public)
- Words with more than one meaning ("sick," "crazy")
- Different languages (Spanish, English, German, etc.)

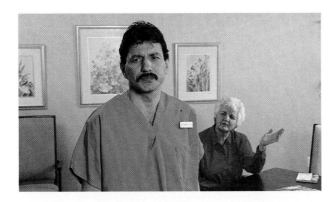
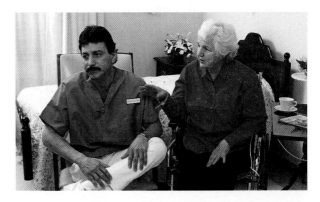
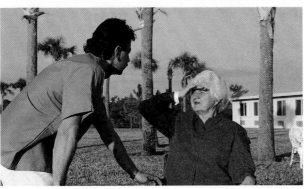
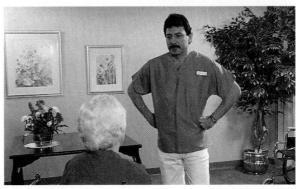

FIGURE 19-8 ■ Can you identify the barriers to communication in each photograph?

- Speaking too fast
- Failure to listen
- Feelings (anger, defensiveness, embarrassment)
- Daydreaming
- Distractions (bright light, noise, odors)
- Being unable to ask questions
- Illness
- Loss of hearing, vision, or speech
- Dementia (confusion)

Communicating with the resident who speaks a different language requires special skills. Using and observing body language and hand gestures often are the primary methods. Being able to point to or draw pictures is sometimes helpful. Listen carefully for poorly pronounced words. It is important to consider cultural differences. Because of these differences, the resident's reactions may be misunderstood. The best communication plan would include the help of a person who speaks the resident's native language.

Many barriers can be avoided if you learn to communicate clearly and skillfully. Both the speaker and receiver should make sure the message is understood. Be aware of signs of misunderstanding, such as frowns or doubtful expressions.

GUIDELINES

COMMUNICATING WITH THE VISION-IMPAIRED RESIDENT

- Before touching the resident, announce your presence as you approach.
- Allow the resident to touch and handle unfamiliar objects.
- Provide a predictable schedule to help the resident feel a sense of security and control.
- Provide good lighting and avoid glare.
- Face the person you are talking to.
- Explain everything that you are going to do.
- Be sure the resident's glasses are clean (see Figure 19-9 ■).
- Describe surroundings when appropriate to do so.
- Describe the location of personal items.
- Describe the location of food by using the clock method at mealtime.
- Describe the new location of furniture if it must be moved.
- Allow the resident to take your arm while walking.

COMMUNICATION IMPAIRMENTS

A resident may have a **communication impairment**. This means that the resident has difficulty communicating because of one or more disabilities. These impairments or disabilities may include problems with vision, hearing, speech, sense of touch, or movement. All these are important to successful communication.

The Vision-Impaired Resident

A person with a vision impairment may have limited vision or may be blind. Those who have vision impairments are more dependent upon the use of their other senses to maintain contact with their world. Touch and hearing are very important communication methods for the vision impaired resident.

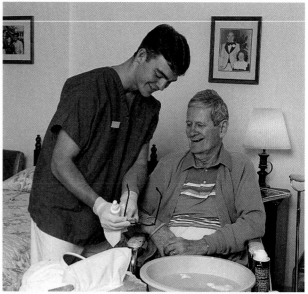

FIGURE 19-9 ■ Be sure the resident wears clean glasses.

The Hearing-Impaired Resident

The hearing-impaired resident is also dependent upon the other senses for communication. It is very important to emphasize the use of sight and touch in communicating with this resident.

Assisting Residents with Hearing Aids

Hearing loss can lead to withdrawal, suspicion, depression, and isolation. It is important for the nursing assistant to be sure that the resident with a hearing aid is able to benefit from its use. There are many types of hearing aids that are designed to amplify sound. Basic parts of a hearing aid include

---

GUIDELINES

COMMUNICATING WITH THE HEARING-IMPAIRED RESIDENT

- Stand in front of the hearing-impaired resident and make eye contact.
- Speak into the better ear, if possible.
- Be sure the resident wears a hearing aid, if required. Check the batteries (see Figure 19-10 ■).
- Face the resident to whom you are speaking. Because the resident may depend on lip reading, provide the opportunity to see your face and lips clearly.
- Do not exaggerate lip movements.

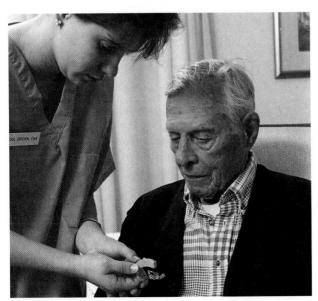

FIGURE 19-10 ■ Be sure the resident's hearing aid is working properly.

GUIDELINES (Continued)

- Carefully explain everything, one step at a time.
- Speak slowly and clearly. Do not shout.
- Stimulate the senses of vision, touch, and smell.
- Use written messages, if necessary.

---

a tiny microphone, amplifier, speaker and a battery (see Figure 19-11 ■). The more modern aids are very small and fit into the ear canal so that they are barely visible, but they usually are not helpful for residents with severe hearing loss. Residents with hearing aids may need assistance to insert, adjust, remove, and care for them.

The Speech-Impaired Resident

Aphasia is the loss of ability to talk or express oneself. The most common cause of aphasia is brain damage. Some chronic diseases also can cause aphasia. This impairment can take many forms.

GUIDELINES

ASSISTING THE RESIDENT WITH A HEARING AID

- Place the hearing aid into the ear with the volume on low.
- After positioning the hearing aid in the ear, slowly turn the volume up until it is comfortable for the resident.
- If whistling occurs, turn the volume down until it stops. Check for proper positioning of the ear-piece in the ear.
- To remove the hearing aid, turn it off with the volume set at low. Pull it toward you by holding the earpiece.
- Check the resident's ear for irritation or wax buildup.
- Check the tubing for ear wax and carefully use the appropriate tool to remove the wax.
- Clean the earpiece by wiping it with soap and water. Do not place it in water and keep water out of the tubing.
- Check the battery regularly. Battery life varies from approximately 1 week to 1 month.
- Keep the hearing aid away from heat.

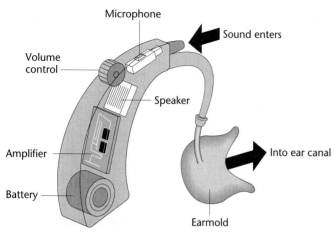

FIGURE 19-11 ■ Basic parts of a hearing aid.

- The aphasic resident may not be able to understand what is said.
- Aphasia may allow the resident to understand what is said but may interfere with the ability to communicate accurately.
- The aphasic resident may speak with a normal rhythm, but without the use of meaningful words.
- Aphasia may involve the loss of control of the muscles needed for speech.
- Aphasia may leave the muscle control intact, but the memory of how to form words is lost.

Some aphasic residents are not confused but may not be able to speak clearly and correctly. Other aphasic residents may be confused.

Be patient with anyone who has a communication impairment and develop empathy. Think about how you might feel if you could not see, hear, or speak. The world would be a lonely place if you lost your ability to communicate.

GUIDELINES

COMMUNICATING WITH THE SPEECH-IMPAIRED RESIDENT

- Remember that the resident hears and responds emotionally, although speech is not possible.
- Treat the resident as an adult.
- Speak in a normal voice, not loudly.
- Don't speak or fill in words for the aphasic resident. Help only if the resident is overly tense or under pressure.
- Allow time for response (at least 10 to 30 seconds).
- Do not correct or criticize. Repeat what is said so that the resident may hear errors.

GUIDELINES (Continued)

- Don't talk about aphasic residents as if they were not there.
- Maintain a relaxed atmosphere.
- Ask questions that can be answered with simple words.
- Use key words. If you want the resident to go to the dining room, say "eat."
- Encourage drawing or writing if the resident is able.
- Stand where the resident can see you when you are talking.
- Don't assume that the resident understands.
- If the resident has difficulty understanding you, speak slowly in short, simple sentences.
- Include the resident in your conversation when he or she is present (see Figure 19-12 ■).
- Be sensitive to the resident's emotions.
- Remember that the resident is an adult. Do not speak as if speaking to a child.

Communicating with the Developmentally Disabled Resident

An individual who has not developed normally due to a birth defect, an injury, or an illness is developmentally disabled. Some of the developmentally disabled are mentally retarded, and many have difficulty communicating.

GUIDELINES

COMMUNICATING WITH THE DEVELOPMENTALLY DISABLED RESIDENT

- Consider each resident as an individual.
- Treat each resident with respect and dignity.
- Remain calm and use touch if acceptable.
- Find opportunities to offer praise and encouragement.
- Treat residents as adults regardless of their behavior. Avoid "baby" talk.
- Use short, simple sentences.
- Repeat actions and words to ensure that the resident understands.

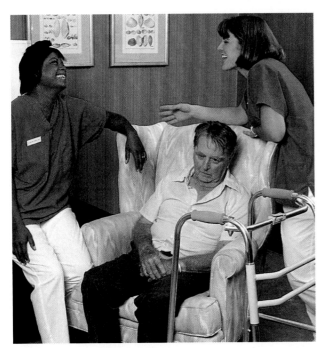

FIGURE 19-12 ■ Include the resident in your conversation when he is present.

COMMUNICATING WITH THE RESIDENT'S FAMILY AND FRIENDS

You will be an important link between the facility and the resident's visitors. You may be the staff member whom the resident's family and friends see first or most often. Their opinion of the facility often will be affected by their impression of you. When staff members have good relationships with visitors, it creates a positive impression of the facility. They will be reassured when they believe that you care about the residents and if you are helpful in responding to their concerns and needs. Family members often experience anxiety about the resident and his or her care. If they trust you, their nervousness will be relieved.

A visitor needs to be listened to when angry or upset. Knowing that someone cares enough to listen to a problem is often the key to solving it and calming the anger. Do not become defensive. Remind yourself that listening is the key to helping another person deal with problems. Mentally separate yourself from blame while you listen attentively to what is being said. Even if the problem is not related to you, listen carefully. Show concern and take the visitor to the nurse, who will continue to assist (see Figure 19-13 ■).

No matter with whom you are communicating, be pleasant, polite, and considerate. Be aware of your body language. A successful relationship depends upon the quality of communication that takes place within it. Communication skills can be learned and are worth every effort to do so.

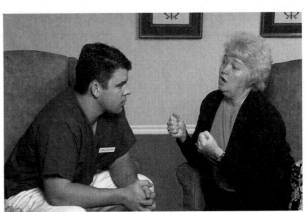

FIGURE 19-13 ■ It is important to be concerned when someone is upset.

CHAPTER HIGHLIGHTS

1. Communication is the sharing of information and is an important part of providing quality care.

2. A restorative approach must be taken when communicating with the resident of the long-term care facility.

3. Encouraging the resident to talk about topics of interest helps to maintain and/or restore a sense of self-worth.

4. A skillful communicator avoids using conflicting verbal and nonverbal messages.

5. Listening is giving your attention to what you are hearing.

6. Verbally announce your presence before touching the vision-impaired resident.

7. Face the hearing-impaired resident when communicating.

8. Check the battery and volume on the resident's hearing aid.

9. Allow the speech-impaired resident time for response.

10. The nursing assistant has a responsibility to communicate with the resident's family and friends.

11. The quality of relationships depends upon the quality of the communication that takes place within them.

VOCABULARY REVIEW

Fill in the blanks with the vocabulary term that best completes the sentence.

1. _____ helps keep the residents in touch with reality.

2. Giving your attention to what you are hearing is _____.

3. _____ is the sharing of information.

4. The loss of ability to talk or express oneself is called _____.

5. _____ is the use of words to share information.

6. Sharing of information without the use of words is _____.

7. _____ means that the resident has difficulty communicating because of a disability.

8. Problems that interfere with communication are called _____.

9. _____ is understanding how you would feel if you were in another person's place.

10. The opinion one has of oneself is _____.

CHECK YOUR UNDERSTANDING

The following questions cover the highlights of this chapter. Choose the best answer for each question.

1. Which of the following is a communication barrier when talking to the resident?
   A. listening very attentively
   B. speaking slowly
   C. asking questions
   D. using medical terminology

2. Which of the following is *not* a communication impairment?
   A. aphasia   C. listening
   B. poor hearing D. blindness

3. Which is the *best* way to communicate with a vision-impaired resident?
   A. Talk loudly and exaggerate lip movements.
   B. Verbally announce your presence before touching.
   C. Touch the resident before you begin talking.
   D. Use hand gestures and body movements.

4. Which is your best response when a resident tells you she's feeling sad?
   A. "Cheer up, things could be worse."
   B. "I'm sorry."
   C. "Everything will be better tomorrow."
   D. "Would you like to talk about it?"

5. A visitor is very angry about her mother's nursing care and is expressing her anger to you. What is your best response?
   A. Tell her it isn't your fault.
   B. Quickly ask her to tell the administrator.
   C. Listen and tell her she'll need to find the nurse.
   D. Listen and encourage her to talk about the problem.

6. Your resident with a speech impairment is having difficulty telling you what she wants you to do. How can you best respond?
   A. Help her by pronouncing the words that you think she means.
   B. Tell her you will be back after she has had time to think.
   C. Tell her not to try to talk.
   D. Wait patiently for at least 30 seconds for her to speak.

7. Which is the *best* way to communicate with the hearing-impaired resident?
   A. Turn the volume high on the resident's hearing aid.
   B. Touch the resident before you start talking.
   C. Raise your voice and shout.
   D. Speak slowly and clearly.

8. Which is the *best* way to communicate with a speech-impaired resident?
   A. Fill in words for the resident.
   B. Allow time for response.
   C. Talk for the resident.
   D. Correct mistakes immediately.

9. How do you clean a hearing aid?
   A. Use alcohol to clean all the parts.
   B. Wipe the earpieces with soap and water.
   C. Soak the tubing in soapy water.
   D. Place the hearing aid in warm water.

COMMUNICATION CENTRAL

AGE-SPECIFIC TIP

Encourage the elderly resident to talk about his interests, family, and history. This helps build self-esteem and confirm the resident's value to society.

CULTURALLY SENSITIVE TIP

Because of cultural differences, the resident's communication may be misunderstood. Listen carefully and observe hand gestures and body language.

EFFECTIVE PROBLEM SOLVING

The resident's son angrily says, "My father hasn't been bathed in a week." The nursing assistant protests and says, "I bathed your father this morning. I don't like being accused of neglect. You shouldn't say things like that."

Was the nursing assistant's communication appropriate? If not, what would have been more appropriate?

_____

_____

_____

_____

_____

_____

_____

_____

_____

INTERPERSONAL COMMUNICATION

The following are attempts to communicate with Mr. Brown, who is speech- and hearing-impaired. Check the examples that are appropriate.

_____ Loudly announce your presence.
_____ Face the resident while speaking.
_____ Exaggerate your lip movements.
_____ Use key words to communicate.

OBSERVING, REPORTING, AND RECORDING

In order to observe and report changes and problems of the residents, you must listen carefully. List four guidelines for listening.

_____

_____

_____

_____

_____

_____

_____

_____

_____

_____

_____

EXPLORE MEDIALINK

Check out www.prenhall.com/grubbs for additional chapter-specific interactive study and review activities.

20

*U*SING THE LANGUAGE OF MEDICINE AND USING COMPUTERS

*O*BJECTIVES

1. List six guidelines for observing.
2. Describe six guidelines for reporting.
3. Identify 10 guidelines for recording information about the resident.
4. List four guidelines for correcting a charting error.
5. Explain the purpose and use of the resident's care plan.
6. List five guidelines for answering the telephone in the long-term care facility.
7. Explain the use of computers in health care.
8. Define and give examples of a word root, a prefix, and a suffix.
9. Define medical terms by dividing them into their elements.
10. Identify abbreviations commonly used in the long-term care facility.

*V*OCABULARY

The following words or terms will help you to understand this chapter:

Report	Care plan	Root
Observation	Mouse	Prefix
Symptom	Central processing unit (CPU)	Suffix
Objective reporting	Software	Abbreviation
Recording	Glossary	

This chapter explains and provides guidelines for communication to be used by the health-care team. Medical terms are defined and the basics of computer use are summarized.

INTRODUCTION TO THE USE OF THE MEDICAL LANGUAGE

The medical field has a language of its own, one that the nursing assistant must be able to understand in order to perform safely and prevent medical errors. Medical language may be used in your assignment, and in your reporting and recording of information about your residents.

OBSERVATION, REPORTING, AND RECORDING

Observation, reporting, and recording are methods of communication that are used by the health care team. Every shift begins with a report. A **report** is the communication of resident information and assignments to those who are coming on duty.

Each resident is discussed briefly. The nurse may give this information verbally to the nursing assistant or include the information on the assignment sheet.

The information about the residents must include the care that is to be provided and changes that have taken place. Remember that you are responsible for providing the proper care for your residents. If you have any questions or doubts about your assignment, you must ask for additional information and make sure you understand clearly. Be familiar with the resident's plan of care.

Observation

Observation is a means of gathering information. The nursing assistant's observation is very important to the prevention of medical errors and to the safety and well-being of the resident. The person who notices early changes in the resident's condition is often the nursing assistant. Some problems become worse very quickly, and early detection may prevent them from becoming life-threatening.

Using all your senses to recognize change is a skill. As you learn about the elderly resident, the changes that take place with aging, and what is

normal for the resident, you will have a better understanding of which observations are important. Figure 20-1 ■ lists some general observations you should make. Sometimes the changes that occur in the resident's body, behavior, or mood may be very slight and difficult to observe.

Bath time is an excellent time to communicate and to perform a thorough observation (see Figure 20-2 ■). Not only is it a time to observe the entire body, but it is also usually the longest period of time that is spent with the resident. This extra time

---

Making Observations By Using the Senses

VISUAL OBSERVATIONS are made by the use of sight. Notice:

Resident Activities such as eating, drinking, walking, dressing, socializing, and toileting
Body Posture and Movement
Shape and Form of Body Parts
Skin: color, perspiration, injuries, and swelling
Breathing: depth and difficulty
Bowel Movement: consistency, color, amount, frequency, and control
Urine: consistency, color, amount, frequency, and control
Vomitus: consistency, color, amount, and frequency
Drainage: color, consistency, and amount
Bleeding
Facial Expressions
Unusual Actions
Safety Hazards

AUDITORY OBSERVATIONS are made by the use of hearing. Notice:

Body Sounds such as breathing sounds, coughing, cracking and popping of joints or bones, and bowel sounds
Verbal Complaints
Speech Problems
Confused Speech

TACTILE OBSERVATIONS are made by the use of touch. Notice:

Skin: temperature and texture
Pulse
Response to Touch

OLFACTORY OBSERVATIONS are made by smelling. Notice:

Odors of drainage, vomitus, urine, bowel movement, mouth and breath, and poor hygiene
Any Unusual Odor

FIGURE 20-1 ■ Using your senses to make general observations of the resident.

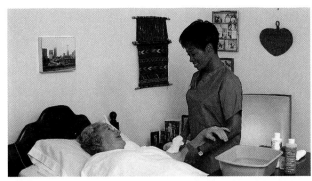

FIGURE 20-2 ■ Communicating during the bath provides an excellent opportunity to observe symptoms.

allows you to use your listening skills to hear complaints and comments. Asking questions also may give you information about how the resident is thinking and feeling. The resident may be experiencing something that cannot be seen or observed by others. Evidence of disease that must be communicated is called a **symptom**. Headaches, nausea, and pain are symptoms.

Staying aware helps to prevent errors. The following guidelines will help you maintain the awareness that is necessary for the well-being and safety of the residents.

GUIDELINES

OBSERVING

- Observe with your senses.
- Remain observant at all times. Avoid allowing your mind to drift or daydream.
- Observe and report any differences that you sense. Sometimes a change may be so vague that you feel unable to describe it, yet it could quickly become life-threatening.
- Observe for problems that often result from the changes of aging. They may include dizziness, stiffness, lack of sensation, dehydration, malnutrition, fragile skin, urinary and bowel problems, and vision or hearing problems.
- Observe for verbal complaints and listen for changes in mood, speech, and mental status. Encouraging communication with the resident will increase your opportunities for this type of observation.

GUIDELINES (Continued)

- Use bath time to observe areas that are usually less visible. These areas include skin creases, such as the abdominal fold, under the breasts, behind the neck, ears and knees, between the fingers and toes, and the genital, rectal, and coccyx areas.
- Observe for nonverbal clues such as facial expressions, movement, and posture.
- Prevent medical errors by close observation and correct identification of residents prior to providing any care.

As you gain experience, your observation skills will improve. In addition to observing the resident's condition, you must also notice any safety hazards in the long-term care facility.

Reporting

Reporting is communicating information to another person. Always report your observations to your nurse. Changes in the resident must be reported immediately so that measures can be taken to prevent a more serious problem. The nurse may have to call the doctor or take some other action.

It is important that you report facts without influencing them with your own ideas and judgment. This reporting of specific factual information is called **objective reporting**. If your statements are not strictly factual, or if they are vague or are influenced by your own opinions, they may not be correct. Some examples of objective reporting are as follows:

Vague Reporting	**Objective Reporting**
The injury is small.	The injury is the size of a dime.
Mr. Smith is combative.	Mr. Smith shoved Mr. Jay.
Mrs. Jones is crying with pain.	Mrs. Jones is crying and says her chest has been hurting for 10 minutes.
Mr. Dye has been in the bathroom for a long time.	Mr. Dye has been in the bathroom for 30 minutes.

Be objective as you report information. Organize your thoughts, use familiar words, be brief, and report only the facts. Do not use words that have more than one meaning, such as the word "sick"; it would be better to say that the resident "complained of nausea and is vomiting." The resident may offer the most accurate description of symptoms being experienced. Use the same words as the resident when reporting complaints.

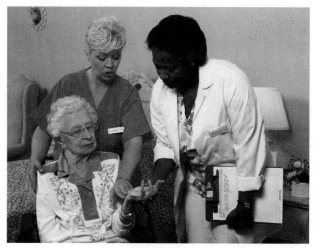

FIGURE 20-3 ■ Thorough observation and prompt reporting helps prevent complications.

GUIDELINES

REPORTING

- Report your observations of accidents or changes to the nurse immediately.
- Procedures and actions should be reported when you complete them.
- Be factual and specific when reporting. Use objective reporting.
- Avoid influencing your reports with your opinions or judgment.
- Choose words that can be clearly understood.
- For accuracy in reporting something that was said to you, repeat the words used by the resident.
- Report any changes that you sense, even though the description may be vague. Slight changes may quickly become life-threatening.
- Organize your thoughts and be brief.
- Continue to observe the resident and check back with the nurse periodically.

Sometimes you may not be able to be specific about the change that you have observed. You may just sense that something is wrong or different about your resident. It is important to report this to the nurse and continue to observe closely.

Nothing is too small or unimportant to report to the nurse. Have you heard the sentence "An ounce of prevention is worth a pound of cure"? It would be better to report more than is necessary than to report too little or too late. You have a responsibility to prevent problems by thorough observation and prompt reporting (see Figure 20-3 ■).

Recording

Writing information about the resident is called **recording** (charting). The purpose of recording is

to create a permanent communication of care given and other resident information. This information can be reviewed to determine if the resident is improving, remaining stable, or getting worse. Information to be recorded includes observations, treatments provided, and the resident's response to treatments. Activities, events, and checklists of items such as clothing also are recorded.

Accurate and timely recording is essential to the safety and well-being of residents. Failure to chart correctly can cause medical errors and incidents. The following guidelines will help you to record properly. There are also guidelines for correcting a charting error.

GUIDELINES

RECORDING INFORMATION ABOUT THE RESIDENT

- Make entries throughout the shift as soon as care is provided.
- Make entries in order of occurrence, and include the date and time.
- Never record on a page that does not contain information identifying the resident.
- Be specific and use objective observations.
- Never omit information or leave blanks, empty spaces, or lines.
- Never chart for another team member.   (continued)

GUIDELINES (Continued)

- Always include your signature and title as required by facility policy (for example, Maria Gonzalez, C.N.A.).
- Use correct grammar and spelling.
- Write with nonerasable ink in the color that is required for your shift.
- Learn and use symbols, abbreviations, and initials that are approved by your facility.
- Maintain the confidentiality of resident information.
- If the resident or a visitor asks to see the chart, politely refer the person to the nurse.

GUIDELINES

CORRECTING A CHARTING ERROR

- Draw a single line through the incorrect entry.
- Write "Error" next to the entry.
- Chart the correct entry.
- Sign your name and title (see Figure 20-4 ■).
- Never erase, use correction fluid, or remove errors from sight. The error and the correct entry must be legible.
- Let the nurse know that you have made a charting error and corrected it.

MEDICAL RECORDS

Medical records contain documentation that allows information to be communicated to other shifts. It preserves important information for future reading. The chart is a legal document and can be used in court. Check your facility's policy regarding the use of the medical record.

Resident Care Forms

The resident's plan of treatment and care depends upon the information that the nursing assistant and other health team members have recorded. Accuracy is very important.

Each section in the medical record has a specific purpose. Some of the forms that might be included are

- Admission sheet
- Nurses' notes
- Doctors' notes and orders
- Resident history and physical examination reports
- Lab and X-ray reports
- ADL sheets (see Figure 20-5 ■)
- Care plan

There are a variety of titles for forms used by nursing assistants to record patient care information. Observations, measurements, care, treatments, and activities usually are recorded by nursing assistants on these forms.

THE CARE PLAN

The **care plan** is a plan of care for the resident. Problems, needs, or concerns of the resident and actions that will be taken by staff members are listed. All departments are involved in creating and following the plan. Meetings are held regularly with representatives from various departments for the purpose of reviewing, evaluating, and revising the plan of care for each resident.

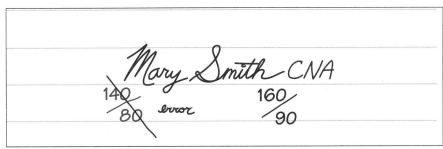

FIGURE 20-4 ■ Errors are corrected by drawing a single line through the error and writing the word "error" with your name and title.

ACTIVITIES OF DAILY LIVING CHECKLIST

Self   Done by resident
Assist   Resident assisted by nursing staff
Total   Done by nursing staff
✔   Check procedure performed
          Include time if appropriate

DATE														
DIET	B'fast	Dinner	Supper	B'fast	Dinner	Supper	B'fast	Dinner	Supper	B'fast	Dinner	Supper	B'fast	Dinner	Supper
Ate all food served															
Ate approx. 1/2 food served															
Refused to eat															
PROCEDURE	11-7	7-3	3-11	11-7	7-3	3-11	11-7	7-3	3-11	11-7	7-3	3-11	11-7	7-3	3-11
A.M. or H.S. Care															
Oral hygiene															
Bath-Bed bath complete															
Bed bath partial															
Shower															
Tub															
Self care															
Back care															
Bed made															
ELIMINATION															
Bowel movement															
Involuntary B.M.															
Voided															
Incontinent															
Foley catheter															
Sitz bath@															
ACTIVITY															
Bed rest complete															
Dangle															
Bed rest–B.R.P.															
Up in chair															
Up in room															
Walk in hall															
Ambulatory															
POSITION CHANGED															
Flat in bed															
Semi-Fowler's															
Deep breathe, cough															
Range of motion															
Turn from side to side															
Side rails–Up															
Down															
Fresh water @															
SIGNATURE & TITLE															

FIGURE 20-5 ■ A flow sheet provides a brief way to record information about the resident.

Nursing assistants can be very helpful with suggestions for care planning. You may be asked to attend and participate in the care plan meeting. By reporting your observations to the nurse, you are contributing to care planning. You may be the source of information regarding new problems, needs, or concerns of the resident. These will be entered into the care plan.

The nursing assistant should read the resident's care plan to be familiar with it. Many of the actions to be taken are the responsibility of the nursing assistant. If your resident has achieved a goal or is failing to meet one, it is important that this information be reported to the nurse. It will affect the care plan.

*U*SING THE TELEPHONE

Check the policies of your facility regarding telephone use. If you are responsible for telephone communication in your facility, you become someone's link to the facility. The impression you make will help form an impression of the facility.

GUIDELINES

WHEN ANSWERING THE TELEPHONE IN THE LONG-TERM CARE FACILITY

- Speak slowly and clearly.
- Always answer by stating your work area, name, and title.
- Be polite and helpful.
- If you must transfer the caller to another extension, watch to be sure it is answered.
- Write messages and include

  Date and time

  Person being called

  Message

  Caller's name

  Your name

---

*U*SING COMPUTERS

Introduction to Computer Use

The use of computers has dramatically changed our lives both at work and at home. Computers provide a method of communicating and recording that is efficient, fast, and accurate. They are used to store information that can be easily recovered. Computers allow individuals to accomplish tasks with more accuracy and speed than is possible without them. These tasks include the research and accessing of information, word processing or typing, and mathematical calculations. Most jobs require the use of a computer. Learning to use a computer will add to your job qualifications.

In health care, computers are used to record, access, and store patient information. The business office uses computers for time cards, the employee payroll, inventory, and bookkeeping. They also are used to exchange information with other facilities and administrative locations. Computers measure and record patients' health status. These measurements include vital signs and blood oxygen levels, among others. Alarms may sound if significant changes occur in a resident's condition.

You may be nervous about learning to use computers because you are unfamiliar with their use. Actually, you already may be using computers without realizing it. Banking ATMs are controlled by computers, and most cars are equipped with them. Bar code scanners and cash registers also are computerized. You may use a computer that records the time when you begin and leave your shift. In becoming computer literate, you become familiar with the major functions of computers. These functions include the input, processing, and output of *data* (information that is stored in a computer). Data is entered by an individual, *processed* by the computer processor, and can be accessed when an individual wishes to retrieve it.

Hardware and Software

Two necessary components of computer use are hardware and software. Computer equipment that is visible is called "hardware." You may find it easier to understand each part if you refer to Figure 20-6 ■ as you read the following list that describes hardware.

- *keyboard* An input device used to enter data and instructions for the computer. This is similar to a typewriter keyboard. *Scanners* and *microphones* also can be used for input (see Figure 20-6A).

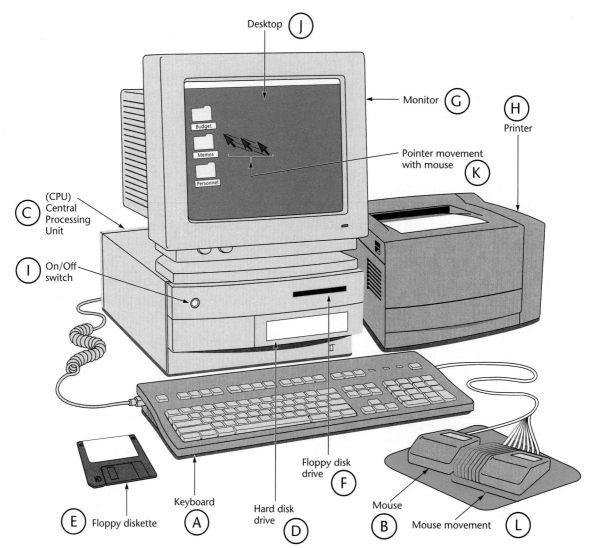

FIGURE 20-6 ■ Computer hardware

- **mouse** A hand-operated input device that also is used to control the computer. It sits on a special pad which allows it to move freely (see Figure 20-6B).
- **central processing unit (CPU)** The controlling part of the computer, or its "brain." The CPU processes information and supervises the entire computer operation (see Figure 20-6C).
- *hard disk* A data storage area of the computer (see Figure 20-6D).
- *floppy disk (diskette)* A piece of magnetically treated plastic that is enclosed in a hard plastic case. The diskette provides portable storage space that is separate from the hard drive (see Figure 20-6E).

- *floppy disk drive* Allows floppy disks (diskettes) to be used in the CPU (see Figure 20-6F).
- *monitor* A device that displays files and text that has been typed on the keyboard. The monitor also provides visible options for controlling the computer (see Figure 20-6G).
- *printer* A device that produces a printed or hard copy of data (see Figure 20-6H).

Software includes the programs or sets of instructions that cause the computer to perform specific actions. Each facility or corporation uses programs that are specific to its needs. Software programs are installed in the computer on the hard disk. Memory is where information and files are stored. Both temporary and long-term memory are available to store data.

Using a Computer

When the computer is turned on, an area called a *desktop* (see Figure 20-6J) appears on the screen. The desktop displays *icons* (symbols) for programs and files that may be used.

A pointer that is visible on the screen may be controlled by sliding the mouse in various directions on its pad (see Figure 20-6K). The pointer moves on the screen in the same direction that the mouse is moved on its pad (see Figure 20-6L). By clicking a mouse button while the pointer is in a specific position, you can start programs and perform specific actions. The mouse should be held gently between the thumb and fingers of the right hand. The index and middle fingers rest lightly on top of the mouse, ready to press the right or left button. If you run out of space on the mouse pad, you may pick the mouse up and place it in another area of the pad. Actions upon the mouse that may be used to control the computer include *Left-Click, Right-Click, Double-Click,* and *Drag-and-Drop.*

A computer keyboard has more keys than a typewriter (see Figure 20-7 ■). These keys perform specific actions that are determined by the software program being used. Unlike a typewriter, the keys

will repeat as long as you hold them down. The numbers "0" and "1" are not interchangeable with the letters "O" and "I." A list describing the functions of some keys follows.

- <←**Enter**> Is used like the carriage return on a typewriter to end a paragraph and begin a new line. It also is used to create blank lines in text (see Figure 20-7A).
- **cursor keys** The *cursor* is a flashing vertical line that appears at the area that may be typed upon. Arrow keys (→←↑↓) allow you to move the cursor around the screen without disturbing what has been typed (see Figure 20-7B). Other keys (*Home, End, Page Up,* and *Page Down*) allow cursor movement in larger jumps such as from page to page, or to the beginning or end of a line or page (see Figure 20-7C).
- <←**Backspace**> Erases the character to the left of the cursor (see Figure 20-7D).
- <**Delete**> Erases characters by deleting them to the right of the cursor. The cursor does not move (see Figure 20-7E).
- <**Caps Lock**>Locks in capital letters (see Figure 20-7F). Some nonalphabetic keys require the

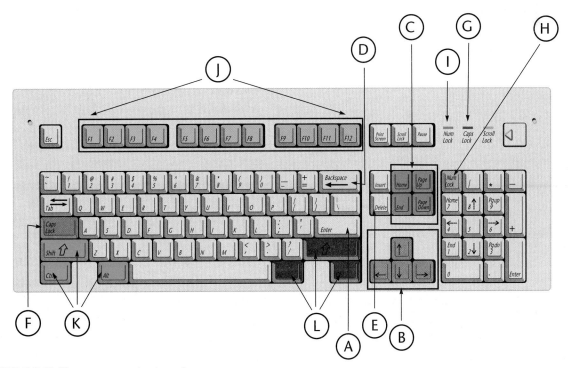

FIGURE 20-7 ■ A computer keyboard

additional use of the <*Shift*> key. This key's use is indicated by a *status light* on the keyboard (see Figure 20-7G).

- <**Num Lock**> Initiates and discontinues the 10-key number pad for numeric calculations (see Figure 20-7H). This key's use is indicated by a status light on the keyboard (see Figure 20-7I).
- <**F₁,**>, <**F₇**> Special "F" keys from *F1* to *F12* initiate commands that are specific to each program used (see Figure 20-7J).
- **booster keys** <*Ctrl*>, <*Alt*>, and <*Shift*> may be used simultaneously with other keys to change the action of specific keys (see Figure 20-7K and L).

Files and documents may be created, saved, renamed, opened, closed, and deleted. When a file is saved, it is placed on the disk for storage. A file manager program provides an organized listing of all files, and enables the user to search for, access, and modify files that are stored in the computer or on diskettes.

A file may be created by activating a program, entering data, and saving the information that was entered. Information can be entered by using the keyboard. Data that is being entered will be displayed on the monitor.

After completing a file, you may save it to either the hard disk or a floppy diskette. The first time work is saved, it becomes a file and must be given a name. (In order to use the data again, you will need to remember the location, folder, and file name.)

Specific actions by the mouse or the keyboard turn the computer off. These actions differ according to the operating system that is controlling the computer. Do not use the on/off switch to discontinue power until the screen indicates that it is safe to turn the computer off. (Some computers may be set to power down automatically.) Help and information for using the computer is available on the screen of the monitor. Manuals also are available to provide instructions for using the operating system installed in the computer.

MEDICAL TERMINOLOGY

Medical terms may refer to body parts, measurements, orders, activities, treatments, diagnoses, time, or place. Some terms are general and can be used in any health care facility, and others are specific to long-term care.

At the back of the book is a glossary. The **glossary** is like a small dictionary that includes definitions of many words that are found in this book.

THE WORD ELEMENTS OF MEDICAL TERMS

Medical words usually are a combination of word elements or parts. There are thousands of medical terms, so you cannot expect to memorize all of them. However, you can learn to identify the elements that define words.

Three elements of medical terms are roots, prefixes, and suffixes. The **root** is the foundation of the word and contains the basic meaning. A **prefix** is the element that is at the beginning of a word. A **suffix** is the element that is at the end of a word. Words can be formed by adding a prefix or a suffix to a root. For example, the root "cardi" means "heart," and the suffix "ology" means "study of," so the medical term "cardiology" means "study of the heart." You will need to learn some commonly used roots, prefixes, and suffixes to understand medical terms.

Root

The root forms the basic meaning of a word. Word roots are the building blocks of medical terminology. A word root can be combined with a prefix, a suffix, or another root to form a medical term. Sometimes the letter "o" or "i" is added to the root to make the word easier to pronounce. Roots commonly used in the long-term care facility include

Root	Meaning	Root	Meaning
arthr(o)	joint	*neur(o)*	nerve
cardi(o)	heart	*oste(o)*	bone
col(o)	colon	*psych(o)*	mind
derma	skin	*pulmo*	lung
gastr(o)	stomach	*septic*	infection
glyc(o)	sugar	*thoraco*	chest
hema	blood	*trache(o)*	trachea
my(o)	muscle	*ven(o)*	vein

Prefix

A prefix is always found at the beginning of a word. A prefix cannot stand alone, but must be combined with another element to become a word. Some prefixes commonly used in the long-term care facility include

Prefix	Meaning	Prefix	Meaning
a, an	without, not	*hyper*	high, above normal
ab	away from	*hypo*	low, below normal
ad	toward	*micro*	small
ante	before	*non*	not
anti	against	*per*	by, through
auto	self	*poly*	many
bi	double, two	*post*	after, behind
brady	slow	*pre*	before, in front
circum	around	*retro*	backward
dys	difficult, abnormal	*semi*	half
epi	on, over	*sub*	under
hemi	half	*tachy*	fast, rapid

Suffix

A suffix is always placed at the end of a word. A suffix must be combined with another element to become a word. Suffixes commonly used in the long-term care facility include

Suffix	Meaning	Suffix	Meaning
algia	pain	*pathy*	disease
ectomy	surgical removal	*phasia*	speaking
emia	blood	*phobia*	fear
gram	record	*plegia*	paralysis
itis	inflammation of	*pnea*	to breathe
meter	measuring instrument	*scope*	examining instrument
ology	study of	*therapy*	treatment
ostomy	surgical opening	*uria*	condition of urine

Combining Word Parts

Medical terms can be formed by several different combinations of word parts. For example, a word might contain a prefix and a root, a root and a suffix, a prefix and a suffix, or two roots. The following list shows some common medical terms that have been divided into their elements.

Medical Term	Prefix	Root	Suffix
antiseptic	*anti*	*septic*	
arthritis		*arthr*	*itis*
colostomy		*colo*	*stomy*
dyspnea	*dys*	*pnea*	
hypoglycemia	*hypo*	*glyc*	*emia*
hemiplegia	*hemi*	*plegia*	

$\mathcal{A}$BBREVIATIONS

An **abbreviation** is a shortened form of a word or phrase. It is developed by leaving out or substituting letters. The purpose of an abbreviation is to save time and space. Abbreviations are an important part of the health care system. Learning some commonly used abbreviations will help you to understand and communicate clearly. Some will be obvious to you; others will have to be memorized. The following guidelines include some suggestions that will help you to learn the meaning of abbreviations.

The following list contains only a few of the thousands of abbreviations that exist. All facilities do not use the same abbreviations. It is your responsibility to find out which ones are acceptable in your facility. Anytime you are not sure how to abbreviate a word or a phrase, you should write it out in full.

GUIDELINES

CLUES TO HELP UNDERSTAND ABBREVIATIONS

An abbreviation may

- Use the first letter of each word (VS = vital signs).
- Use the first and last letter of the word (ht = height).
- Use three or four letters of a word (amb = ambulate).

(continued)

GUIDELINES (Continued)

- Use a chemical symbol that includes a numeral (O_2 = oxygen; H_2O = water).

Remember that

- The letter "q" usually means "every" (qd = every day).

  or

  it may indicate four (qid = four times a day).

- The letter "h" usually means hour (qh = every hour).

It helps to

- Associate ac with am (ac = *before* meals, am = *before* noon) and pc with pm (pc = *after* meals, pm = *after* noon).

- Think of bid, tid, and qid as 2 *in* a day, 3 *in* a day, and 4 *in* a day.

Abbreviation	Meaning
ac	before meals
ADLs	activities of daily living
ad lib	as desired
am	morning
amb	ambulate
amt	amount
bid	twice a day
BM	bowel movement
BP	blood pressure
BR	bedrest/bathroom
BRP	bathroom privileges
BSC	bedside commode
$\bar{c}$	with
CA	cancer
cc	cubic centimeter
C.N.A.	certified nursing assistant
c/o	complains of
CPR	cardiopulmonary resuscitation
CVA	cerebrovascular accident/stroke
dc	discontinue/discharge
D.O.N.	director of nurses
GI	gastrointestinal
GU	genitourinary
H_2O	water
HOH	hard of hearing
hr, h	hour
HS	hour of sleep/bedtime
ht	height
I&O	intake and output
IV	intravenous
liq	liquid
L.P.N.	licensed practical nurse
L.V.N.	licensed vocational nurse
LTC	long-term care
meds	medications
ml	milliliter
NPO	nothing by mouth
O_2	oxygen
OOB	out of bed
OT	occupational therapy
oz	ounce
p	after
pc	after meals
pm	afternoon
po	by mouth
prn	when necessary/as needed
pt	patient
PT	physical therapy
q	every
qam	every morning
qd	every day
qh	every hour
q2h, q3h, q4h, etc.	every 2 hours, every 3 hours, every 4 hours
qhs	every night at bedtime
qid	four times a day
qod	every other day
qs	quantity sufficient or enough
R.N.	registered nurse
ROM	range of motion
$\bar{s}$	without
S&A	sugar and acetone test
SOB	shortness of breath
stat	at once/immediately
tid	three times a day
TLC	tender loving care
TPR	temperature, pulse, and respirations
VS	vital signs
w/c	wheelchair
wt	weight

CHAPTER HIGHLIGHTS

1. The nursing assistant's observations are very important to the safety and well-being of the resident.
2. Observe with all your senses and remain observant at all times.
3. Always report your observations promptly to the nurse.
4. Accurate and timely recording helps prevent medical errors.
5. Never erase, use correction fluid, or cover up an error on a chart.
6. A care plan is a plan of care that lists problems, needs, and concerns of the resident.
7. Nursing assistants can provide valuable assistance in care planning.
8. Answer the telephone politely, and state your work area, name, and title.
9. Computers provide a method of communication and recording that is efficient, fast, and accurate.
10. The central processing unit (CPU) is the controlling part of the computer.
11. You must be able to understand medical terminology in order to perform safely.
12. Most medical terms are a combination of roots, prefixes, and suffixes.
13. It is your responsibility to know which abbreviations are acceptable in your facility.
14. If you are not sure of an abbreviation, write out the term in full.

VOCABULARY REVIEW

Fill in the blanks with the vocabulary term that best completes the sentence.

1. Evidence of disease that must be communicated is a/an _____.

2. The _____ contains a list of definitions of many words found in a book.

3. _____ includes the programs or sets of instructions that cause the computer to perform specific actions.

4. A/an _____ is a shortened form of a word or phrase.

5. The reporting of specific factual information is called _____.

6. A/an _____ is the element at the end of a word.

7. _____ means gathering information.

8. The problems, needs, and information about the care of the resident are listed on the _____.

9. The _____ is the foundation of a word and contains its basic meaning.

10. The controlling part or "brain" of the computer is the _____.

CHECK YOUR UNDERSTANDING

The following questions cover the highlights of this chapter. Choose the best answer for each question.

1. Using the senses to gather information is called
   - A. reporting
   - B. observation
   - C. recording
   - D. objection

2. When should you report a change in the resident's condition?
   - A. every 2 hours
   - B. at the end of the shift
   - C. immediately
   - D. after lunch

3. Which of the following is a proper way to correct an error in charting?
   - A. Draw a single line through it.
   - B. Erase it completely.
   - C. Scribble it out with several lines.
   - D. Use correction fluid.

4. Where is the *best* place to look for information about the resident's care?
   - A. your job description
   - B. the procedure book
   - C. the I&O sheet
   - D. the resident's care plan

5. The nursing assistant senses that something is different about one of the residents. Although she is unable to be specific about the change, what should she do?
   - A. Wait until something specific happens.
   - B. Report her observations to the nurse immediately.
   - C. Talk to her best friend about it.
   - D. Call the resident's family immediately.

6. What is your best response when taking a telephone message at work?
   - A. I'll tell Mary as soon as she returns.
   - B. It will be better if you call back when Mary is here.
   - C. I will be glad to write a message for Mary.
   - D. You should not call Mary at work.

7. The primary use of computers in health care facilities is to
   - A. store and retrieve information
   - B. play games and relax
   - C. send personal e-mail
   - D. surf the Net

8. The computer device that displays files and text that have been typed is the
   - A. mouse
   - B. monitor
   - C. CPU
   - D. keyboard

9. Your instructions are to ambulate the resident bid. What does this mean?
   - A. Walk the resident every 2 hours.
   - B. Feed the resident three times a day.
   - C. Walk the resident two times a day.
   - D. Feed the resident four times a day.

10. The resident is to have a back rub qam and HS. When will you give the back rub?
    - A. every day at breakfast and lunch
    - B. three times a day
    - C. four times a day
    - D. every morning and at bedtime

AGE-SPECIFIC TIP

The elderly resident may be experiencing symptoms that cannot be observed by others. Ask questions to gain information about how the resident is feeling.

CULTURALLY SENSITIVE TIP

Culture may affect the resident's reaction to pain. Observe the resident's face and body language carefully. Ask the resident if he or she is comfortable.

EFFECTIVE PROBLEM SOLVING THROUGH COMMUNICATION

The nursing assistant notices that Mrs. Cook isn't eating her lunch. When asked why she isn't eating, Mrs. Cook responds, "I can't eat this food." The nursing assistant says she will tell the nurse. She reports that Mrs. Cook didn't like her lunch.

Was the nursing assistant's communication appropriate? If not, what would have been more appropriate?

_____

_____

_____

_____

_____

_____

_____

_____

_____

INTERPERSONAL COMMUNICATION

Fill in the blanks.

Medical terms should not be used when communicating with _____ or

_____ .

OBSERVING, REPORTING, AND RECORDING

List 3 visual and 3 auditory observations.

_____

_____

_____

_____

_____

_____

_____

_____

_____

_____

_____

_____

_____

_____

_____

_____

21

THE RESIDENT, AGING, AND PSYCHOSOCIAL NEEDS

OBJECTIVES

1. Describe the geriatric resident.
2. Identify six guidelines for caring for the developmentally disabled resident.
3. Identify the major developmental tasks of each age group.
4. List five factors that affect aging.
5. List the five basic needs of all human beings.
6. Explain the concept of caring for the "whole" person.
7. Describe the effect of culture and spirituality on the resident's needs.
8. List six guidelines for working with culturally diverse residents.
9. Give examples of restorative care in helping the resident meet the needs for love, self-esteem, and self-actualization.

VOCABULARY

The following words or terms will help you to understand this chapter:

Developmentally disabled
Geriatric resident
Disoriented
Adolescence

Puberty
Menopause
Environment
Pollution

Physical needs
Psychosocial needs
Self-actualization
Adapt

It is difficult to identify typical residents of long-term care facilities because they represent assorted age groups and cultures. However, most of the residents are elderly, and the majority are women. Most are widowed. Some have outlived all their immediate family members, and there is no one to care for them. Many require care that no longer can be provided at home. Some of the residents are developmentally disabled. A **developmentally disabled** person is someone who has not developed normally due to a birth defect, an injury, or an illness. Many long-term care residents have difficulty performing ADLs. A person with this problem needs help with bathing, dressing, toileting, and other daily needs.

THE GERIATRIC RESIDENT

A **geriatric resident** is an elderly person who lives in a long-term care facility. The personalities of geriatric residents are as varied as those of people in any other age group (see Figure 21-1 ■). Think about the personalities of the members of your class. Are they all the same? The individual elderly residents are no more alike than are the students. The basic personality that a person has developed over the years does not change with age. However,

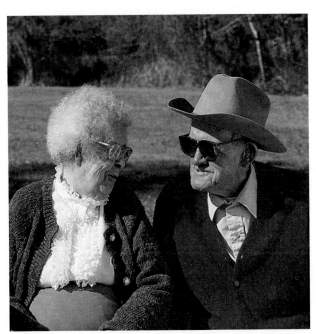

FIGURE 21-1 ■ Geriatric residents come from different backgrounds and have a variety of personalities.

certain characteristics of the personality often get stronger and more noticeable. A pleasant young person usually becomes a pleasant old person, and the older person who is irritable now probably was disagreeable earlier in life.

Geriatric residents may have many health problems. Some are caused by body changes that take place. All the body systems slow as a person gets older and response and coordination decrease. Stiff joints and weak muscles make it difficult to get around. Bones become brittle. Vision and hearing loss may occur. These changes place the elderly person at greater risk of injury from falls and other accidents. The body does not heal as quickly, and rehabilitation may take more time. Some geriatric residents are **disoriented** (confused). Confused residents have a communication problem because they cannot follow directions or understand what is being said to them. Most geriatric residents, however, are mentally alert and are not disoriented.

It is important to develop an understanding of geriatric residents and their problems. They often are frail and likely to catch a disease if they are exposed. Protection of their health and safety is your main concern. Use empathy, and care for the geriatric residents as if they were elderly members of your own family.

THE DEVELOPMENTALLY DISABLED RESIDENT

Persons who are developmentally disabled have a chronic condition that limits normal function. Many are unable to live independently or take care of themselves. They may have trouble communicating, and their learning ability may be reduced (see Figure 21-2 ■).

Some of the developmentally disabled are mentally retarded. Mental retardation occurs early in life, sometimes before birth. These people may have low intellectual and learning skills. The degree of retardation may range from mild to severe. Developmentally disabled persons may have a disease that causes difficulty in controlling muscle activity. They often are in wheelchairs. Developmental disability also may be caused by an

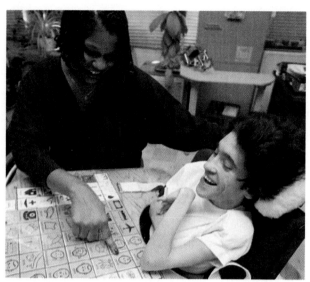

FIGURE 21-2 ■ Developmentally disabled residents may have difficulty communicating.

injury to the brain. Some developmentally disabled persons may be paralyzed or unconscious.

Developmentally disabled residents are at different levels of functioning physically, emotionally, and mentally. Some have behavior problems that interfere with their care and their ability to interact successfully with others. A plan to modify destructive behavior is included in the care plan when needed.

GUIDELINES

CARE OF THE DEVELOPMENTALLY DISABLED RESIDENT

- Follow each residents care plan.
- Encourage independence in self-care.
- Assist with ADLs as necessary.
- Consider each resident as an individual.
- Treat each resident with respect and dignity.
- Look for opportunities to offer praise and encouragement.
- Be familiar with each resident's plan of behavior management.
- Respond appropriately to each resident's behavior.
- Treat residents as adults, regardless of behavior.
- Repeat actions and words to ensure the resident's understanding.

GROWTH AND DEVELOPMENT

Growth and development take place at an orderly rate throughout life. There is a burst of tremendous growth in the first year of life and again in **adolescence** (the teenage years between 13 and 18). By young adulthood, most people have achieved their full physical growth. However, mental, emotional, and spiritual development continues through the different stages of life.

In the 1950s, Erik Erikson, a psychologist, proposed the theory that specific developmental tasks must be accomplished as an individual passes through certain stages of life. The accomplishment of these tasks allow a person to remain emotionally healthy (see Figure 21-3 ■).

Life Stages

Infancy   Body weight doubles in the first 6 months and triples by the end of the first year. The temporary "baby teeth" start appearing, and the infant learns to roll over, sit up, crawl, and walk. Babies soon learn to recognize familiar faces and voices. However, they tend to cling to their mothers or primary caregivers. The major developmental task of infancy is developing trust.

The Toddler (Early Childhood)   By the end of their third year, most toddlers have cut all the temporary teeth. Although growth slows, muscle

ERIKSON'S LIFE STAGES AND DEVELOPMENTAL TASKS	
Stage	Developmental Task
1. Infancy	Develop trust
2. Early childhood	Develop independence and self-direction
3. Play age	Develop initiative
4. School age	Develop competence
5. Adolescence	Develop self-identity
6. Early adulthood	Develop intimacy and love
7. Middle adulthood	Develop concern for others and continue productivity
8. Old age	Develop integrity

FIGURE 21-3 ■ The developmental tasks according to Erik Erikson.

strength and energy increase. Toddlers learn to run, jump, and climb stairs. They are able to move quickly and have little concept of danger. Although toddlers usually are able to speak, understand, and think, they have no clear idea of right or wrong behavior. The developmental task of this age group is to gain independence. The "terrible twos" are a direct result of these efforts toward independence.

Play Age or Preschool Age The 3-year span from 3 to 6 years of age produces many changes. Physical growth is seen more in height than in weight. Muscular development increases throughout this time period. Language and social skills increase, and the child's focus shifts from home to playmates. Play is important because it provides opportunities to practice social skills and improve muscular coordination. The developmental task is to develop initiative, which means trying out new and different things.

School Age The school age years cover a 6-year period from ages 6 to 12. There is a lot of variation in this age group. The arms and legs lengthen, muscle tissue increases, and the child grows stronger. Sex differences become more obvious, with boys having more muscle tissue and girls having more fatty tissue. In the later years of this stage, some children enter **puberty** (the period when sex characteristics appear and the reproductive organs begin to function). Peer group acceptance becomes more important as interests shift from home to school. The major developmental task is to gain competency in intellectual skills such as reading, writing, and arithmetic.

The Teenage Years During this time, the individual changes from a child to an adult. There is a sudden increase in height and weight. Body proportions change and the secondary sex characteristics appear. Girls develop breasts, pubic hair, and underarm hair. Boys develop hair on the face, body, underarms, and pubic area. Sexual maturity takes place and the sex hormones, estrogen and testosterone, play a major role in growth and development. Psychosocial growth is as great as physical growth. These rapid changes in growth and development often result in poor emotional control. The major developmental task is to gain self-identity. This involves separating from parents and developing independence.

The Young Adult There is not much physical growth after adolescence. The body systems usually are fully developed and functioning by this time. The major developmental task is to establish intimacy in a close personal relationship. Dating and building relationships are part of the process of selecting a mate.

Middle Age People who are middle-aged are just what the name suggests—they are in the middle, neither young nor old. The body starts showing signs of aging. Hair grays, wrinkles appear, and strength declines. During these years, most women go through **menopause**, the end of menstruation. Some people experience what is called a "midlife crisis." They think that time is "running out," and some become confused and restless. Divorce is not uncommon. Most people, however, see this as the best time of their lives and enjoy themselves. The developmental task of middle age is to achieve productivity. Interests move from meeting one's own needs to caring for society as a whole.

Old Age Today, people are living longer and healthier lives. Life expectancy has increased tremendously over the years. The physical changes of aging become more obvious during these years. Although aging is individualistic, some general changes appear in most older people. These changes are discussed later in this chapter.

The major developmental task of the elderly is to find meaning in life's experiences. This involves remembering, discussing, and perhaps writing about past events. This "life review" helps the individual let go of the past and adjust to the present. It raises self-esteem and gives life more quality.

THE PROCESS OF AGING

Aging is not a sudden event that begins at a particular age (see Figure 21-4 ■). It begins at birth and continues until death.

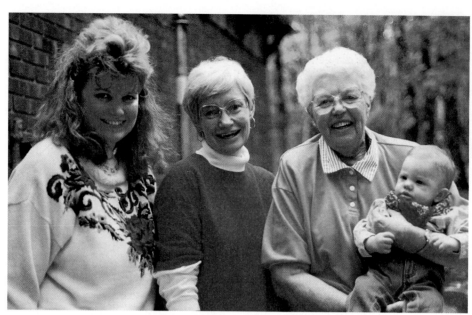

FIGURE 21-4 ■ Growth and development take place at an orderly rate throughout life.

All people do not age at the same rate. Some appear old in middle age, and others seem to age very slowly. Aging is influenced greatly by one's state of mind. The person who feels old often will look, feel, and act old.

Many factors, such as heredity, environment, lifestyle, physical health, and mental health, affect aging. Heredity refers to all the characteristics that a person inherits from parents and other ancestors. One of those characteristics is life span, or length of life. In some families, many members live to be very old.

Environment is also important. **Environment** means all the conditions and influences around us. These include air, water, and noise level in the home, neighborhood, and workplace. **Pollution** occurs when we contaminate the environment with such things as trash and cigarette smoke. Automobiles, insecticides, and garbage contribute to pollution. People live longer in an environment that is clean, quiet, and less polluted.

Lifestyle directly affects how long and how well a person will live. Smoking and the abuse of alcohol and other drugs shorten life. A person's social, emotional, or sexual activities may contribute to a destructive lifestyle. Many people have too much stress in their lives or are not able to cope well with stress. Good nutrition, adequate sleep, and regular exercise contribute to a healthy lifestyle. Developing this type of lifestyle helps to lengthen the life span.

People who are in good health usually do not age as quickly. They are able to be more active and involved in meaningful activities. This allows them to feel useful and independent. Those who have either physical or mental health problems often do not feel well enough to remain active. Although the discovery of new medicines and treatments has extended life, many diseases still have no cure.

Facts About Aging

There are some common beliefs about aging that are not true. These include the following: age 65 is old; the elderly see themselves as sick and helpless; all old people are confused; most of the elderly live in nursing homes.

The true facts about aging are as follows:

- Many people over 65 are working and leading productive lives. They do not consider themselves old, nor does society.
- The majority of older people see themselves as physically healthy, mentally alert, and independent.
- Confusion is not a normal change of aging.

- Most of the elderly in the United States live at home with family or friends. Only a small percentage live in nursing homes.

Having a purpose, being useful, and being independent delay the aging process. People who have a purpose in life are still setting goals. They are making plans for the future. They have a reason for living as they look forward to what tomorrow might bring. We all have a need to be useful. People who age early often complain that "Nobody needs me; I'm just in the way." Being useful means that what you are doing is worthwhile. This increases the feeling of self-worth.

Independence also helps to keep us young. The ability to take care of oneself and to make choices and decisions is important. Even a slight amount of independence helps. The person who is able to do only a little will feel better than the person who is totally dependent. A more positive self-image usually will result in a more youthful appearance.

It is important to remember that aging is a normal process. It is not a disease. However, there are some changes of aging that may affect the ability to maintain complete independence. These changes are described in the next chapter.

*B*ASIC NEEDS

Physical needs and psychosocial needs are basic needs shared by all human beings. **Physical needs** are the needs of the body. **Psychosocial needs** are emotional, social, and spiritual needs. "Psycho" refers to thoughts and emotions; "social" refers to contact and involvement with others. Many psychosocial needs are met through interaction with others. Basic human needs include

- Physical needs
- Safety and security needs
- Love and belonging needs
- Self-esteem needs
- Self-actualization needs (the need to prove oneself)

The quality of life depends upon the fulfillment of all of these basic needs.

Abraham Maslow, a scientist, listed the five basic needs in the order of their importance. As

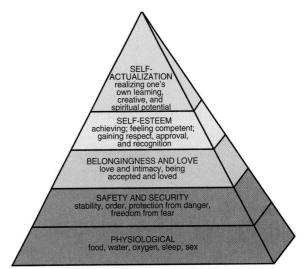

FIGURE 21-5 ■ Physical needs are the foundation for all other human needs.

you can see in Figure 21-5 ■, he illustrated these needs by using a pyramid. The most basic needs are the foundation that supports all other needs. If the physical needs of the foundation are not met, the pyramid will crumble and the upper levels will fall.

The Whole Person

In nursing, it is important to care for the whole person, which includes caring for both the physical and the psychosocial needs of the resident. You will spend much time learning procedures for the care of the resident's body because physical care is very important. However, it is also important to provide care that fulfills the resident's emotional, social, and spiritual needs. To have a good quality of life, the psychosocial needs must be met. Perfect physical health does not mean much if it is not accompanied by emotional health.

Physical Needs

The most basic needs are the physical needs, which include oxygen, food, water, and rest. If the physical needs are not met, other, higher needs become less important. An individual can be concerned with higher needs only when physical needs have been met and life is not in danger. For example, a resident who is having difficulty breathing may not want to leave the room to socialize. When breathing improves, the need for love and belonging will become important again.

The Need for Safety and Security

The second level of basic needs is the need for safety and security. Being safe and secure means that an individual is free from harm. Having money, a job, and a safe place to stay meet a person's need for security. Being able to trust others and to trust one's environment increases a person's feelings of safety and security.

The Need for Love and Belonging

The need for love and belonging is the need for affection and to feel connected with others. This need may be met by belonging to a group such as a family, a church, or an organization. Meaningful relationships with other people fulfill the need for love and belonging.

The Need for Self-Esteem

This is the need to feel good about oneself. Feeling important and useful helps to meet the need for self-esteem. Self-esteem is fulfilled by the roles we hold throughout life. When we are needed by others, we feel that we are important. Being independent also improves self-esteem.

The Need for Self-Actualization

This is the highest need and can be met only when all other needs are fulfilled. When something is "actual," it is "real" and has been proven by facts. With this definition in mind, you might think of **self-actualization** as "proving yourself." Accepting challenges and meeting goals are examples of self-actualization. Spiritual fulfillment is self-actualization, too. Learning, creating, and striving to achieve all help to meet the need for self-actualization. Completion of a class is an example of self-actualization.

The resident's unmet needs are included in the care plan. Many of the approaches that are used to meet these needs will be the responsibility of the nursing assistant. Be familiar with the resident's care plan, and review it often, to fulfill your role in ensuring that all basic needs are met.

CULTURE AND SPIRITUALITY

"Cultural diversity" refers to the differences that exist between individuals from various cultures or ethnic groups. Customs, values, and beliefs are influenced by a person's culture and spirituality. A person's needs and methods for meeting those needs also are influenced by them. The following guidelines will help you to care for culturally diverse residents. America is a "melting pot" of cultures, and you may care for residents from a variety of backgrounds (see Figure 21-6 ■).

GUIDELINES

WORKING WITH CULTURALLY DIVERSE RESIDENTS

- Learn about other cultures. This will help you to understand and be comfortable with all residents (see Figure 21-7 ■).
- Understand your own feelings. This will help you to accept the differences of others.
- Realize how your attitude may affect residents.
- Help the residents feel accepted and comfortable.
- Be aware that culture and religion influence a person's beliefs and practices in regard to health.
- Observe for individual reactions to pain, which often are influenced by culture.
- Strive for understanding when communicating with residents who speak a different language.
- Be aware of differences in body space requirements, privacy issues, family interactions, and levels of formality.
- Realize that hand gestures may have different meanings to residents of other cultures.
- Be aware that *you* may seem strange to the resident.
- Remember that being different does not change a person's worth.
- Understand how you would feel in similar circumstances and be sensitive to the resident of another culture. Have empathy.

You may gain better understanding of cultures by considering the differences that exist worldwide.

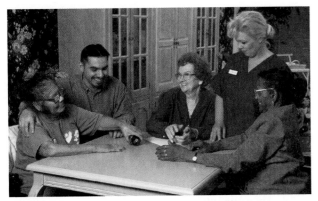

FIGURE 21-6 ■ America is a melting pot of cultures.

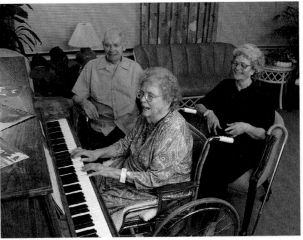

FIGURE 21-8 ■ Music is an expression of spirituality, joy, and emotional energy.

Religion and spirituality are part of one's cultural background. Religion, however, is not the only type of spiritual expression. Expressing spirituality gives a sense of fulfillment, joy, and emotional energy (see Figure 21-8 ■). Each person will express spirituality in a unique and individual way. This may be accomplished by creative efforts, by service to others, or by religious practices. A group of people with similar beliefs and spiritual needs may join to form an organized religion. Religion also may be practiced through personal beliefs without participation in a group.

Respect and accept each resident's spiritual beliefs. Be respectful of clothing and objects that may have religious importance to the resident. Do not attempt to influence the resident with your beliefs. Requests for visits by religious representatives should be reported to the nurse without delay. Provide privacy for the visit. Assist the resident who wants to attend religious services and activities.

PSYCHOSOCIAL CHANGES AFFECTING THE ELDERLY

In the course of a lifetime, each of us fills many roles that help us meet our psychosocial needs and form our personalities. As we proceed through life, our circumstances and roles change, and we must adapt. To **adapt** means to change or adjust.

Major adjustments are necessary as a person ages (see Figure 21-9 ■). The elderly must adapt to

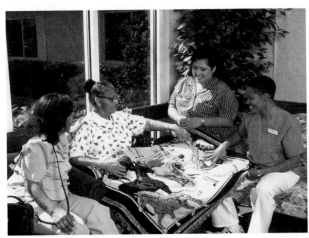

FIGURE 21-7 ■ It is important to develop an understanding of other cultures.

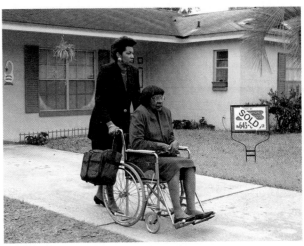

FIGURE 21-9 ■ As a person ages, major adjustments are necessary.

many stressful role changes. Significant psychosocial changes such as retirement, loss of income, loss of a spouse, loss of health, or loss of home may have a severe effect upon the emotional health of the elderly person. Psychosocial needs may become difficult to meet. For example, being unable to drive or to afford a car makes it difficult to socialize and be independent.

In America, we have been taught to value youth and usefulness. Growing old, without an important role to play, leaves some elderly individuals with low self-esteem and a poor sense of self-worth.

PSYCHOSOCIAL NEEDS OF THE RESIDENT IN THE LONG-TERM CARE FACILITY

Some elderly people who become chronically ill and dependent must be admitted to a long-term care facility. Leaving one's own environment to enter a facility increases a person's potential for unmet psychosocial needs. It is difficult to feel loved when you are separated from your loved ones. Being dependent upon others affects self-esteem. Sharing living quarters with many others makes it difficult to maintain privacy and individuality.

It is your responsibility as a nursing assistant to help the resident be independent and maintain, or regain, a sense of self-esteem. The resident's safety and security are always your primary concern. You are a daily source of love, and you are the one who will help to accomplish goals. Report any signs of unmet needs that you observe so that they can be addressed in the resident's care plan. You are the resident's lifeline to health, happiness, and well-being.

RESTORATIVE MEASURES TO MEET THE RESIDENT'S PSYCHOSOCIAL NEEDS

Helping the resident to regain independence is a basic step toward helping to meet many other psychosocial needs. Self-esteem, privacy, and freedom to socialize are influenced by the ability to do things for oneself. Encouraging the resident's independence is an invitation to use your creativity.

Allowing and encouraging residents to make decisions, assist with their own care, and be as active as possible are restorative measures that can challenge your imagination. Noticing and praising even the smallest successes of the resident's efforts is important. Successfully assisting the resident to achieve independence and improve self-esteem will meet your own need for self-actualization. Your self-esteem will increase by helping another succeed.

Safety and Security

Being in control of your own safety is reassuring, whereas having to depend on others for safety and security is frightening. Many of the residents are totally dependent upon the staff for survival. Their need for safety and a sense of security can be met by following safety rules. Safety measures are discussed in Chapter 6.

It is important to encourage a sense of security by developing trusting relationships with residents. If you fulfill your promises to them, they will feel more secure. They will know that they can count on you when it is necessary. Showing concern for their welfare, encouraging them to discuss their concerns, and listening carefully will help to reassure them of their safety.

Love and Belonging

Nursing assistants help to meet the residents' needs for love by caring about them and being sensitive to their needs. Taking time to talk with residents, giving encouragement and praise, and listening attentively helps them to feel loved and appreciated. While you are using verbal communication skills, remember the importance of nonverbal skills. A smile, a touch on the shoulder, and a hug all communicate love. Love usually is returned to you through the residents' responses to your care.

The family is basic to meeting the resident's psychosocial needs. Being an accepted part of a family is the foundation for meeting the resident's need for love and belonging. Encourage family members to visit and help them to be as comfortable as possible. Arrange your care to allow time and privacy for visits (see Figure 21-10 ■).

Some residents have very few visitors. Communicating with others and participating in social activities helps to restore their sense of belonging. For many residents, staff members and other residents become "family." Remember to introduce residents to people they don't know.

Be sure the residents have clean glasses and hearing aids that function properly. Without these, some residents would be alone in a crowd. Help residents to attend activities. Assisting with ambulation or providing a wheelchair or walker may be necessary to help the resident socialize. The resident who feels the most unloved and isolated may not be able to be with others unless you help.

Self-Esteem

The resident's self-esteem is improved by many of the same things that help you feel better about yourself. Helping the resident to be well groomed, to keep things in order, and to feel loved and useful are self-esteem builders. You can support residents' self-esteem by encouraging independence, treating them as individuals, and recognizing their accomplishments (see Figure 21-11 ■).

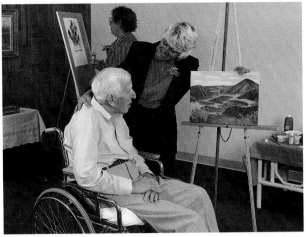

FIGURE 21-11 ■ Giving praise helps the resident feel valued.

If others' reactions are positive toward people, they tend to feel good about themselves. If those reactions from others are negative or unkind, self-image may be affected in a negative way. Be aware of your attitudes and interactions with residents, and make sure you send positive messages to them.

Self-Actualization

Provided that basic needs have been met, the resident may be ready to pursue some higher goals that will increase their self-actualization. Your creativity will be useful in helping the resident find ways to meet the need for self-actualization. Helping the resident achieve goals will be rewarding for both of you.

Social activities provide many opportunities for self-actualization. Creative projects provide a way for residents to feel that they have accomplished something. Remembering and sharing life stories and events helps restore a sense of pride in their accomplishments earlier in life. Religious expression is also an important part of meeting the need for self-actualization.

A positive self-image contributes to a person's motivation. Can you recall a time when you felt so good about yourself that you wanted to take on a new challenge or do something exciting? You had a need for self-actualization. As you help the residents to succeed, be aware of your own

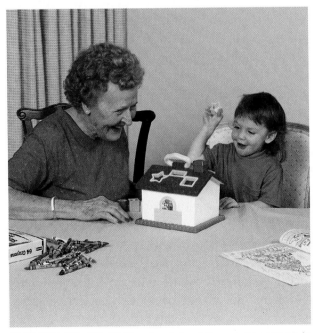

FIGURE 21-10 ■ The family's visits are important in meeting the resident's psychosocial needs.

feelings of pride, joy, and success. This is an opportunity for one of the most satisfying rewards of nursing.

SEXUALITY AND THE ELDERLY

Sexuality is as much a part of the whole person as spirituality. Sexual fulfillment is not only physical, but also includes a need for closeness, love, and affection. Most sexual relationships include a warm and caring attitude between the partners (see Figure 21-12 ■).

Sex and intimacy are important and acceptable for the elderly. Both elderly men and women have sexual interests. Elderly men and women are attracted to each other, and appearance is important.

Sexuality is a very individual need. The sexual needs of a person continue throughout life. Patterns of sexual fulfillment generally remain the same. The need for the warmth, caring, and security of a close relationship with another may increase.

Changes in the elderly person's sexual activity may occur. The physical changes of aging in the reproductive system cause some problems. Chronic illness, fatigue, and immobility or pain may interfere with sexual function. Loss of a sexual partner is a common problem for elderly individuals.

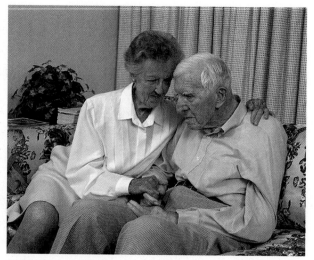

FIGURE 21-12 ■ Love and affection are satisfying.

Sexuality in the Long-Term Care Facility

When an elderly person becomes a resident of a long-term care facility, the need for sexual fulfillment is more difficult to meet. Even though married partners may share a room, they often sleep in separate hospital beds. Privacy becomes a problem for elderly residents who develop intimate relationships.

One of the greatest problems in dealing with sexuality in the long-term care facility is the discomfort of staff members. You may become embarrassed when confronted with the sexuality of another person. It is not unusual to feel uncomfortable.

It is important to be able to manage your reactions to the residents' behavior. Being knowledgeable about sexuality in the elderly will help. Comfort with your own sexuality and concern for the residents' quality of life also will help you to handle these situations correctly.

Encouraging and assisting the resident in grooming is important, and your compliments are helpful. Personal appearance and a positive self-image support a person's sexual identity. Makeup or shaving, fragrance, and clothing make a statement about a person's sexuality.

Protect the resident's privacy by preventing exposure of the body during care. Close the door if it seems appropriate to do so, and knock before entering a resident's room. Allow time for the resident to respond before entering. Advise other staff members when you know that the resident wants time alone.

Accept displays of affection between residents as a natural part of human relationships. Also, accept the residents' individual preferences of sexual expression. Do not be judgmental or gossip. Accept the resident's individuality. Think of elderly couples in the same way that you would think of younger couples.

Some residents may be sexually aggressive and make advances toward you or other residents. Guidelines for managing sexually aggressive behavior are located in Chapter 24.

CHAPTER HIGHLIGHTS

1. Most of the residents of a long-term care facility are elderly.

2. Most of the elderly in the United States live at home, or with family or friends. Only a small percentage live in nursing homes.

3. Your main concern with geriatric residents is to protect their health and safety.

4. It is important to treat the developmentally disabled person with dignity and respect.

5. Growth and development take place at an orderly rate throughout life.

6. According to Erik Erikson, there are specific developmental tasks that must be accomplished during certain stages of life.

7. Physical health, mental health, heredity, environment, and lifestyle affect aging.

8. The basic needs of all human beings are physical, safety and security, love and belonging, self-esteem, and self-actualization.

9. The most basic needs are physical.

10. Fulfillment of basic needs affect the quality of one's life.

11. Culture and spirituality influence an individual's basic needs and the way in which those needs are fulfilled.

12. Cultural diversity refers to the differences that exist between individuals from various cultural or ethnic groups.

13. The many psychosocial changes and losses experienced by the elderly cause emotional stress.

14. Independence helps the resident gain self-esteem, privacy, and the freedom to socialize.

15. The nursing assistant's interest in the resident's accomplishments helps to meet the resident's need for self-actualization.

16. Sexual fulfillment helps meet the needs for closeness, love, affection, and belonging.

VOCABULARY REVIEW

Fill in the blanks with the vocabulary term that best completes the sentence.

1. _____ are the teenage years between 13 and 18.

2. To _____ means to change or adjust.

3. The end of menstruation is _____.

4. A _____ person is someone who has not developed normally due to a birth defect, an injury, or an illness.

5. Proving yourself and meeting goals is called _____.

6. _____ needs are the emotional, social, and spiritual needs.

7. A _____ is an elderly person who lives in a long-term care facility.

8. _____ means confused.

9. _____ occurs when we contaminate the environment with such things as trash and cigarette smoke.

10. The needs of the body are the _____ needs.

CHECK YOUR UNDERSTANDING

The following questions cover the highlights of this chapter. Choose the best answer for each question.

1. The major developmental task of the elderly is to
   A. develop trust
   B. gain competence in intellectual skills
   C. establish intimacy
   D. find meaning in life's experiences

2. Which of the following statements about developmentally disabled residents is true?
   A. Many are unable to care for themselves.
   B. All are mentally retarded.
   C. All have muscular difficulties.
   D. Most live in nursing homes.

3. A mentally retarded resident is having difficulty eating her roast beef. What is your best response?
   A. Feed the resident yourself.
   B. Cut the meat into small pieces.
   C. Let her do it all herself.
   D. Take away the roast beef.

4. The most basic of all human needs is
   A. Love   C. Physical
   B. Self-esteem   D. Safety

5. You are caring for a resident who speaks Spanish. Which of the following statements would be most helpful?
   A. "I'm sorry, I don't understand Spanish. Let me get someone who does."
   B. "You'll have to speak English. I don't speak Spanish."
   C. "Your daughter will have to stay here and interpret for you."
   D. "I'm sorry, I don't speak Spanish. Can it wait until later?"

6. Which statement about geriatric residents is most *true*?
   A. They heal quickly.
   B. Their personalities change significantly with aging.
   C. Body systems work faster.
   D. Their health and safety is your main concern.

7. Which fact about the sexuality of the elderly is *true*?
   A. The elderly are unattractive to each other.
   B. Chronic illness may interfere with sexual function.
   C. Sexual patterns change with aging.
   D. Elderly women have no interest in sex.

8. Which would meet the need for a resident's self-actualization?
   A. Learning to walk again.
   B. Being fed by the nursing assistant.
   C. Receiving a complete bed bath.
   D. Emptying the urinary drainage bag.

9. According to Maslow's list of human needs, which is *not* a basic need?
   A. Physical.   C. Self-actualization.
   B. Entertainment.   D. Self-esteem.

AGE-SPECIFIC TIP

To help maintain elderly residents' self-esteem, address them by their proper names and titles. Do not use nicknames or first names unless requested to do so by the resident.

CULTURALLY SENSITIVE TIP

Eye contact, use of touch, and personal space requirements differ among different cultures. Stay aware of and honor the resident's need for personal space.

EFFECTIVE PROBLEM SOLVING

June Grannell is a 50-year-old resident who is developmentally disabled. She is crying, shouting, and pounding her fists because she wants to go for a ride in the car. The nursing assistant heaves a sigh of frustration and says, "June, don't act like a child! I would have to call your mother to come and take you for a ride. I can't do everything you ask of me."

Was the nursing assistant's communication appropriate? If not, what would have been more appropriate?

_____

_____

_____

_____

_____

_____

_____

_____

INTERPERSONAL COMMUNICATION

Communication patterns differ as an individual moves through the stages of life. Place the letter of each item of Column 2 beside the matching item in Column 1.

	Column 1	Column 2
_____ 1.	"All my friends are doing it."	A. Infancy
_____ 2.	"I want to do it myself."	B. Toddler
_____ 3.	"That's not the way we used to do it."	C. School age
_____ 4.	Crying and kicking	D. Old age

OBSERVING, REPORTING, AND RECORDING

Specific behavior and characteristics are evident with each age group. You must be able to recognize what is normal and what is abnormal. List the common behavior and characteristics that may be observed in each age group.

_____

_____

_____

_____

_____

_____

_____

_____

EXPLORE MEDIALINK

22

BODY STRUCTURE AND FUNCTION: CHANGES OF AGING

OBJECTIVES

1. Describe the structure and function of cells, tissues, organs, and systems.
2. Identify two changes of aging in each system of the body.
3. Identify and describe the special senses.
4. Describe the relationships of all the body systems.

VOCABULARY

The following words or terms will help you to understand this chapter:

Anatomy	System	Peristalsis
Physiology	Appendage	Colon
Cell	Respiration	Feces
Tissue	Diastole	Hormones
Organ	Systole	Metabolism

This chapter discusses the function and structure of the human body and describes common body changes that occur with aging.

*B*ASIC BODY STRUCTURE

The human body is composed of many parts that work together in an amazing way. Body "structure" refers to how the body parts are arranged, and "function" refers to how the body works. **Anatomy** is the study of body structure. **Physiology** is the study of body function. In order to care for residents safely, it is best to understand the body and how it works. For more detailed information, refer to the physiology and anatomy insert.

Cells

The smallest unit, the basic building block of the body, is the **cell**. A cell is a living organism that needs food, water, and oxygen. The basic parts of the cell are the membrane, cytoplasm, and nucleus (see Figure 22-1 ■). The membrane is the outer protective covering. It permits food, water, and oxygen to enter and allows waste products to exit. Cytoplasm is the material inside the cell, and the nucleus directs and controls the cell.

Cells are so small that they can be seen only through a microscope. The human body contains millions of cells that differ in size, shape, and function. Most cells do not work alone, but combine with other cells that are alike in size, shape, and function.

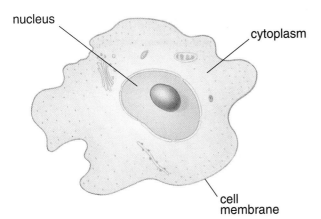

FIGURE 22-1 ■ Structure of the cell

Tissues

A **tissue** is a group of cells that work together to perform a certain function (see Figure 22-2 ■). Tissues can be divided into four types:

* Connective
* Epithelial
* Muscle
* Nerve

Blood and lymph are special types of connective tissue.

Mucous membranes are thin sheets of tissue that line certain parts of the body. They produce mucus, a thick, sticky fluid that lubricates and protects the membranes. Your mouth and nose are two of the body parts that are lined with mucous membranes.

Organs

An **organ** is a group of tissues that work together to perform a certain function. Organs are located in compartments of the body called "cavities." See Figure 22-3 ■ for the location of some major organs and cavities of the body.

Systems

A group of organs that work together to perform a function is called a **system**. The systems of the body include

* Integumentary system
* Musculoskeletal system
* Respiratory system
* Circulatory system
* Digestive system
* Urinary system
* Nervous system
* Endocrine system
* Reproductive system

The human body is a combination of all these systems. No system of the body works independently; therefore, a change in one system will affect the others. Although you will study the systems separately, remember that a healthy body requires the combined function of all systems. Figure 22-4 ■ provides a summary of the structure and function of

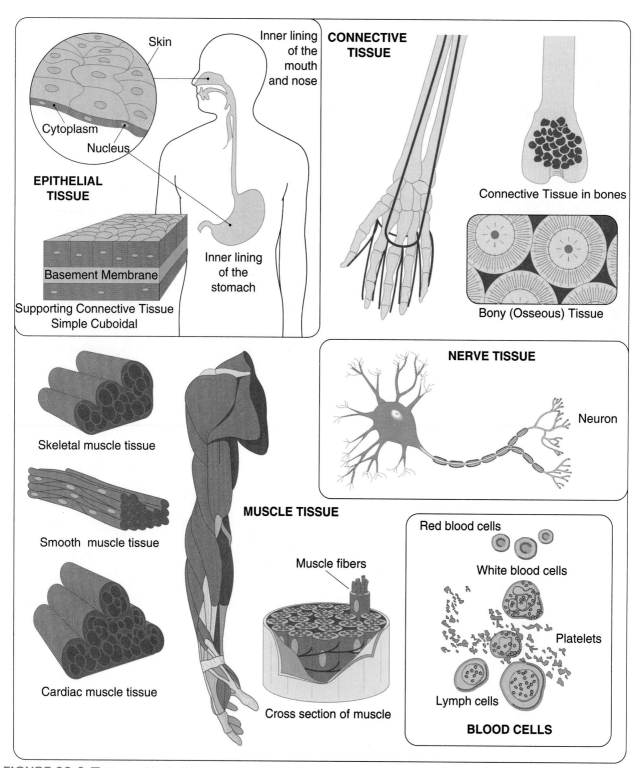

EPITHELIAL TISSUE

Skin

Cytoplasm

Nucleus

Inner lining of the mouth and nose

Basement Membrane

Inner lining of the stomach

Supporting Connective Tissue
Simple Cuboidal

CONNECTIVE TISSUE

Connective Tissue in bones

Bony (Osseous) Tissue

NERVE TISSUE

Neuron

Skeletal muscle tissue

Smooth muscle tissue

Cardiac muscle tissue

MUSCLE TISSUE

Muscle fibers

Cross section of muscle

Red blood cells

White blood cells

Platelets

Lymph cells

BLOOD CELLS

FIGURE 22-2 ■ Types of body tissues

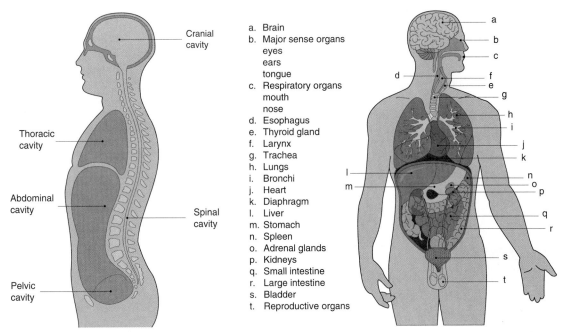

a. Brain
b. Major sense organs
    eyes
    ears
    tongue
c. Respiratory organs
    mouth
    nose
d. Esophagus
e. Thyroid gland
f. Larynx
g. Trachea
h. Lungs
i. Bronchi
j. Heart
k. Diaphragm
l. Liver
m. Stomach
n. Spleen
o. Adrenal glands
p. Kidneys
q. Small intestine
r. Large intestine
s. Bladder
t. Reproductive organs

FIGURE 22-3 ■ Major organs and cavities of the body

each system. A summary of the changes of aging is shown in Figure 22-5 ■.

THE INTEGUMENTARY SYSTEM

Structure

The integumentary system is composed of the skin and its appendages. An **appendage** is an extension of a body part. Appendages of the skin include fingernails, toenails, hair, sweat glands, and oil glands.

The outer layer of skin is called the "epidermis." It is very thin and contains the pigment that determines skin color. The dermis is the inner layer of skin that contains blood vessels and nerve endings. Cells flake off the epidermis and are replaced by new ones from the dermis. A layer of subcutaneous fatty tissue separates the skin from the underlying structures. It provides a shock-absorbing cushion for insulation and protection (see Figure 22-6 ■).

Function

The main functions of the integumentary system are to

- Protect internal parts of the body.
- Form a barrier against germs and protect from infection.

- Help regulate water balance.
- Help maintain normal body temperature.
- Eliminate body waste through pores in the skin.
- Provide lubrication through oil glands.
- Allow the sensations of heat, cold, pleasure, and pain through nerve endings in the skin.

Changes of Aging

The first signs of aging often are seen in the integumentary system. Hair thins and loses its color or turns gray. Brown spots, sometimes called "liver spots," may develop. As the skin loses elasticity, wrinkles appear. Less active sweat and oil glands cause the skin to be dry. The skin gets thinner and more fragile, which means it is easily damaged.

The fatty tissue that provides padding between the skin and bones gets thinner, leaving the skin with less protection and less insulation. Because of these changes, the elderly often complain of feeling cold.

A decrease of sensitivity in nerve endings causes the elderly person to be less able to identify sensations. The sense of touch may not be dependable. Fingernails and toenails become thick, hard, and yellowed. Torn cuticles and ingrown nails can occur. The nails may become diseased because they are hard to clean.

System	Structure	Function
Integumentary	Skin and appendages.	Protects against infection. Protects internal organs. Regulates body temperature. Helps regulate water balance and eliminate waste. Provides lubrication. Allows sensations such as heat, cold, pleasure, and pain.
Musculoskeletal (combination of muscular and skeletal systems)	Bones, joints, muscles, tendons, ligaments, bursa, and cartilage.	Provides structure and framework. Produces movement. Protects vital organs.
Respiratory	Nose, pharynx, larynx, trachea, bronchi, lungs and alveoli.	Brings oxygen into the body and removes carbon dioxide.
Circulatory (cardiovascular)	Heart, blood, and blood vessels.	Transports food, water, and oxygen to the cells and waste products away from the cells. Helps regulate body temperature. Helps protect the body from disease.
Digestive	Mouth, pharynx, esophagus, stomach, small intestine, and large intestine.	Prepares food for the body's use and eliminates waste products.
Urinary	Kidneys, ureters, bladder, and urethra.	Filters wastes from blood, produces urine, and eliminates waste products from the body. Helps maintain fluid and chemical balance.
Nervous	Brain, spinal cord, and nerves.	Controls and coordinates body activities.
Endocrine	Pituitary, thyroid, thymus, parathyroid, and adrenal glands. Pancreas and gonads.	Secretes hormones that regulate and coordinate body functions.
Reproductive	*Female:* Ovaries, fallopian tubes, uterus, and vagina. *Male:* Testes, scrotum, penis, seminal vesicles, and prostate gland.	Reproduction of the species.

FIGURE 22-4 ■ Summary of the structure and functions of body systems.

Changes of aging in the integumentary system leave the elderly person less protected from the environment.

THE MUSCULOSKELETAL SYSTEM

Structure
The musculoskeletal system is composed of bones, joints, and muscles. Although bones are hard and rigid, they are made of living cells that grow and harden slowly. The human skeleton contains 206 bones. The four most common types of bones are long bones, short bones, flat bones, and irregular bones (see Figure 22-7 ■).

Joints connect the bones and are composed of ligaments, tendons, bursa, and cartilage. Ligaments connect bone to bone, and tendons connect muscle to bone. Bursa are small sacs of fluid that lubricate and prevent friction in the joints. Cartilage

Physical Changes of Aging

Integumentary System
Hair thins and loses color
Dry, thin, fragile skin
Wrinkles and liver spots
Loss of fatty tissue
Decrease of feeling
Thick, hard nails

Musculoskeletal System
Weakening muscles and loss of tone
Slowing of body movements
Stiff joints
Brittle bones
Changes in posture, loss of height

Respiratory System
Rib cage more rigid
Weakening of muscles
Decreased elasticity of lungs
Weakening of voice

Circulatory System
Heart pumps with less force
Hardening and narrowing of blood vessels

Digestive System
Decrease in saliva and taste buds
Decrease in digestive juices

Digestive System (Cont.)
Difficulty in chewing and swallowing
Slowing of peristalsis
Reduced absorption of vitamins and minerals

Urinary System
Decrease in kidney filtration
Decrease in bladder muscle tone.

Nervous System
Decrease in nerve cells
Slowed message transmission
Slowed responses and reflexes
Decreased sensitivity of nerve endings
Short-term memory loss
Decrease in vision
Hearing loss
Loss of smell receptors

Endocrine System
Decrease in hormones
Reduced regulation of body activities

Reproductive System
Menopause in women
Drying and thinning of vaginal walls
Enlargement of male prostate gland
Change in male hormone levels

FIGURE 22-5 ■ Physical changes of aging

provides padding between bones. There are several types of joints that allow a variety of movements (see Figure 22-8 ■).

There are three types of muscles: voluntary, involuntary, and cardiac. Voluntary muscles are muscles that are controlled by will. For example, you can move the muscles in your arms or legs by thinking about doing so. Involuntary muscles work automatically, without conscious thought. These muscles help you to breathe and digest food. Cardiac muscle is a special type of involuntary muscle that controls the heartbeat.

Muscles work together in groups. Some muscles, like those in your upper arm, work in pairs. A muscle

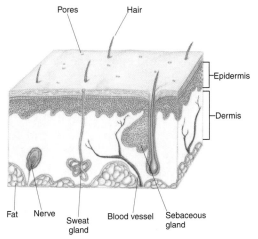

FIGURE 22-6 ■ The layers of the skin

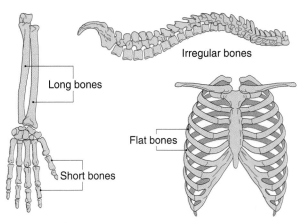

FIGURE 22-7 ■ Types of bones

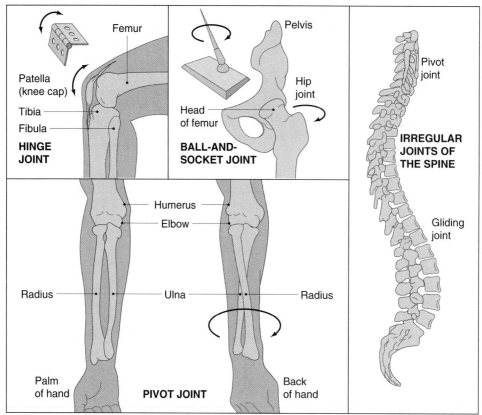

FIGURE 22-8 ■ Types of joints

in the front of the arm contracts (shortens) while the one in the back relaxes (lengthens); this allows you to bend your arm (see Figure 22-9 ■). Working muscles use food for energy and produce body heat.

Functions

The main functions of the musculoskeletal system include the following:

- Produce movement
- Protect vital organs
- Provide support and framework for the body

Muscles and bones must work together to move the body. The musculoskeletal system must work with other body systems to allow you to accomplish even a small movement such as lifting one finger.

Changes of Aging

As a person gets older, many changes occur in the musculoskeletal system. Muscles weaken and lose their tone. Strength and endurance decrease, while body movement slows.

Joints become stiff as cartilage deteriorates and tissue hardens. This can make movement difficult, which may lead to decreased activity and further loss of muscle tone.

Bones become porous and brittle. Because they are not as hard as they once were, bones are broken easily. Many older people lose calcium, so their bones become even more fragile. Changes in

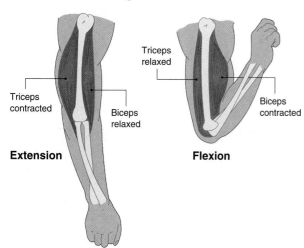

FIGURE 22-9 ■ Coordination of muscles

the spinal column (the bony structure that protects the spinal cord) can result in stooped posture and a loss of height.

Changes of aging in the musculoskeletal system may interfere with the ability of elderly people to care for themselves and remain independent. These changes also place the resident at increased risk of injury.

THE RESPIRATORY SYSTEM

Structure

Structures of the respiratory system include the nose, pharynx, larynx, trachea, bronchi, lungs, and alveoli (see Figure 22-10 ■). Air enters the body through the nose and pharynx. The pharynx (throat) is a passageway for both air and food. The larynx ("voice box") contains the vocal cords and is located at the opening to the trachea (windpipe). After leaving the pharynx, air enters the trachea and flows through the bronchi, or bronchial tree. The left bronchus and right bronchus branch out into smaller tubes, much like branches on a tree.

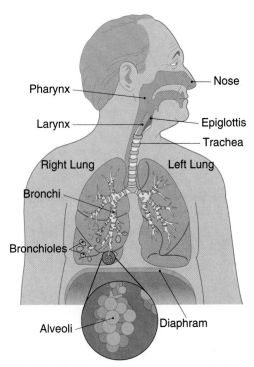

FIGURE 22-10 ■ The major structures of the respiratory system

Tubes of the bronchial tree lead to small air sacs of the lungs, called "alveoli."

A piece of cartilage, called the "epiglottis," covers the trachea to prevent food in the throat from entering the airway. It lifts when you breathe or talk and closes when you swallow. Have you ever choked while trying to talk and eat at the same time? That happened because the epiglottis opened to allow you to talk and food went down the wrong way, into the trachea.

Functions

The main functions of the respiratory system are

* To bring oxygen into the body
* To remove carbon dioxide from the body

Oxygen is a colorless, odorless gas found in the air. Each cell of the body needs oxygen to survive. Carbon dioxide is a gas that is a waste product of the body.

The respiratory system provides a pathway for oxygen to enter the body and carbon dioxide to leave. This process is accomplished by **respiration** (breathing). During respiration, blood vessels in the alveoli exchange carbon dioxide that has been brought to the lungs for oxygen. Oxygen is then carried to the heart to be circulated to the cells.

The lungs are located in the chest cavity and are protected by the rib cage. The diaphragm, a muscle that separates the chest cavity from the abdominal cavity, is immediately below the lungs. Inhalation (breathing in) occurs when the diaphragm flattens, enlarging the chest cavity. This causes the lungs to expand and fill with oxygen. Exhalation (breathing out) occurs when the diaphragm expands, decreasing the size of the chest cavity. Air containing carbon dioxide is then forced out of the lungs.

The center that controls respirations is in the brain. The rate of respirations is affected by the amount of carbon dioxide in the blood. The faster you move, the more carbon dioxide you produce, and the faster you must breathe to eliminate it.

Changes of Aging

The rib cage, which normally expands, becomes more rigid, and muscles weaken. These changes limit the lungs' ability to fill. With increased activity, the older person has to breathe harder and faster to get enough air. There is a decrease in the elasticity of the lungs. The ability to resist disease is lowered. Changes in the larynx may weaken the voice and cause it to sound different. Any change in the respiratory system that reduces the amount of oxygen brought into the body will affect all the systems.

*T*HE CIRCULATORY SYSTEM

Structure

The circulatory (cardiovascular) system includes the heart, blood, and blood vessels. Together, they form the body's transportation and delivery system. The heart moves blood through the blood vessels, carrying oxygen and other substances to and from the cells. The blood delivers products to and from the cells by traveling through the blood vessels.

Function

The main functions of the circulatory system are to

- Transport food, water, and oxygen to the cells
- Transport waste products away from the cells
- Help regulate body temperature
- Protect the body against disease

The Heart

The heart is an organ about the size of your fist that is composed of cardiac muscle. It is located in the chest slightly to the left of the midline, between the two lungs. The rib cage protects the heart, as it does the lungs. The function of the heart is to pump blood throughout the body. The heart is divided into four chambers that are separated by muscular walls and one-way valves. The two upper chambers are the right and the left atria. The function of the atria is to receive blood from the body. The two lower chambers are the right and left ventricles. Their function is to pump blood out of the heart to other parts of the body.

The Cardiac Cycle

The heart moves blood through the body. It does this in precise, coordinated movements, called the cardiac cycle. The cycle is divided into two stages: diastole and systole. **Diastole** is the stage of the cardiac cycle when the heart is resting and filling with blood. **Systole** is the stage when the heart is contracting and pumping out the blood.

The blood returning from the body is low in oxygen and high in carbon dioxide. Most of the oxygen has been delivered to the cells and exchanged for carbon dioxide. The blood enters the right atrium of the heart through large veins called the inferior and superior vena cava. From the right atrium, the blood enters the right ventricle. The right ventricle contracts and pumps unoxygenated blood into the pulmonary artery, through which it flows to the lungs. In the alveoli of the lungs, the carbon dioxide is exchanged for oxygen.

The blood returns from the lungs to the left atrium of the heart and passes into the left ventricle. The left ventricle contracts and pumps the blood into the aorta, the largest blood vessel in the body. The blood then circulates through a series of blood vessels to all parts of the body before returning to the heart. Look at Figure 22-11 ■, and trace the flow of blood through the heart.

The Blood

Blood is the part of the body that actually carries oxygen, food, wastes, and other substances. The

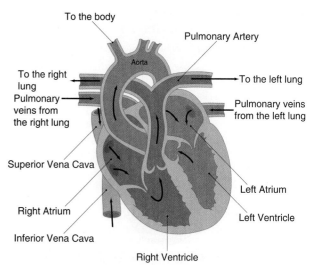

FIGURE 22-11 ■ The flow of blood through the heart

average adult has 4 to 6 quarts of blood, which is composed of plasma and cells. Although plasma is mostly water, it also contains many other important substances.

The three main types of blood cells are

- Red blood cells
- White blood cells
- Platelets

Red blood cells carry oxygen. They give blood its red color. White blood cells help to fight disease and are a part of the body's immune or defense system. Platelets help the blood to clot. Blood cells live for only a short time and must be replaced by new ones.

The Blood Vessels

Blood vessels are tubes that transport blood throughout the body. They are the "roadways" of the circulatory system. The major types of blood vessels are arteries, veins, and capillaries:

- Arteries carry blood away from the heart.
- Veins carry blood back to the heart.
- Capillaries connect arteries to veins, and exchange substances.

Arteries carry oxygen-rich blood, except for the pulmonary artery. The pulmonary artery carries blood from the heart to the lungs, where it receives oxygen. Veins carry oxygen-poor blood, except for the pulmonary veins, which return oxygenated blood from the lungs to the heart. Capillaries are very small blood vessels that allow food, oxygen, and other substances, including waste products, to enter and exit the bloodstream.

The circulatory system, the respiratory system, and the nervous system are essential to life. A malfunction of any one of the three can cause immediate death.

Changes of Aging

Changes of aging slow the movement of blood throughout the body. Heart muscle weakens with age, causing the heart to pump with less force. Although the heart works harder to keep the blood moving, it is less effective. This results in a decrease in blood flow. Changes in the blood vessels also

slow the flow of blood. Blood vessels that harden and lose their elasticity become narrow. Fatty deposits and other substances may clog the narrowed vessels. Changes in the circulatory system are the cause of many physical and mental problems of the elderly.

THE DIGESTIVE SYSTEM

Structure

The primary organs of the digestive system are the mouth, pharynx (throat), esophagus, stomach, small intestine, and large intestine. These structures form a long, continuous tube that extends from the mouth to the anus (the opening to the rectum) (see Figure 22-12 ■). This tube, called the "alimentary canal," is lined with mucous membrane. The accessory organs of the digestive system are the teeth, tongue, salivary glands, liver, gallbladder, and pancreas. The

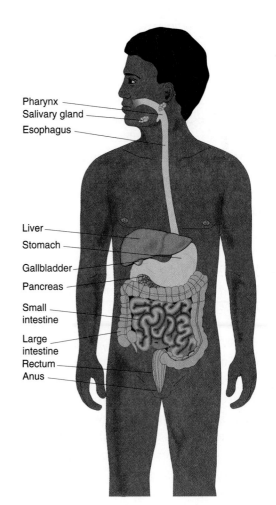

FIGURE 22-12 ■ The digestive system

"gastrointestinal (GI) system" is another name for the digestive system.

Function

The main functions of the digestive system are to

- Prepare food for the body's use
- Eliminate solid wastes

The process of preparing food for the body's use is called "digestion." Digestion begins in the mouth, with the assistance of the teeth, tongue, and salivary glands. The teeth bite and chew the food into pieces that are small enough to be swallowed. The salivary glands secrete saliva to add moisture and chemicals. Taste buds on the tongue allow a person to enjoy the food. The tongue also helps during swallowing by pushing the food into the pharynx, which contracts and moves the food into the esophagus. Peristalsis moves the food from the esophagus to the stomach. **Peristalsis** is the muscular contractions that move food through the digestive system.

The stomach churns the food into smaller pieces. Gastric juices from the stomach help to digest the food. The food mixture moves from the stomach into the small intestine, where digestive juices from the liver, gallbladder, and pancreas are added. Digestion is completed in the small intestine, where projections called "villi" absorb the digested food particles and release them into the bloodstream. The rest of the food mass moves into the **colon** (large intestine). The purpose of the colon is to remove water from the food for the body's use. The material that remains forms a solid waste product that is called "**feces**." The feces is stored in the rectum until it leaves the body through the anus (the opening of the rectum).

Changes of Aging

Many changes of aging occur in the digestive system. A decrease in saliva and in the number of taste buds leads to a decrease in appetite. The elderly often have difficulty chewing and swallowing. Muscles weaken and lose their tone. A reduction in digestive juices makes food harder to digest. The absorption of vitamins and minerals is reduced. Peristalsis slows. These changes cause the process of digestion to be less efficient in the elderly.

THE URINARY SYSTEM

Structure

The main structures of the urinary system (see Figure 22-13 ■) are the kidneys, ureters, bladder, and urethra. The kidneys are two bean-shaped organs located in the upper abdomen, toward the

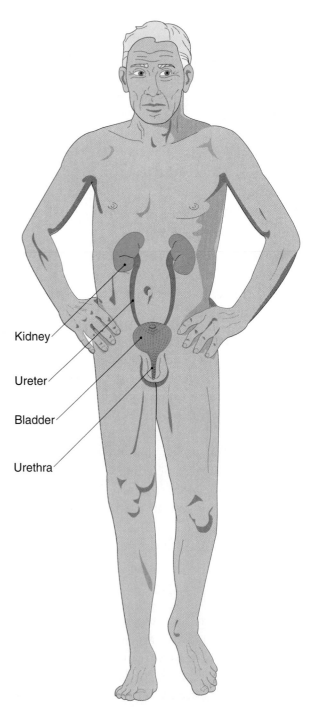

Kidney

Ureter

Bladder

Urethra

FIGURE 22-13 ■ The urinary system

back, on either side of the spine. A ureter leads from each kidney to the bladder. The bladder is a muscular sac that is located in the front of the lower abdomen. The tube that leads from the bladder to the outside of the body is called the "urethra." The external (outside) opening of the urethra is called the urinary meatus.

Function

The main functions of the urinary system are as follows:

- Filter waste from the blood
- Eliminate liquid waste (urine) from the body
- Help maintain the body's fluid and chemical balance

The major function of the kidneys is to filter and remove waste from the blood. This is accomplished through a complicated system of tubes and blood vessels. Filtration takes place in the nephrons, which are located in the outer layer of each kidney. Each kidney may have a million or more nephrons. The kidneys produce urine from filtered wastes and water. The ureters carry the urine from the kidneys to the bladder.

The bladder is a muscular, expandable sac. Urine, which is continuously produced by the kidneys, is held in the bladder until it is eliminated from the body. The average adult bladder can hold about one quart of urine. When the bladder is approximately one-third full, the brain sends a signal causing an urge to urinate. The amount the bladder can hold without discomfort, and the length of time between signals from the brain, vary from one person to another.

The urethra allows urine to pass from the bladder to the outside of the body through the urinary meatus. The elimination of water and waste products by the urinary system help to maintain the fluid and chemical balance of the body.

Changes of Aging

The kidneys do not filter as efficiently in the elderly person because there is a decrease in the number of functioning nephrons. Slowed circulation also delays the filtering of the blood. This can

cause waste products and toxins (poisonous substances) to build up in the body.

A decrease in the muscle tone of the bladder leads to a loss of elasticity. The bladder holds less urine for shorter periods of time and may not empty completely. The muscle that keeps urine in the bladder weakens and may allow urine to escape involuntarily.

The urinary, integumentary, digestive, and respiratory systems are all involved in eliminating waste products from the body.

THE NERVOUS SYSTEM

Structure

The nervous system (see Figure 22-14 ■) is composed of the brain, spinal cord, and nerves. It is divided into the central nervous system and the peripheral nervous system. The central nervous system is made up of the brain and spinal cord. The brain is divided into sections that each control specific functions. The right side of the brain controls the left side of the body, and the left side of the brain controls the right side of the body. The brain is protected by the skull. The spinal cord is protected by the vertebral (spinal) column.

The peripheral nervous system consists of all the nerves that are outside of the brain and spinal cord. There are 12 pairs of cranial nerves that carry messages into and out of the brain. There are 31 pairs of spinal nerves that carry messages to and from the spinal cord. Nerves are composed of bundles of nerve fibers. The basic unit of the nervous system is the neuron (nerve cell). There are billions of neurons transmitting messages throughout the body.

Function

The function of the nervous system is to control and coordinate the body's activities. It is the body's communication center. The special senses of sight, hearing, smell, taste, and touch receive messages from the environment. Nerves carry those messages along the spinal cord to the brain, where they are processed. The brain then sends instructions for a response through the nerves to the appropriate

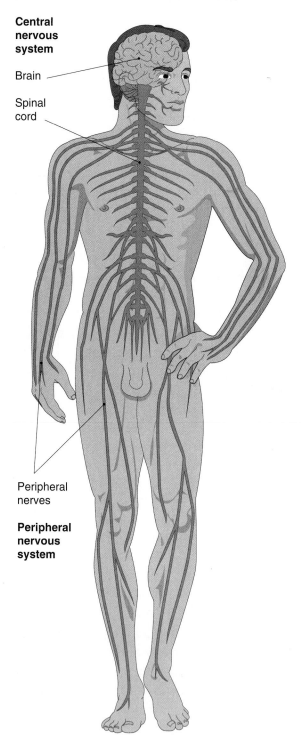

Central nervous system

Brain

Spinal cord

Peripheral nerves

Peripheral nervous system

FIGURE 22-14 ■ The nervous system

body part. For instance, if you put your finger against a hot iron, nerves take that message to the brain. The brain then directs you to remove your finger from the iron. The entire process may take only a fraction of a second.

Changes of Aging

The number of neurons decreases with aging. Slowed circulation also affects the nervous system. These factors of aging delay the transmission of messages through the body, resulting in slower responses and reflexes.

There is a decrease in the sensitivity of nerve endings in the skin. Numbness may interfere with the ability to handle small objects and the sense of touch is not as accurate.

Elderly persons often are more forgetful. They may forget information that is stored in short-term memory, such as names, dates, telephone numbers, or items on lists. It once was thought that there was a decrease in intelligence and awareness with aging because of a decrease in brain cells. Later studies showed that elderly people who stay active and involved with others do not experience this decline.

*T*HE SPECIAL SENSES

The five special senses are sight, hearing, smell, taste, and touch. Nerve endings (receptors) in certain parts of the body transmit received information to the brain. For example, receptors in the eye allow you to see.

The Eye

The eye (see Figure 22-15 ■) is the sense organ for vision. The structure of the eye includes the eyeball, orbit, muscles, eyelids, conjunctiva, and optic nerve.

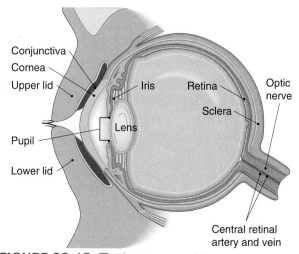

Conjunctiva
Cornea
Upper lid
Iris
Retina
Optic nerve
Sclera
Lens
Pupil
Lower lid
Central retinal artery and vein

FIGURE 22-15 ■ The structure of the eye

The eyeball, the globe-shaped part of the eye, is composed of three layers. The outer layer contains the sclera (the white part of the eye) and the cornea (which helps to focus light rays). The middle layer contains the iris (the colored part of the eye). In the center of the iris is the pupil, a round, dark opening that changes size to control the amount of light that can enter. Behind the iris is the lens, which focuses light images onto the retina. The inner layer of the eyeball is the retina, which contains sight receptors called "rods" and "cones."

All these structures work together to allow you to see. Light images enter through the cornea and the pupil and pass through the lens, which projects the images onto the retina. These sight messages are received by the rods and cones of the retina and are carried to the brain by the optic nerve.

The Ear

The ear (see Figure 22-16 ■) is the sense organ for hearing and balance. It is divided into three parts: the outer ear, the middle ear, and the inner ear. The auricle (pinna) and auditory canal compose the outer ear. The auricle is the outer part that surrounds the opening to the auditory canal. The tympanic membrane (eardrum) separates the outer ear from the middle ear. Located in the middle ear are three small bones, the malleus, the incus, and the stapes. These bones are called the "ossicles." The inner ear contains semicircular canals filled with fluid and nerve receptors.

Sound waves are received by the auricle, which reflects them into the auditory canal. They flow through the auditory canal to the eardrum, causing it to vibrate. The vibrations of the eardrum set the ossicles into motion. The motion of the ossicles moves fluid in the semicircular canals of the inner ear, causing waves of fluid to stimulate tiny nerve receptors. Nerve impulses are initiated and travel to the brain by way of the auditory nerve.

The semicircular canals also contain nerve receptors for balance. Changes in the position of your head cause the fluid in the semicircular canals to move. The nerve impulses for balance are initiated by this fluid movement and are transmitted to the brain.

The Nose

Although the major function of the nose is to bring oxygen into the body, it also contains the receptors for smell. Messages from the receptors in the upper part of the nose are carried by the olfactory nerve to the brain. Although the senses of smell and taste are closely related, smell is the more accurate.

The Tongue

The receptors for taste are located on the tongue. They are called "taste buds." The taste buds for sweet and salty are on the tip of the tongue. Sour receptors are on the sides of the tongue, and those for bitter are located on the back of the tongue. The taste buds help you to enjoy food.

The Skin

Nerve cells located in the dermis layer of the skin act as receptors for pressure, heat, cold, pain, pleasure, and touch. The tactile (touch) receptors permit you to identify objects by touching them. They send messages to the brain, which directs a response. The sense of touch increases your awareness of the environment, allowing you to protect yourself and stay comfortable.

Changes of Aging

Aging affects the special senses in many ways. The eyes take longer to adjust to changes in light, distance, and direction. Some people have trouble reading small print and must have brighter light to see. Many older people wear glasses to correct their

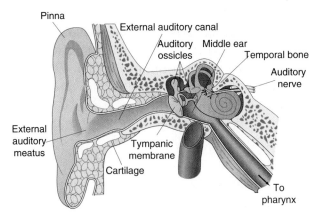

FIGURE 22-16 ■ The structure of the ear

vision. Atrophy of nerve fibers and receptors in the ear cause hearing loss. The receptors become less sensitive, causing sound to be distorted. The sense of balance may be affected. Smell receptors deteriorate with age, reducing the accuracy of smell. Taste becomes less distinct because there is a decrease in the number of taste buds. A decrease in the sensitivity of receptors in the skin means that the sense of touch may be changed.

These sensory changes may interfere with the elderly persons' ability to communicate, protect themselves, and enjoy life.

THE ENDOCRINE SYSTEM

The endocrine system works with the nervous system to regulate and control the activities of the body. The nervous system uses electrical impulses and chemicals for control, while the endocrine system acts only by chemicals called **hormones**.

Structure

The endocrine system is composed of glands that secrete hormones directly into the bloodstream. The major endocrine glands are as follows:

- Pituitary gland
- Thyroid gland
- Parathyroid glands
- Thymus
- Pancreas (islets of Langerhans)
- Adrenal glands
- Gonads (testes in the male; ovaries in the female)

See Figure 22-17 ■ for the location of the major endocrine glands in the body.

Function

The function of the endocrine system is to control and regulate body functions by secreting hormones. Each gland produces different hormones, and each hormone has a specific purpose.

The Pituitary Gland

The pituitary gland is often called the "master" gland because it regulates other glands. It produces hormones that regulate growth, water balance, and reproduction.

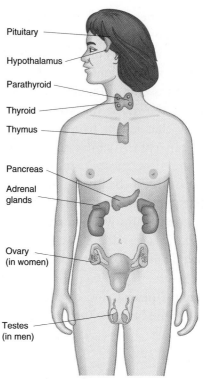

FIGURE 22-17 ■ The major endocrine glands

The Thyroid Gland

The thyroid gland, located in the neck, secretes hormones that affect body growth and development. This gland also regulates metabolism. **Metabolism** is the combination of all body processes. All body functions are affected by changes in metabolism.

The Parathyroid Glands

The parathyroids are located on the back of the thyroid gland. They secrete a hormone that regulates calcium in the body. Calcium levels affect nerve and muscle function.

The Thymus

The thymus produces a hormone that assists in the immune process. The immune system helps the body resist germs and disease. White blood cells that regulate the immune function also develop in this gland. They are called "T cells."

The Pancreas

The pancreas produces hormones that are necessary for the metabolism of sugar. Clusters of cells in the pancreas, called "the islets of Langerhans," produce insulin and glucagon. These hormones are needed to convert sugar to energy.

The Adrenal Glands

The adrenal glands are located on top of the kidneys. These glands produce hormones that help regulate water balance and the metabolism of some foods. Small amounts of sex hormones also are secreted. The adrenals produce hormones that control the body's response to stress. One of these hormones is epinephrin (adrenalin), which allows the body to quickly produce great amounts of energy in an emergency.

The Gonads

The gonads control human reproduction. In the male, the testes produce testosterone. The ovaries of the female produce estrogen and progesterone. These hormones are involved in reproduction, and in the development of male and female characteristics.

Changes of Aging

Changes of aging in the endocrine system affect the levels of hormones in the body. For example, there is a decrease in the production of estrogen and progesterone. Some hormones, like insulin, become less effective. The changes in hormone levels decrease the endocrine system's ability to regulate body activities.

The Exocrine Glands

All glands are not part of the endocrine system. Exocrine glands secrete substances into organs or outside the body, not directly into the bloodstream. The sweat glands, oil glands, and parotid glands, for example, are exocrine glands.

*T*HE REPRODUCTIVE SYSTEM

All living things must have a method to reproduce themselves. A single cell does this by splitting or dividing itself. Human beings reproduce by sexual reproduction, a method requiring a male and a female. Each has special cells, organs, and hormones that work together to accomplish reproduction.

The Female Reproductive System

The major structures of the female reproductive system are the ovaries, fallopian tubes, uterus, and vagina. See Figure 22-18A ■ for the location of the structures of the female reproductive system. The breasts also are considered part of this system.

The ovaries are located on either side of the uterus in the pelvic cavity. The major function of the ovaries is to produce ova (eggs), the female reproductive cells. They also secrete the female hormones, estrogen and progesterone. The fallopian tubes are attached on each side of the uterus and end near each ovary. Their functions are to carry the ova to the uterus and to assist in uniting the male and female sex cells. The uterus is a hollow, muscular organ in the pelvic cavity, above the bladder and in front of the rectum. The functions of the uterus are

* To protect and nourish the fetus during pregnancy
* To expel the fetus during childbirth
* Menstruation

The vagina acts as a passageway for birth of the fetus and menstruation. It is also a receptacle for the penis during sexual intercourse. During intercourse, the sperm enters through the vagina into the uterus and the fallopian tubes. If it unites with an ovum (egg), pregnancy occurs, and the fertilized ovum passes from the fallopian tube to the uterus. If pregnancy does not occur, the ovum will die and be discharged from the body with the menstrual flow.

The Male Reproductive System

The major structures of the male reproductive system are the testes, scrotum, penis, seminal vesicles, and prostate gland. The external sex organs include the penis and the scrotum, which contains the testes. The functions of the testes are to produce sperm (the male reproductive cells) and to produce the male hormone testosterone. The scrotum contains two sacs and is located behind the penis. The penis becomes enlarged and erect when sexually stimulated. Semen, the fluid that contains the sperm, is released from the penis during sexual intercourse. The seminal vesicles and the prostate gland both secrete fluids that become part of the semen. See Figure 22-18B ■ for the location of the male reproductive system.

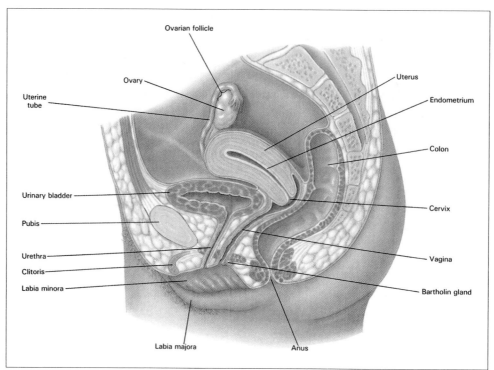

A   The organs of the female reproductive system. *Frederic Martini,* Fundamentals of Anatomy and Physiology, 2e, © *1992, pp. 918, 929. Reprinted by permission of Pearson Education, Upper Saddle River, NJ.*

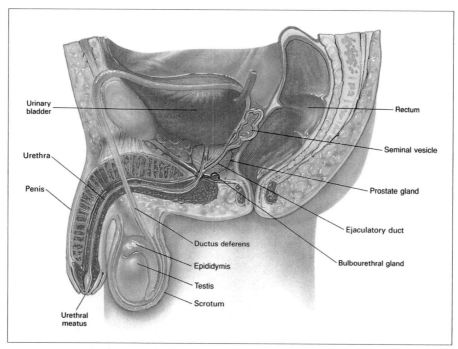

B   The organs of the male reproductive system. *Frederic Martini,* Fundamentals of Anatomy and Physiology, 2e, © *1992, pp. 918, 929. Reprinted by permission of Pearson Education, Upper Saddle River, NJ.*

FIGURE 22-18 ■ The reproductive system

Changes of Aging

In women, menstruation ends with menopause, and natural pregnancy can no longer occur. A decrease in the production of estrogen leads to a loss of calcium, causing the bones to become more brittle. Decreased estrogen also contributes to a thinning and drying of the vaginal walls. Weakened muscles cause the breasts to be less firm. In men, there is a change in hormone levels and a decrease in sperm. The prostate gland enlarges and hardens, causing pressure on the urinary urethra. Regardless of changes in the reproductive system, sexual needs continue for both men and women.

CHAPTER HIGHLIGHTS

1. The basic building block of the body is the cell.
2. All the body systems are interdependent. A change in one body system will affect the others.
3. All body systems tend to slow with aging.
4. The skin provides a barrier for germs and protects against infection.
5. Muscles work with bones and joints to allow body movement.
6. The main functions of the respiratory system are to bring oxygen into the body and to remove carbon dioxide.
7. The primary functions of the circulatory system are carrying oxygen to the cells and assisting in the elimination of waste.
8. Slowed circulation occurs with aging and affects all the body systems.
9. The functions of the digestive system are to prepare food for the body's use and to eliminate waste.
10. The functions of the urinary system include removing waste products and maintaining fluid and chemical balance.
11. The nervous system is the body's communication center.
12. The five special senses are sight, hearing, smell, taste, and touch.
13. The endocrine system secretes hormones that regulate body functions.
14. The immune process helps the body to resist germs and disease.
15. Changes in the reproductive system do not eliminate sexual needs.

VOCABULARY REVIEW

Fill in the blanks with the vocabulary term that best completes the sentence.

1. _____ is the study of body structure.

2. Glands of the endocrine system secrete chemicals called _____.

3. A/An _____ is an extension of a body part.

4. The combination of all body processes is called _____.

5. _____ is the study of body function.

6. The large intestine is also called the _____.

7. _____ is the stage of the cardiac cycle when the heart is contracting and pumping out blood.

8. A group of organs that work together is called a/an _____.

9. _____ is the muscular contractions that push food through the digestive system.

10. _____ means breathing.

CHECK YOUR UNDERSTANDING

The following questions cover the highlights of this chapter. Choose the best answer for each question.

1. The basic building block of the body is
   A. an organ   C. a cell
   B. a tissue   D. a system

2. Which of the following statements about slowed circulation is *false*?
   A. The integumentary system will be affected.
   B. No other systems will be affected.
   C. The urinary system will be affected.
   D. The respiratory system will be affected.

3. Thinning of the fatty layer under the skin is likely to cause the resident to
   A. feel cold
   B. lose appetite
   C. having difficulty moving
   D. be less protected against infection

4. The major function of the musculoskeletal system is
   A. respiration   C. movement
   B. circulation   D. elimination

5. The exchange of oxygen and carbon dioxide takes place in the
   A. diaphragm   C. bronchi
   B. trachea   D. alveoli

6. A major function of the circulatory system is to
   A. transport food, water, and oxygen to the cells
   B. bring oxygen into the body
   C. prepare food for the body's use
   D. control and coordinate body activities

7. Urine is produced in the
   A. urethra   C. bladder
   B. ureters   D. kidneys

8. Which systems control and coordinate body activities?
   A. nervous and endocrine systems
   B. muscular and skeletal systems
   C. circulatory and respiratory systems
   D. urinary and reproductive systems

9. Which of the special sense organs controls balance?
   A. eye   C. nose
   B. ear   D. fingertips

10. The stage of the cardiac cycle when the heart is resting and filling with blood is called
    A. Diastole   C. Systole
    B. Aorta   D. Peristalsis

11. The outer layer of skin is called the
    A. Dermis   C. Fatty layer
    B. Epidermis   D. Third layer

12. Which type of blood cells fight infection?
    A. Red blood cells   C. Capillaries
    B. Platelets   D. White blood cells

AGE-SPECIFIC TIP

Many elderly residents experience vision and hearing impairment. Encourage and assist with the use of hearing aids and glasses to facilitate communication.

CULTURALLY SENSITIVE TIP

Be aware that cultural background affects the resident's attitude toward aging. Avoid being judgmental.

EFFECTIVE PROBLEM SOLVING

A resident with a severe respiratory disorder says he feels too weak to walk today. The nursing assistant replies, "Your breathing problems have nothing to do with your ability to walk. Exercise will make you feel better."

Was the nursing assistant's communication appropriate? If not, what would have been more appropriate?

_____

_____

_____

_____

_____

_____

_____

_____

_____

INTERPERSONAL COMMUNICATION

The following changes of aging may affect communication with the resident. Place the letter of each item in Column 2 beside the matching item in Column 1.

_____ 1. Short-term memory loss may occur.

_____ 2. Hearing loss may occur.

_____ 3. The voice may weaken.

_____ 4. The sense of touch may not be dependable.

_____ 5. Decreased blood flow may lead to confusion.

A. Circulatory system

B. Integumentary system

C. Nervous system

D. Respiratory system

E. Special senses

OBSERVING, REPORTING, AND RECORDING

List six physical changes of aging that you may observe.

_____

_____

_____

_____

_____

_____

_____

EXPLORE MEDIALINK

Check out www.prenhall.com/grubbs for additional chapter-specific interactive study and review activities.

23

COMMON HEALTH PROBLEMS OF THE ELDERLY RESIDENT

OBJECTIVES

1. Describe three basic types of illness.
2. List six guidelines for caring for residents with musculoskeletal problems.
3. Identify six guidelines for caring for residents with respiratory problems.
4. List five guidelines for caring for residents with circulatory problems.
5. Describe six guidelines for caring for a resident who has had a stroke.
6. List five guidelines for caring for residents with diabetes.
7. Identify six guidelines for caring for residents with cancer.

VOCABULARY

The following words or terms will help you to understand this chapter:

Acute illness
Chronic illness
Complications
Terminal illness
Inflammation
Fracture
Amputation
Dyspnea

Cyanosis
Aspiration pneumonia
Aspiration
Edema
Hypertension
Dementia
Paralysis
Hemiplegia

Paraplegia
Quadriplegia
Seizure
Comatose
Obese
Hyperglycemia
Hypoglycemia

Although residents in long-term care may suffer from many diseases, some health problems are more common than others. This chapter explains types of illnesses and groups health problems according to systems for easier understanding. Guidelines for resident care are provided throughout the chapter. Keep in mind as you study this material that no system works independently; a problem in one system may affect other systems as well.

Some health problems occur more frequently within certain ethnic groups. For example, diabetes is more common in Hispanics, Native Americans, and African Americans. Be aware of the variety of cultural beliefs that influence health care behavior. There may be differences in health care practices, gender roles, and communication styles. Remember that individuals within a culture may also differ. Avoid making assumptions. Respect their values and beliefs and let the nurse know if there are any problems.

TYPES OF ILLNESSES

Illnesses can be divided into three categories—acute, chronic, and terminal. They are classified according to onset, length, and expected outcome. All three types of illnesses can be found in a long-term care facility.

An **acute illness** is an illness that begins suddenly and lasts for a short time. This type of illness is usually severe, but can often be treated and be cured. Appendicitis is an example of an acute illness. The best response to an acute illness is to seek medical assistance immediately.

A **chronic illness** is an illness that usually begins slowly and lasts for a long time. Although most chronic illnesses are not curable, they can be controlled by treatment. In fact, correct treatment and care are necessary to prevent **complications** (additional problems that can occur as a result of a disease or other condition). Diabetes is an example of a chronic illness. The appropriate response to chronic illness is to seek treatment and prevent complications.

A **terminal illness** is an illness that is expected to end in death. There is very little hope of recovery. Many diseases become terminal when treatment is not successful. The key to caring for a person who has a terminal illness is to provide comfort for the resident and support to the family.

MUSCULOSKELETAL PROBLEMS

Diseases and injuries of the musculoskeletal system create special problems because they often interfere with the ability to move. Decreased mobility results in further problems or complications such as atrophy or contractures (see Figure 23-1 ■). Complications of limited mobility are discussed in Chapter 11.

Arthritis

Arthritis is a chronic disease that causes inflammation of the joints. **Inflammation** means that the body part is red, swollen, hot, and painful. Although there are several types of arthritis, the two most common are osteoarthritis and rheumatoid arthritis.

Osteoarthritis   Osteoarthritis causes breakdown of cartilage in the joints. The weight-bearing joints, such as the knee and hip, are most often affected. Joints are stiff and sore as a result of tissue damage. Because movement causes pain, people who have this condition may be less active. Osteoarthritis affects many elderly people and can lead to a loss of function and independence.

Rheumatoid Arthritis   Rheumatoid arthritis can affect people of any age. It usually begins in the

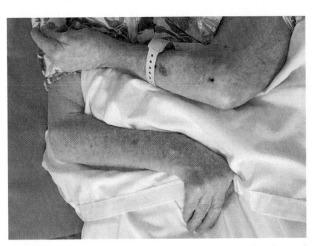

FIGURE 23-1 ■ Contractures are a complication of arthritis.

hands and fingers. The inflammation may spread to other tissues.

Sometimes arthritic joints are replaced in surgery by a prosthesis (an artificial body part). A person who has had this type of surgery may be admitted to a long-term care facility to recover from the surgery.

Osteoporosis

Osteoporosis is a disease in which loss of calcium causes bones to become brittle. The spine usually is affected, causing curvature and a loss of height. The major complication of osteoporosis is a **fracture** (broken bone). Hip fractures are often seen in the elderly. Brittle bones break easily when a person falls. Sometimes the brittle bone breaks first, causing a fall. Osteoporosis is more common in women because of hormonal changes.

Fractures

There are many types of fractures, but the most common are open fractures and closed fractures. In an open fracture, the skin is open, the bone is broken, and there may be severe tissue damage. This type of fracture (also called a "compound fracture") requires surgical repair. In a closed fracture, the bone is broken, but the skin is intact or closed.

A fractured bone must be immobilized (kept from moving) until it heals. This often is done by applying a cast. Cast care is discussed in Chapter 18.

Amputation

Amputation is the removal of a body part, usually by surgery. Amputation may be the result of an injury or a disease such as diabetes. The amputee may wear a prosthesis, such as an artificial leg. The person with an amputated leg may use crutches or a wheelchair.

GUIDELINES

CARING FOR RESIDENTS WITH MUSCULOSKELETAL PROBLEMS

- Follow each resident's plan of care.
- Assist with ADLs as necessary.

GUIDELINES (Continued)

- Encourage the resident to do as much as possible independently.
- Allow the resident to move at his or her own speed.
- Encourage and promote activity.
- Position and support the body properly and maintain good body alignment.
- Provide range-of-motion exercises as ordered.
- Provide assistive equipment as needed.
- Assist the resident to move safely.
- Report changes in the resident's mobility promptly.

RESPIRATORY PROBLEMS

The term "chronic obstructive pulmonary disease (COPD)" is used to describe many of the problems that affect the respiratory system. It is a chronic, progressive disease in which the airway is obstructed. Symptoms may include fever, **dyspnea** (difficult breathing), cough, wheezing, and fatigue. Some respiratory problems require the administration of oxygen.

Emphysema

Emphysema is a chronic disease in which changes in the structure of the lungs cause breathing problems. Lung tissue loses its elasticity, and the alveoli remain expanded. Mucus obstructs or plugs the bronchi and bronchioles, making it difficult to get air into and out of the lungs. These changes lead to a decrease in the exchange of oxygen and carbon dioxide. The person with emphysema breathes harder and faster in an attempt to get more air. Dyspnea is common.

A decrease in the amount of oxygen affects all systems of the body. Residents with emphysema may be too weak to eat or care for themselves. Nutrition is affected as appetite decreases. A person with breathing difficulty must assume a body position that allows maximum lung expansion. This usually is a sitting or upright position (see Figure 23-2 ■). Fear and anxiety are common. Unfortunately, the more upset a person becomes, the more difficult it is for him or her to breathe.

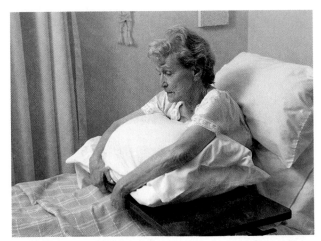

FIGURE 23-2 ■ An upright position helps the resident with COPD to breathe easier.

Coughing and wheezing are common. The skin is usually pale or there may be **cyanosis** (a blue color caused by a lack of oxygen). Emphysema can result in restlessness, confusion, respiratory failure, coma, and death.

Pneumonia

Pneumonia is an acute infection of the lungs. It often follows a cold or other upper respiratory infection. Symptoms include chills, fever, chest pain, cough, headache, and weakness. Pneumonia can progress to coma and death.

Pneumonia can be treated with antibiotics and other medications. If diagnosed and treated early, it usually is curable. Pneumonia can be serious or fatal in the elderly resident who already may be weakened from some other condition.

Aspiration Pneumonia   Aspiration pneumonia is caused by food or fluid entering the airway, instead of the stomach. **Aspiration** means choking. This can happen to someone who is not alert and oriented or to a person who is vomiting. Residents with feeding tubes also are at risk for this type of pneumonia. Residents who have difficulty swallowing may aspirate. The food or liquid causes irritation of the respiratory tract and leads to infection.

Hypostatic Pneumonia Hypostatic pneumonia results from fluid collecting in the lungs. This type of pneumonia often is a complication of limited

activity. Failure to turn and move allows fluid to collect in the lungs.

GUIDELINES
CARING FOR RESIDENTS WITH RESPIRATORY PROBLEMS

- Follow each resident's plan of care.
- Position the resident for easier breathing (usually an upright position).
- Provide frequent rest periods and watch for signs of fatigue.
- Provide mouth care frequently.
- Keep clothing and linen clean and dry.
- Use standard precautions when in contact with body fluids.
- Follow safety rules if oxygen is in use.
- Recognize the resident's fears and provide emotional support.
- Encourage fluid intake and proper nutrition.
- Observe closely and report observations promptly.

CIRCULATORY PROBLEMS

Diseases of the heart and blood vessels can range from mild to severe. They can be acute or chronic and may involve all age groups. Some people are born with heart disorders. Heart disease is a leading cause of death in the United States.

Coronary Artery Disease

Coronary artery disease (CAD) causes a narrowing of the coronary arteries in the heart. Changes in the lining of the arteries obstruct the blood vessels. Arteriosclerosis (hardening of the arteries) contributes to coronary artery disease. In these situations, the blood supply to the heart muscle is reduced. The heart muscle requires more oxygen than the blood vessels can supply. Blood pressure may be affected by coronary artery disease.

Angina

Angina is an episode of chest pain that occurs when narrowed blood vessels do not allow enough oxygenated blood to reach the heart muscle. The pain often occurs after exercise, eating, or an emotional experience.

Symptoms of angina begin with a sudden, acute pain in the chest. Pain sometimes travels or radiates down the left arm. It usually lasts only a few minutes. This pain can range from mild to agonizing. Treatment is aimed at relieving pain. Rest, diet, and a healthy lifestyle help to reduce the frequency of attacks. During an angina attack, the person is anxious and fearful that a serious heart attack may be occurring.

Myocardial Infarction

A myocardial infarction (MI) is a heart attack that often results in death. It occurs when there is a sudden blockage of blood flow to the heart, causing heart muscle to die. This can be caused by a blood clot or other material blocking the blood vessel.

Symptoms of an MI generally begin with a sensation of pressure or a sudden, severe, crushing pain in the chest and dyspnea. The skin is pale or cyanotic (bluish-colored). Although the person may be sweating, the skin feels cold to touch. There may be nausea and vomiting. Fear and anxiety may be present.

An MI is a life-threatening situation that requires immediate medical attention. The person usually will be taken to a hospital for intensive treatment. Death can occur suddenly. If a resident complains of chest pain, stay with the resident, and call the nurse immediately.

Congestive Heart Failure

Congestive heart failure (CHF) occurs when the heart fails to pump efficiently. Blood and other body fluids tend to pool or congest in the body. One of the first signs observed in CHF is edema. **Edema** is the accumulation of fluid that leads to swelling (see Figure 23-3 ■). It is most noticeable in body parts that are farthest from the heart, such as the hands and feet. There usually is weight gain. Because the heart and lungs are congested (filled with fluid), breathing is labored, and the pulse may be irregular. Urine output usually is decreased because the body is holding fluid. Pain, nausea, and vomiting may be present.

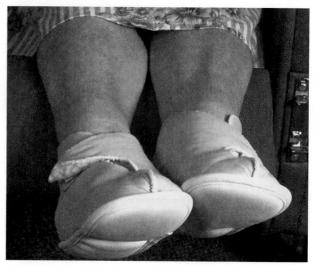

FIGURE 23-3 ■ Edema can result from poor circulation.

CHF can become a chronic illness, with acute episodes. An acute attack can result in death.

Hypertension

Hypertension is high blood pressure. A blood pressure of 140/90 or above is considered high. Although the exact cause of hypertension is not known, factors that contribute to it include heredity, diet, weight, and lifestyle. Hypertension is common in heart disease and diabetes and can lead to other complications, such as a stroke.

GUIDELINES

CARING FOR RESIDENTS WITH CIRCULATORY PROBLEMS

- Follow each resident's plan of care.
- Observe the resident carefully and report changes promptly.
- Report complaints of pain immediately and be aware of indications of pain.
- Provide reassurance and emotional support.
- Encourage the resident to follow fluid and diet instructions.
- Measure and report vital signs accurately.
- Encourage activity while being alert for signs of fatigue.
- Provide good skin care and observe for problems.
- Observe for and report respiratory problems.

NERVOUS SYSTEM PROBLEMS

Problems of the nervous system may involve the brain, spinal cord, or nerves. These structures control and regulate the activities of the body. Diseases of the nervous system may interfere with thinking, talking, and moving. People with mental or nervous disorders may or may not have other physical problems as well. Because care of residents with nervous system problems varies according to the condition, guidelines will focus on caring for the resident who has had a stroke.

Dementia

Dementia is an impairment of mental function. Mental illnesses such as schizophrenia cause dementia. It also can be caused by a severe stroke or a series of small strokes. The death of brain cells due to interruption of blood flow leads to a loss of mental function. The most common form of dementia is Alzheimer's disease.

Residents with dementia are disoriented. Their ability to cope is decreased. They often are irritable and angry. Their inability to understand what is happening causes them to focus on themselves. As their world narrows, they may appear demanding and thoughtless. It is frightening to lose control of both self and environment. While mental illness usually is treated in mental health facilities, many people with dementia are residents in long-term care facilities. See Chapter 24 for care of residents with Alzheimer's disease and related disorders.

Cerebrovascular Accident

Cerebrovascular accident (CVA) is the correct term for what is commonly called a stroke. "Cerebro" means brain; "vascular" means blood vessels. A CVA is an accident in the blood vessels in the brain. Either something blocks a blood vessel or the vessel ruptures (breaks open). Frequently, the cause is a blood clot. The affected area of the brain is left without a blood supply and, therefore, without oxygen. The oxygen-deprived brain cells die.

A stroke may occur because the blood pressure is too high. In this situation, the person may complain of a headache and dizziness. This might continue for hours or days before the pressure damages the blood vessel. However, a stroke also may happen suddenly, with no warning. Symptoms may vary from a mild dizzy spell to coma and death.

Strokes not only are a leading cause of death in the United States, but they also cause a large number of illnesses and disabilities. The type of disability depends on the area of the brain involved and the amount of damage to the area. A CVA in one side of the brain will affect the opposite side of the body. There are areas of the brain that control speech, thinking, and movement. A CVA in the speech center will affect the ability to speak. A CVA in the area that controls movement will affect the ability to move. **Paralysis**, the inability to move a body part, is common.

The resident who has had a stroke can have many problems affecting any of the body systems (see Figure 23-4 ■). Difficulties in swallowing, digestion, and elimination are common.

GUIDELINES

CARING FOR A RESIDENT WHO HAS HAD A STROKE

- Follow each resident's plan of care.
- Encourage activity and self-care.
- Provide a calm environment.
- Allow time for activities and do not rush the resident.
- Feed the resident on the unaffected side.
- When dressing the resident, put clothes on the affected side first; remove clothes from the unaffected side first.
- Position the resident in correct body alignment and provide support for affected limbs.
- Provide range-of-motion exercise as ordered.
- Encourage the resident to use rehabilitation training in daily activities.
- Provide assistive equipment as needed.
- Have patience and empathy.
- Follow guidelines for communicating with residents with sensory impairments.
- Observe nonverbal communication.
- Remind the resident and family that recovery takes time.
- Observe and report changes in the resident's condition.

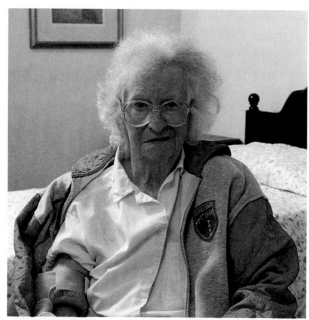

FIGURE 23-4 ■ A stroke can cause many problems for the resident.

Multiple Sclerosis

Multiple sclerosis (MS) is a progressive disease that primarily affects the brain and spinal cord. Myelin, the substance that insulates nerve fibers, deteriorates and is replaced by scar tissue. The scar tissue interferes with the transmission of nerve impulses. This results in numbness, tremors, staggering gait, weakness, paralysis, and loss of balance and coordination. The resident with MS may be in a wheelchair. There may be vision and speech problems. Although intelligence usually is not affected, there may be emotional instability. Because of these problems, residents with MS may be unable to care for themselves.

MS usually begins at an early age, between 20 and 40. Although the person's condition gets progressively worse, there may be periods of time when the disease symptoms level off or seem to disappear.

Parkinson's Disease   Parkinson's disease is a chronic disease that causes loss of control of motor function. Because it is a progressive disease, the symptoms become more severe over the years. Although Parkinson's disease is usually thought of as a disease of old age, it can strike people in their 30s and 40s.

The most noticeable symptoms are trembling, stiffness, and a shuffling walk. The trembling may be so severe that involuntary movements of the arms and legs prevent the person from performing ADLs independently. There may be difficulty swallowing and handling secretions. Communication problems are common. Some people with advanced Parkinson's disease are unable to show facial expression, causing the face to look like a mask. Anger and frustration are common because the resident cannot control movements or facial expressions but remains aware of these problems.

Nervous System Injuries   Most injuries of the nervous system involve either the brain or the spinal cord. Many of the younger residents of a long-term care facility are there because of an injury to the nervous system.

An injury to the nervous system may result in one of the following forms of paralysis:

- **Hemiplegia** (paralysis of one side of the body)
- **Paraplegia** (paralysis of the lower half of the body)
- **Quadriplegia** (paralysis of both arms and legs)

"Plegia" means paralysis. "Quad" means four. You have four extremities (arms and legs). That makes understanding quadriplegia easy. "Hemi" and "para" both mean "half," so how do you tell them apart? A "paraplegic" puts on a "pair of pants" over the legs, so a paraplegic has both legs paralyzed. A hemiplegic is paralyzed on one side.

Symptoms of a brain injury depend on the location and severity of the damage. Any part of the body may be affected. Weakness, dizziness, headache, loss of coordination, spasms, or seizures may occur. A **seizure** (convulsion) is a sudden spasm of muscle contractions and relaxations. Partial or complete paralysis may occur. Vision and hearing problems are common. Mental changes may include irritability, restlessness, confusion, or amnesia (loss of memory). The person with a brain injury may be comatose. **Comatose** means unconscious or unable to respond.

Symptoms depend on whether the spinal cord is damaged or severed (cut in two). If the cord is damaged, there may be weakness, spasms, or paralysis.

There may not be complete paralysis in this situation. However, if the cord is severed, the result will be total paralysis of body structures below the injury. Paralysis can result in the inability to control urine or bowel movements. Most paraplegics and quadriplegics in long-term care have suffered a spinal cord injury.

SENSORY PROBLEMS

The most common problems of the sensory system involve loss of vision or hearing. The majority of elderly people are affected to some degree by one or both of these disorders. This can result in communication difficulty and a loss of independence.

Ears

Hearing problems can range from slightly hard-of-hearing to total deafness. One or both ears may be affected. The loss might involve inability to hear low-, medium-, or high-pitched sounds or a combination. There are two basic types of hearing loss. One kind can be helped by a hearing aid (see Figure 23-5 ■), which makes sounds louder. The other type of hearing loss usually is not helped by a hearing aid.

Hearing loss can be caused by disease, noise, or injury. It also is affected by the changes of aging.

Eyes

People of all ages may have vision problems. They may be nearsighted (they can see things that are nearby but their distant vision is poor) or farsighted (they can see things that are far away but they have difficulty with close vision). Many people who have good vision in their younger years become farsighted as they get older. They have difficulty seeing small print and tend to hold reading material at a distance in an attempt to see better. Although some of these conditions may respond to surgery, people who have these problems usually wear glasses or contact lenses. Individuals who are vision-impaired still can maintain independence (see Figure 23-6 ■).

There are two other eye conditions that frequently are seen in elderly people.

Cataracts   A cataract is a clouding of the lens of the eye. As the lens loses its transparency, there is a gradual loss of vision that can lead to blindness. A person may have a cataract in one or both eyes.

Cataracts can be caused by disease, injury, or aging. The main symptom is a gradual decrease in vision. The condition usually is not painful. As the cataract progresses, the pupil of the eye appears white and cloudy.

Treatment of cataracts includes corrective glasses, contact lenses, or surgery. Surgery involves removing the diseased lens and implanting a new one.

Glaucoma   Glaucoma is a disease in which pressure within the eye gradually destroys the optic

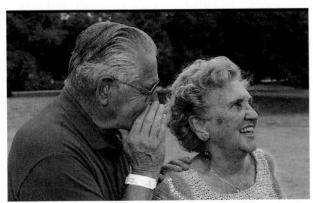

FIGURE 23-5 ■ A hearing aid makes communication easier for the resident who is hearing impaired.

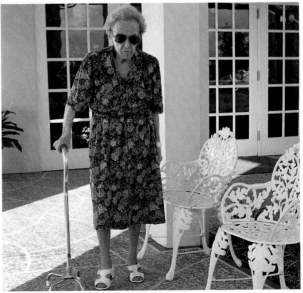

FIGURE 23-6 ■ Individuals who are vision-impaired still can maintain independence.

nerve. Although the cause is unknown, high blood pressure and diabetes are related factors. It tends to occur in members of the same family, and the chance of developing glaucoma increases with age.

Symptoms of glaucoma include headaches and a decrease in the field of vision. Some complain of seeing "halos." However, in early glaucoma there may be no symptoms at all. Treatment includes eye drops and other medications. Surgery is sometimes helpful.

Guidelines for communicating with residents with sensory problems are located in Chapter 19.

DIABETES MELLITUS

Diabetes mellitus is a chronic disease that results when insulin is not produced or used properly by the body. Insulin is a hormone, produced in the pancreas, that changes sugar to energy for the body's use. When the body can't use sugar, it will use fat. The breakdown of fat produces acetone (ketones). The ketones and unused sugar can build to toxic levels in the blood and spill over into the urine. The disease is commonly called "diabetes."

Types of Diabetes

There are several types of diabetes, but the most common are Type 1 and Type 2.

Type 1 Diabetes   Type 1 diabetes causes the diabetic to be insulin-dependent. Because the body produces little or no insulin, it must be given by injection. Type 1 used to be called "juvenile diabetes" because it primarily affected young people. Only a small percentage of diabetics are Type 1.

Type 2 Diabetes   Type 2 diabetes does not always cause insulin dependence. A normal amount of insulin is produced, but for some reason, the body can't use it. Type 2 diabetes often is controlled with diet and exercise. Oral medication or insulin also may be needed. This type of diabetes generally affects an older age group. The majority of diabetics are Type 2.

Cause of Diabetes

The exact cause of diabetes is not known. However, there are certain factors that contribute to the development of the disease. It is hereditary and runs in families. Although anyone can develop diabetes, it is more common in certain ethnic groups such as Native Americans. Women are more at risk than men, and the risk increases with age. However, the primary risk factor is obesity. **Obese** means overweight. With the increase in obesity in the United States, there has been an increase in the incidence of diabetes.

Symptoms of Diabetes

The symptoms of diabetes include frequent urination, thirst, and hunger. The diabetic tires easily and may have weight loss, even though food intake has increased. There may be vision problems or sores that won't heal. Some diabetics are depressed. Women may complain of vaginal itching. Tests show a high level of sugar in the blood.

Treatment of Diabetes

Although there is presently no cure for diabetes, many complications can be prevented. Treatment for diabetes includes diet, exercise, oral medication, and insulin. Treatment begins with an individually planned diet and exercise program. Oral medications sometimes are effective. Some diabetics must have insulin injections. The goal in managing diabetes is to keep the blood sugar level within a normal range.

Complications

There are many complications of diabetes. Some are short-term, occur quickly, and may be relieved by prompt treatment. Hyperglycemia and hypoglycemia are examples of short-term complications.

When the blood sugar is high, or above normal, it is called **hyperglycemia**. ("Hyper" means high, "glyc" means sugar, and "emia" means blood). It can result from eating too much, eating the wrong foods, or not exercising enough. High blood sugar also may lead to diabetic coma. Hyperglycemia is treated with medications to decrease the amount of sugar in the blood.

Low blood sugar is called **hypoglycemia**. It can be caused by skipping a meal, not eating enough, too much exercise, too much medication, or an

SIGNS AND SYMPTOMS	Hyperglycemia (Diabetic Coma)	Hypoglycemia (Insulin Shock)
Behavior	Sluggishness	Irritable, excited, dizziness, coma
Skin	Hot, dry, flushed	Cold, clammy, pale
Breathing	Deep, fruity odor	Shallow
Pulse	Slow to normal	Rapid, thready
Speech	Slurred	Normal
Urine	Glucose and acetone present	No glucose or acetone
Possible Causes	Overeating, infection, vomiting, not enough insulin	Not eating enough, excessive exercise or activity, too much insulin

FIGURE 23-7 ■ Signs and symptoms of hyperglycemia and hypoglycemia

illness. People with low blood sugar may go into insulin shock. The treatment for hypoglycemia is simple sugar, such as candy, sweetened orange juice, or administration of glucose.

Either of these reactions to the blood sugar level can result in coma or death. It is important that you know the symptoms of hyperglycemia and hypoglycemia. The chart in Figure 23-7 ■ will help you to understand the difference in the two reactions.

Long-term complications occur gradually and may go unnoticed for some time. Most problems occur as a result of years of uncontrolled diabetes. They can lead to blindness, amputation, and death.

One of the most serious long-term complications involves the circulatory system. Changes in the blood vessels slow the flow of blood throughout the body. Because of this, the diabetic is more prone to heart attacks, high blood pressure, and strokes. Kidney problems often occur. Slowed circulation means that sores don't heal and infection frequently occurs. Impaired circulation to the feet and legs results in infection that may turn to gangrene (a serious infection that causes tissue death). Gangrene can lead to amputation.

Nerve damage results in a loss of sensation in the nerve endings. A feeling of numbness may occur, placing the diabetic at risk for burns and other injuries. Diabetics have vision problems that can lead to blindness. Personality changes, confusion, and disorientation may occur. Diabetics who control their disease can avoid many of these complications.

Nursing Care

The nursing assistant plays an important role in the care of the diabetic resident. You will have many opportunities to encourage the resident to follow the plan of nursing care and treatment. Because of poor circulation, special skin care, especially of the legs and feet, will be necessary (see Figure 23-8 ■). This care is described in Chapter 12. Although blood testing is usually done by nurses, you may be asked to test the resident's urine for S&A. These tests are discussed in Chapter 18. The following guidelines will help you care for residents with diabetes and help prevent complications.

GUIDELINES

CARING FOR RESIDENTS WITH DIABETES

- Follow each resident's plan of care.
- Encourage the resident to follow dietary guidelines.
- Serve meals on time and provide snacks as ordered.
- Observe, report, and record diet intake accurately.

(continued)

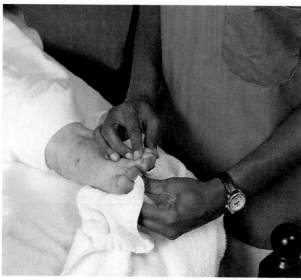

FIGURE 23-8 ■ Proper foot care can help prevent some of the complications of diabetes.

Guidelines (Continued)

- Encourage exercise and activity.
- Provide good skin care.
- Observe and report skin problems promptly.
- Take care and prevent injuries when providing care.
- Provide special foot care as described in Chapter 12.
- Report S&A test results promptly and accurately.
- Observe and report any mental, emotional, and physical changes.

CANCER

Cancer is a disease that can affect any system of the body. It begins with a body cell that changes to a cancer cell. Cancer cells grow and divide rapidly. They use food and oxygen that are needed by normal cells. Cancer cells group to form tumors. A tumor is a mass of tissue that grows in the body and performs no useful function. Tumors can be benign or malignant. A benign tumor is not cancerous and does not spread. A malignant tumor grows rapidly and spreads to other body tissues. Cancer cells form malignant tumors and can metastasize (spread to other parts of the body). As they grow and spread, they interfere with normal body functions. For example, a malignant tumor in the lung will interfere with breathing.

Cancer affects all age groups, from newborn babies to the very old. However, over 50 percent of cancer patients are elderly. While cancer can be treated and sometimes cured, it remains one of the leading causes of death in the United States. Although the cause of cancer is unknown, research indicates that a number of factors are involved. These factors include viruses, immune response, diet, and heredity.

Exposure to certain substances (carcinogens) is known to cause cancer. Some carcinogens include tobacco smoke, asbestos, pesticides and other chemicals, sunlight, X-rays, and other types of radiation. We are exposed to many carcinogens in our normal, everyday life. They are found in the environment—in our food, water, and air. Some carcinogens are present because human activities have polluted the environment. Cigarette smoke has been shown to cause lung cancer, not only in the smokers but also in the people around them. When people stop smoking, there is a decrease in the occurrence of lung cancer in them and those around them. Prevention of pollution reduces the number of carcinogens in the environment.

A resident with cancer may have many problems. Weakness, loss of appetite, and skin breakdown can occur. A decrease in mobility and independence are common. Some cancers cause pain. Confusion may result.

A diagnosis of cancer causes many fears and anxieties. Anxiety concerning treatment, fear of death, and fear of the unknown can affect the resident, the family, and the health care workers. They may be influenced by some of the false beliefs about cancer. For example, some may be afraid that cancer is contagious. The person with cancer may question many things such as pain, disfigurement, and the effects of treatment. There is a concern about independence, control, and death.

Cancer can be treated by surgery, radiation, chemotherapy, or a combination of those methods. The goal of treatment is to prevent the spread of cancer cells by destroying them. Both radiation and chemotherapy can harm normal tissue. The side effects of these types of treatment include nausea, diarrhea, and hair loss.

Today, many types of cancer can be cured. Early diagnosis and treatment can mean the difference between life and death. According to the American Cancer Society, early warning signs of cancer are:

- A change in bowel or bladder habits
- A sore that does not heal
- Unusual bleeding or discharge
- A lump or thickening in the breast or elsewhere in the body
- Indigestion or difficulty swallowing
- An obvious change in size or shape of a wart or mole
- A nagging cough or hoarseness

It is your responsibility to observe early warning signs of cancer in the resident. You may be the first to notice them. You can help prevent cancer by careful observation and reporting.

GUIDELINES

CARING FOR RESIDENTS WITH CANCER

- Follow each resident's plan of care.
- Encourage a proper diet.
- Encourage exercise while avoiding fatigue.
- Promote comfort in all care provided.
- Provide good skin care.
- Provide assistance with ADLs as necessary.
- Encourage self-care and independence.
- Encourage the resident to express feelings and concerns.
- Provide emotional support and empathy.
- Observe for and promptly report signs and symptoms of pain.
- Report changes in the resident's condition immediately.

CHAPTER HIGHLIGHTS

1. A problem in one system will affect other systems.
2. Illnesses can be divided into three categories—acute, chronic, and terminal.
3. Diseases and injuries of the musculoskeletal system often interfere with mobility.
4. The most common problem of the respiratory system is chronic obstructive pulmonary disease.
5. Heart disease is a leading cause of death in the United States.
6. The most common form of dementia is Alzheimer's disease.
7. The resident who has had a stroke can have problems affecting many of the body systems.
8. The most common problems of the sensory system involve loss of vision or hearing.
9. Diabetes mellitus is a chronic disease that affects the body's ability to use insulin to change sugar to energy.
10. Many of the complications in diabetes are the result of impaired circulation.
11. The feet of the diabetic resident require special attention to prevent complications.
12. Cancer can affect any system of the body.
13. Everyone should be aware of the seven early warning signs of cancer.

VOCABULARY REVIEW

Fill in the blanks with the vocabulary term that best completes the sentence.

1. A/An _____ is an illness that begins slowly and lasts for a long time.

2. _____ is an impairment of mental function.

3. When the blood sugar is high or above normal, it is called _____.

4. A/An _____ is an illness that begins suddenly and lasts for a short time.

5. _____ are additional problems that can occur as a result of an illness or another condition.

6. Paralysis of the lower half of the body is called _____.

7. _____ means overweight.

8. Paralysis of both arms and legs is called _____.

9. _____ means that the body part is red, swollen, hot, and painful.

10. Low blood sugar is called _____.

CHECK YOUR UNDERSTANDING

The following questions cover the highlights of this chapter. Choose the best answer for each question.

1. Arthritis is most likely to affect the resident's
   A. digestion
   B. mobility
   C. circulation
   D. breathing

2. A severe infection in the foot of a diabetic resident may result in
   A. amputation
   B. a cast
   C. traction
   D. a fracture

3. What kind of pneumonia can result from choking on food or fluids?
   A. aspiration pneumonia
   B. hypostatic pneumonia
   C. bacterial pneumonia
   D. viral pneumonia

4. A resident complains of severe, crushing chest pain. What should you do?
   A. Stay with the resident and urge him to relax.
   B. Stay with the resident and call the nurse immediately.
   C. Go get the nurse immediately.
   D. Call the family immediately.

5. A resident's blood pressure measures 180 over 92. This is an example of
   A. hyperglycemia
   B. hypoglycemia
   C. hypertension
   D. hypotension

6. A stroke has left a resident paralyzed on the left side. This condition is called
   A. paraplegia
   B. quadriplegia
   C. hemiplegia
   D. none of the above

7. A clouding of the lens of the eye is a symptom of what condition?
   A. a cataract
   B. glaucoma
   C. nearsightedness
   D. farsightedness

8. A diabetic resident has hot, flushed skin, slurred speech, and a fruity odor to the breath. These are symptoms of:
   A. hyperglycemia
   B. hypoglycemia
   C. hypertension
   D. hypotension

9. Which of the following is one of the early signs of cancer?
   A. sudden paralysis
   B. hot, flushed skin
   C. a change in personality
   D. a change in the size of a mole

10. Appendicitis is an example of what kind of illness?
    A. An acute illness
    B. A chronic illness
    C. A complicated illness
    D. A terminal illness

11. What is the best way to put a shirt on a resident who is paralyzed on one side?
    A. Put the shirt on over his head.
    B. Place the affected arm in the sleeve first.
    C. Place the unaffected arm in the sleeve first.
    D. Drape the shirt over the resident's shoulders.

AGE-SPECIFIC TIP

An individual's response to chronic illness may be influenced by age. Be aware of and respect generational differences.

CULTURALLY SENSITIVE TIP

Culture affects a person's decisions regarding health care and treatment of disease. Stay aware of your feelings so that you will be able to accept differences in others.

EFFECTIVE PROBLEM SOLVING

Mrs. Gray has severe arthritis. Using her walker, she is walking very slowly down the hall. The nursing assistant, hoping to motivate her, says, "You can go a lot faster than that. The walker will help keep you from falling."

Was the nursing assistant's communication appropriate? If not, what would have been more appropriate?

_____

_____

_____

_____

_____

_____

_____

_____

_____

_____

INTERPERSONAL COMMUNICATION

Some of the following impairments are likely to interfere with communication. Check the examples that are appropriate.

_____ Osteoporosis
_____ A fractured arm
_____ Emphysema
_____ Alzheimer's disease

OBSERVING, REPORTING, AND RECORDING

List four important observations of the diabetic resident that should be reported to the nurse.

_____

_____

_____

_____

_____

_____

_____

_____

_____

_____

_____

_____

_____

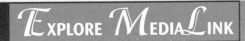

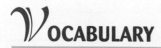

24

ALZHEIMER'S DISEASE AND RELATED DISORDERS

OBJECTIVES

1. Explain the difference between normal aging and memory loss from Alzheimer's disease and related disorders.

2. Identify eight characteristics of Alzheimer's disease and related disorders.

3. List 19 guidelines for communicating effectively with residents who have Alzheimer's disease and related disorders.

4. Identify four conditions that mimic Alzheimer's disease and related disorders.

5. List six causes of Alzheimer's disease and explain how it is diagnosed.

6. Describe the progress, symptoms, and behaviors at each stage of Alzheimer's disease.

7. Identify six guidelines for managing inappropriate behavior.

8. List 10 guidelines for providing personal care.

9. Assist residents to participate in activities; explain the effects of stress upon confusion.

10. List six guidelines for assisting family members and friends of residents with Alzheimer's disease.

11. Explain the importance of a safe, secure, and supportive environment; list four common ethical issues with Alzheimer's disease and related disorders.

VOCABULARY

The following words or terms will help you to understand the chapter:

Alzheimer's disease (AD)
Dementia
Paranoid

Sundowner's syndrome
Aphasia
Hallucinations

Agitation
Autonomy

This chapter will focus on Alzheimer's disease and related disorders (ADRD). **Alzheimer's disease (AD)** is a progressive disorder of the brain that eventually destroys all mental function. This chapter is written in response to recent trends and legislation aimed at helping health care workers better understand, care for, and communicate with individuals with ADRD. It can be used as an outline for presenting mandated training of health care workers having contact with individuals affected by ADRD. A review of Chapter 19 will help you as you study the information in this chapter.

All confused residents do not have AD; for example, a resident with a high fever may be temporarily confused. When the temperature returns to normal, the confusion disappears. Most of the guidelines that are used for residents with AD will be appropriate to use with any confused resident.

Alzheimer's disease was first discovered in 1906. It is a fatal illness that affects 4–5 million Americans and is the most common form of **dementia**, an impairment of mental function. The beginning of AD is the first step of a 2- to 25-year difficult journey for victims of AD, their families, and caregivers. It can affect anyone of any race, nationality, and economic or social standing.

DIFFERENCES BETWEEN NORMAL AGING AND ADRD

Mild memory loss commonly occurs with normal aging and may begin as early as middle age. Memorization becomes more difficult and dates, names, and numbers are often forgotten, while important information is remembered most easily. Memory techniques may be employed to associate new information with past memories. The use of lists, calendars, and journals is helpful. The following guidelines will be helpful in improving memory for people who experience normal forgetfulness as they age.

GUIDELINES

IMPROVING MEMORY

- Take time to process information.
- Focus on the details of new information.

GUIDELINES (Continued)

- Associate new information with past memories.
- Verbalize information repeatedly.
- Practice recalling and using the new information.
- Use reminders and other memory techniques.

While remembering and recalling may take more time, the ability to think clearly is not lost in normal aging. The forgetfulness is mild and does not worsen with time. This type of memory loss does not indicate Alzheimer's disease.

In contrast, memory loss in dementia differs from normal memory loss. Dementia is not a specific disease. Injury, disease, or another condition may lead to dementia. In addition to memory loss, dementia affects mood, personality, thinking, and reasoning. These effects are severe enough to interfere significantly with daily life. The ability to perform ADLs independently declines, and assistance is required.

While many dementias are reversible and curable, AD is not. In the beginning, those with AD may seem normal, while the disease is slowly destroying brain tissue and brain function. There is a reduction in the amount of brain chemicals, cells are destroyed, nerve fibers tangle, and there appears to be a change in the size and shape of the brain. These changes are accompanied by a decline in mental function. Total body function gradually declines as the disease progresses.

CHARACTERISTICS OF ADRD

In addition to long- and short-term memory loss, ADRD leads to confusion and disorientation. Residents with ADRD may not remember where home is or who family members are. Eventually they may lose self-identity. They may be anxious or **paranoid** (overly suspicious), have difficulty reasoning, and can no longer learn. Their attention span is short because the ability to concentrate is decreased, and impaired judgment prevents them from knowing right from wrong or safe from unsafe.

Many behavior problems are seen in residents who are suffering from AD. They become restless, chronic wanderers, constantly on the move, stopping for a few minutes without purpose (see Figure 24-1 ■). In the long-term care facility, they may enter other residents' rooms or staff areas. When an outer door opens, they may be outside in a flash, with no regard for traffic or other dangers. Wandering, restlessness, and confusion may increase as evening occurs. This is called **sundowner's syndrome**. It may be caused by fatigue and frustration from a day full of challenges and stimulation.

Communication skills decrease in AD, and in later stages, conversation and the ability to listen disappear (see Figure 24-2 ■). All that may remain of speech are echoed phrases or mumbled, meaningless words. Socialization becomes difficult or impossible. The physical symptoms of AD include decreased appetite, weight loss, weakness, sleep disturbance, and loss of mobility. Eventually motor tasks become impossible.

There is no typical resident with ADRD. Some are angry and agitated, and others are sweet and gentle. Some endlessly pace the floor, while others sit in one spot for hours. Personality and behavior can change quickly. Much depends upon the progression of the disease.

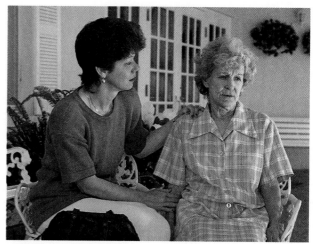

FIGURE 24-2 ■ Confused residents may not understand what is being said.

COMMUNICATING WITH RESIDENTS WHO HAVE ADRD

As residents with ADRD lose their ability to communicate verbally, they begin to depend upon nonverbal communication. You also will need to depend upon nonverbal communication, not only to convey information but also to recognize their needs and feelings. It is important to be aware of your own body language and the message it sends to the resident. As verbal communication skills decline, the resident with ADRD will be less able to follow a conversation and understand directions.

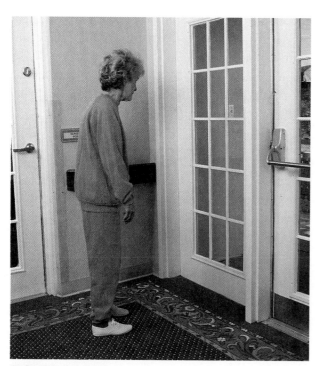

FIGURE 24-1 ■ Protecting the resident with Alzheimer's disease is challenging.

GUIDELINES

COMMUNICATING WITH RESIDENTS WITH ADRD

- Use all of the senses when communicating.
- Be sure your body language agrees with what you are saying.
- Observe for nonverbal messages from the resident.
- Initiate conversation by making eye contact and speaking the resident's name. Repeat the name throughout the conversation as needed.
- Introduce yourself and speak your name each time you communicate.
- Be sure that your nonverbal communication is pleasant and positive.

GUIDELINES (Continued)

- It may be necessary to call the resident by a name that family and friends use.
- Use short, simple sentences. You may need to use key words rather than sentences, especially if the resident speaks in single words.
- Speak slowly, distinctly, and in a soothing tone of voice.
- Be specific, brief, and to the point.
- Use familiar words or phrases to which the resident is accustomed.
- Point to objects and act out messages if necessary.
- Use touch to focus the resident's attention (see Figure 24-3 ■).
- Reassure and explain frequently.
- Use encouragement and praise.
- Visual aids, such as word cards, may be helpful.
- Be sure the resident is wearing clean glasses and a hearing aid if needed.
- Reduce distractions such as radio, TV, or other conversations.
- Attempt to understand what the resident is communicating by confused or repetitive statements.
- Don't assume that because communication is difficult, it is useless.
- Look for clues that the resident has understood you.
- Use smiles to create a friendly atmosphere and to reduce the resident's fear.
- Use positive statements when communicating.

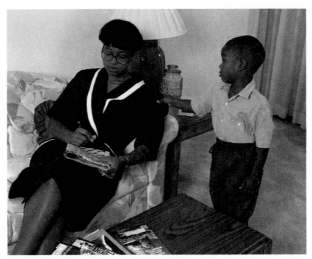

FIGURE 24-3 ■ Touch is important to communication.

Communicating with residents with ADRD can be frustrating. It is important that you use effective skills to control your reactions. Control your emotions, stay calm, and use positive self-talk. Take a moment to think about what is really happening and why. Never argue, threaten, or frighten a resident. It would be very easy to cause the resident to distrust you. You may offer simple reminders of reality, however, do not force issues. Explore the resident's confused statements rather than correcting them. Be aware of the resident's emotions and reassure the resident that you are there to help. If the resident is upset, change the subject or the activity. Remember to use good communication skills. It will be necessary to modify communication as the disease progresses. Even in the late stages, continue to communicate and give explanations for every step. Remember, communication is important for all residents, including those who are comatose.

RELATED DISORDERS

Many chronic diseases cause symptoms that mimic Alzheimer's disease. These include reversible dementia, irreversible dementia, depression, and relocation stress. The most common symptoms of these conditions are failing health, confusion, disorientation, and loss of ability to perform self-care.

Reversible dementias can be treated and cured. Some examples include alcohol abuse, depression, side effects of medications, dehydration, infection, vision and hearing impairments, and malnutrition. Some irreversible dementias include multi-infarct dementia (a series of small strokes), Parkinson's disease, Lewy disease, some palsies, Binswanger's disease, Pick's disease, and Huntington's disease. Many of the symptoms of depression such as decreased energy, fatigue, sleep problems, eating disorders, and poor concentration also occur in AD. Moving to a new location can cause similar symptoms in vulnerable elderly residents.

POSSIBLE CAUSES AND DIAGNOSIS OF AD

While the cause of AD is unknown, extensive research is being conducted. Possible causes being researched include heredity, head injury, and immune system defects. Age, gender, and family history are possible risk factors. Diagnosis of AD can be definite only by examination of brain tissue after death. However, as signs and symptoms begin to appear, a fairly accurate diagnosis of probable AD can be reached. Memory disorder clinics specialize in diagnosis, using a team approach to determine the difference between AD and other forms of dementia. An evaluation is performed that includes a medical, social, and family history, lab tests, a physical exam, psychological testing, and a psychosocial assessment. Medications are reviewed for side effects that might cause dementia. If a probable diagnosis is determined, a plan of care, including community resources, is developed for managing AD. No cure has been found, but there are drugs that help residents to function at somewhat higher levels.

STAGES AND PROGRESSION OF AD

While there is no predictable progression of AD, it is usually divided into three stages: early, middle, and late. Individual progression of the disease is highly variable.

Early Stage of AD

- Memory loss—only short-term memory loss of which the resident usually is aware, problems with recall, repetitive words or statements, misplaced items, inability to say the correct word or names of people
- Personality change—withdrawal, irritability and anger, frustration, depression, anxiety
- Restlessness and wandering
- Loss of ability to perform simple ADLs—decline in hygiene and grooming, short attention span, inability to perform regular routines, inability to participate in normal activities
- Disorientation—poor sense of time and direction, lack of judgment, reduced reading comprehension, inability to follow directions

Middle Stage of AD

- Increased severity of symptoms
- Severe memory loss—both long- and short-term
- Language impairment—problems finding words, confused sentences, slowed speech, difficulty understanding, **aphasia** (inability to speak or express oneself)
- Disorientation
- Decreased ability to perform ADLs—more severe than in the early stage; the resident may need help starting or completing tasks
- Social withdrawal—discomfort in groups, dependence on caregiver, depression
- Restlessness—pacing and fidgeting
- Wandering—may get lost
- Catastrophic reaction—overreaction to situations, paranoia, **hallucinations** (seeing or hearing things that don't exist), angry outbursts, physical violence
- Changes in eating habits—unpredictable eating, weight changes; may try to eat items that are not food
- Sleep disturbance—slow and sleepy most of the time or may sleep very little, mixing up days and nights
- Hiding and hoarding—may include food or objects
- Inappropriate behavior—sexual or social

Late Stage of AD

- Severe memory impairment—little or no memory
- Difficulty communicating—may be unable to speak or understand language
- No recognition of family or friends
- No self-recognition in the mirror
- Inability to eat
- Significant weight loss
- Bowel and bladder incontinence
- Loss of coordination
- Decline in immune function—more susceptible to infection
- Muscle weakness
- Insomnia
- Coma

In the final stages, the resident needs constant supervision and total care. Death is often caused by pneumonia.

BEHAVIOR MANAGEMENT IN ADRD

As the resident progresses through the stages of AD, various problem behaviors may occur. They may include **agitation** (a state of restlessness and excitement with no apparent cause), aggression (a forceful attitude or action expressed physically or verbally), and wandering. Before you can manage the problem, you must control your own reactions to the behavior and use appropriate communication, including nonverbal forms. No matter what the behavior is, the first step is to identify the cause. Determine if there is physical or emotional discomfort that is causing the behavior. For example, a resident who needs to go to the bathroom may become restless and agitated. Meeting his need for toileting may solve the problem.

You may be required to record behaviors over a period of time in order to discover if a pattern exists. This record may be called a "behavior log" and will include the behavior, the situation at the time of the behavior, measures taken, and results achieved. Recording must be accurate and consistent. All staff and visitors should be made aware that a record is being kept, and visitors should be asked to report any incidents immediately. The recorded information is evaluated periodically to determine the progress and effectiveness of the measures that are taken. These measures will be included in the resident's care plan.

Causes of Problem Behavior in Confused Residents

- Physical discomfort or emotional concerns—fear, anxiety, depression, pain
- Environmental factors—noise, crowds, glare, darkness, uncomfortable temperature, overstimulation, change in location.
- Unmet needs—physical or psychosocial, incontinence, hunger, constipation, toileting, thirst, boredom, loneliness
- Fatigue—not enough rest or sleep, too much activity.

Managing Problem Behavior in ADRD

The confused resident requires much empathy, patience, and reassurance. There are some general approaches that can be used in all problem behaviors.

The following guidelines will help you work effectively with residents with ADRD.

GUIDELINES

MANAGING PROBLEM BEHAVIOR

- Observe for causes of behavior
- Provide distraction—change the activity, offer food.
- Provide activities—regular exercise program.
- Maintain a calm environment—reduce stimulation, turn down radios and TV, move away from crowds and noisy individuals.
- Protect the resident from injury.
- Build a trusting relationship.
- Be consistent with care and approaches—provide a regular routine.
- Keep people who have conflicts away from each other.
- Prevent frustration.
- Use alarms and monitoring devices.
- Use signs, labels, or objects to identify rooms.
- Limit choices—avoid overwhelming the resident.
- Be prepared—come to work rested and stay aware of your reactions.

Treatment and Medication

Although there is no cure for AD, some medications are used to slow the disease progression and modify behaviors. There are also medications used to treat psychiatric conditions. Most of these medications have multiple side effects including drowsiness, rashes and hives, constipation, changes in appetite, blurred vision, changes in vital signs, dry mouth, thirst, urinary problems, abnormal movements, muscle spasms, restlessness, dizziness, insomnia, headache, fatigue, agitation, tremors, changes in body weight, seizures, nightmares, nausea, slurred speech, fever, abdominal cramps, jaundice, diarrhea, indigestion, unusual eye movements, clumsiness, joint pain, weakness, salivation, and drooling. Many of these side effects are also symptoms of ADRD. Report any observed changes that take place in a resident. The resident's well-being and safety depend on your close observation and reporting. Report immediately if you find medications in the resident's room.

Inappropriate Sexual Behavior

Mental changes that takes place in ADRD, such as loss of judgment and confusion, may result in inappropriate sexual behavior. Illness, medication, poor self-image, and cultural differences may cause the resident to act this way. The resident may be responding to the caring, nurturing individual that you are. He or she may have difficulty drawing a line between caregiving and affection. Because of poor vision or confusion, the resident may have mistaken you for a spouse, a loved one, or a sexual partner. Some sexual behavior may be the result of mental changes.

Care should be taken to avoid misinterpreting the resident's behavior. Some inappropriate behaviors, such as removing or unfastening clothing, may not be sexual in nature. The confused resident may have simply forgotten to finish dressing or is unaware that he is not wearing clothing.

Some residents may approach confused or unconsenting residents. These residents must be protected by staff members. Sometimes, residents knowingly make inappropriate sexual advances.

The Aggressive/Combative Resident

Residents may be physically or verbally aggressive. A combative resident is one who struggles and fights. Some residents interfere with their care because they are so combative. It is difficult to work with them and provide appropriate care.

Recognizing Signs of Aggressive Behavior

Awareness of the cause of combative behavior will help you develop empathy and understanding. The basis for dealing with aggressive behavior is understanding it. Recognizing the signs of anger will help you to protect yourself and the resident (see Figure 24-4 ■). Often, combative behavior occurs very suddenly, although the tension and anger usually are visible before action occurs. When you are working with an aggressive resident, always trust your intuition or "gut" feelings. Those feelings are usually correct.

GUIDELINES

MANAGING SEXUALLY AGGRESSIVE BEHAVIOR

- Avoid misinterpreting the resident's behavior.
- Be knowledgeable about sexuality in the elderly.
- Observe for causes and patterns of sexual behavior.
- Be aware of and accept your own sexuality and reactions.
- Maintain a professional attitude.
- Be aware that your behavior may affect the resident's behavior.
- Firmly and calmly tell the resident to stop the objectionable behavior.
- Explain that the behavior is not acceptable and that it makes you uncomfortable.
- Never scold, embarrass, shame, or belittle the resident.
- Remain calm and matter-of-fact.
- Distract the resident with food or another activity.
- Provide privacy for a resident who is sexually aroused.
- Check the care plan for approaches to be used.
- Report and record inappropriate behavior.

GUIDELINES

MANAGING AGGRESSIVE BEHAVIOR IN ADRD

- Use a consistent approach in all care.
- Constantly observe for signs of aggression.
- Use communication skills to be sure that the resident understands what you are going to do.
- Repeat steps and explanations frequently.
- Allow the resident to make decisions without overwhelming him or her.
- Provide a predictable schedule for the resident.
- Move calmly and slowly.
- Avoid standing above or talking down to the resident.
- Be respectful and control your reactions.
- Don't take the resident's angry words or actions personally.

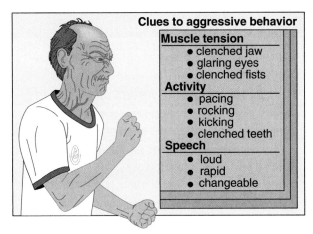

Clues to aggressive behavior

Muscle tension
- clenched jaw
- glaring eyes
- clenched fists

Activity
- pacing
- rocking
- kicking
- clenched teeth

Speech
- loud
- rapid
- changeable

FIGURE 24-4 ■ Learn to recognize signs of anger.

GUIDELINES (Continued)

- Use body language that is nonaggressive.
- Distract the resident with food or another activity.
- Maintain rapport (a mutually trusting relationship) with the resident or involve someone who can do so.
- Maintain a safe, secure environment. Restraints should not be used.
- Protect yourself from a combative resident.
- Don't turn your back, and stay an arm's length away if possible.
- Avoid "cornering" the resident.
- Allow pacing.
- Get help when necessary.
- Report all signs of anger and aggression to the nurse.

The Depressed Resident

Many elderly residents are depressed. Facing the losses they have suffered often overwhelms their emotional strength. Being unable to be independent and run their own lives, in addition to having physical illness and impairment, may burden them to the point of giving up. They may lose the motivation to participate in any part of life.

Symptoms of depression include deep sadness, low self-esteem, a feeling of worthlessness, lack of interest in activities, social withdrawal, negative reactions, and difficulty in decision making. Physical

symptoms resulting from decreased energy include poor hygiene, slow movement, sleep problems, altered appetite, and weight change. Constipation and fatigue also occur with depression.

GUIDELINES

CARING FOR THE DEPRESSED RESIDENT

- Encourage the resident to talk about feelings (see Figure 24-5 ■).
- Listen attentively.
- Allow the resident to cry. Crying may be helpful.
- Provide activity to stimulate and remotivate.
- Encourage the resident to prepare for and attend activities.
- Help the resident to feel accepted and appreciated.
- Compliment the resident's special qualities and individual characteristics.
- A visit out of doors may be helpful.
- Encourage the resident to socialize with other residents.
- Encourage hygiene and grooming, and praise efforts and results.

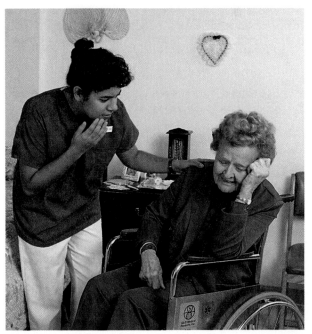

FIGURE 24-5 ■ When a resident cries, you may feel helpless.

RESTORATIVE ADLs

Maintaining the independence of the resident with ADRD should be the basis of all personal care. This can be challenging because the resident may not only be unable to function, but also may resist your assistance. For example, think of the difficulty that you would encounter while attempting to provide oral hygiene for a person who will not open her mouth. All of the care techniques and procedures presented previously will be used with ADRD residents. However, they will need to be adapted.

Personal Care and Hygiene

Although the resident with ADRD may be confused, appearance and hygiene continue to be important concerns. Grooming and hygiene often are neglected by the resident and decline as the confusion worsens. Meeting these needs for the confused resident can be very challenging. You may encounter agitation, resistance, hostility, depression, and restlessness that require behavior management before the basic tasks can be performed. Hygiene is important to maintain healthy skin and prevent infection.

GUIDELINES

ASSISTING WITH PERSONAL CARE AND HYGIENE

- Use simple, short directions such as "Pick up the wash cloth. Wash your face."
- Adapt for special needs of each resident.
- Maintain a regular routine—same time of day, same order of steps.
- Ask the family about the resident's former hygiene routine and follow it as closely as possible.
- Provide privacy and maintain safety.
- Adapt your assistance as needed.
- Avoid forcing or arguing.
- As clothing is removed, place it out of sight and focus on the clothing to be worn.
- When the resident grabs the clothing, offer something to distract him or her.

GUIDELINES (Continued)

- Be sure clothing is easy to put on, wear, and remove.
- Arrange clothing in the order of use.
- Reduce the danger of falls by assisting with dressing while the resident is seated or lying in bed.
- Make sure that clothing is fastened and is appropriate for the location and activity. Check frequently to be sure that clothing is in place.
- Help the resident maintain a simple hairstyle.
- It may be necessary to use an electric razor for shaving.
- Avoid leaving small electrical appliances in the resident's room.
- Continue to assist with makeup.
- It may be easier to trim fingernails while the resident is watching TV.
- Observe dentures for fit and be sure they belong to the resident.
- Be flexible and willing to try new approaches.

Eating and Nutrition

Nutrition becomes an increasing problem from the beginning of ADRD. As the brain deteriorates, chewing and swallowing decline, and food and fluid intake decrease. The ability to use utensils is lost, and the senses of hunger and thirst may not be responded to or understood. Medications may affect the appetite and the sense of taste. Malnutrition and dehydration occur as the resident becomes unable to feed himself. Even eating is impossible (see Figure 24-6 ■).

GUIDELINES

ASSISTING WITH NUTRITION

- Encourage residents with ADRD to feed themselves as much as possible.
- Encourage the resident to hold finger foods such as bread and fruit.
- Maintain a calm atmosphere at mealtime.
- Meals should always be eaten in the same location.
- If necessary, present one food at a time to prevent distress over choices.

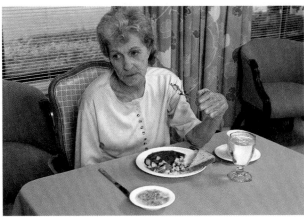

FIGURE 24-6 ■ The confused resident may not remember to feed herself.

<table>
<tr><td>

GUIDELINES

ASSISTING WITH BOWEL AND BLADDER PROBLEMS

- Encourage toileting on a regular basis.
- Recognize nonverbal cues for toileting.
- Respond quickly to requests for toileting.
- Answer call signals promptly.
- Follow all of the guidelines included in Chapter 17 for assisting residents with toileting.
- Observe for patterns of incontinence.
- Report and record all incontinent episodes.

</td></tr>
</table>

GUIDELINES (Continued)

- Use assistive equipment such as plate guards and built-up utensils.
- Season the food for the resident.
- Remove wrappers and packages to prevent distraction.
- Offer frequent snacks.
- Follow all of the guidelines in Chapter 15 for assisting residents to eat.
- Encourage family members to visit at mealtime if it doesn't distract the resident.
- Weigh the resident according to the care plan.
- Do not try to feed a person who is agitated or sleepy. Be sure to report this to the nurse.
- Do not hurry the resident.
- Consider the resident's former eating habits, likes, and dislikes.

Incontinence and Toileting

Changes in both physical and mental function contribute to bowel and bladder incontinence. It is important for all residents, regardless of their mental state, to maintain normal elimination routines as long as possible. They may not recognize the need to toilet, be able to express this need, or be able to find the bathroom. Incontinence may cause emotional problems such as embarrassment or shame. Promote independence and dignity when managing incontinence. Medications may cause incontinence.

Sleep Problems and Sundowner's Syndrome

Sleep problems may involve too much or too little sleep, and the sleep/wake cycle may be confused. Provide activities to prevent boredom and help sleepy residents stay awake. Sundowner's syndrome may be decreased by using more light as evening approaches. Provide a safe environment and allow pacing. Avoid naps, caffeine, and stimulation late in the day.

Afternoon exercise may help prevent nighttime wandering. A warm bath or soothing backrub may help the resident relax. Plan care to avoid waking the resident unnecessarily. Assist with toileting at bedtime. Promote quiet in the halls. Make regular rounds during the night to see if residents are sleeping. Be quiet and avoid turning on bright lights.

MEETING PSYCHOSOCIAL NEEDS

Psychosocial needs include emotional, social, and spiritual needs. One of the best ways to meet these needs of the resident is through activities. Residents with ADRD have the same psychosocial needs as everyone else. However, meeting those needs becomes increasingly difficult. Communication is very important. The sharing of information and creative ideas assures continuity of care, and reporting and recording complete the communication process.

Organize and collect supplies before beginning an activity. Structure and consistency are important. Knowing what to expect and when it will happen help to prevent stress. Activities for residents with

AD should be predictable and routine, and should be based on a written plan of care. Positive activities are planned that provide for both group and individual experiences. Rewarding experiences will help to prevent inappropriate behavior and enhance the quality of life.

Planned activities should consider, and be adapted to, the current functional level, and should be based on former interests of the resident. Skills learned long ago are more likely to be remembered, while impaired learning may interfere with the ability to do new things. Therefore, activities must be based on the remaining ability and knowledge of the individual resident. Avoid assuming that the resident with ADRD can continue to perform tasks just because he once knew how. Be aware that interests and ability change from moment to moment. Limit the length of the activity.

Limit the number of activities. Choose tasks that require few steps, and lead the resident, step by step, through the activity. Choices to be made should be limited to a decision between two items rather than many. Give clear directions and repeat them as many times as necessary. Visual instructions, such as pointing at an object or demonstrating, may be effective. Encourage and compliment the resident's efforts. Avoid negative statements.

Activities should be based on the resident's enjoyment. Avoid activities that the resident sees as childish. Remember, an activity that would bore you may not be meaningless to the resident. Repetition is soothing, and boredom is not usually a problem. Repetitive "busy" work, like folding a piece of linen repeatedly, may be rewarding. Doing something independently leads to satisfaction and self-esteem.

Do not force a resident to participate. If the resident refuses, offer another activity or return later and ask again. Discontinue the activity if the resident becomes agitated or fatigued. Ensure safety and maintain a calm environment. Remain aware of your communication techniques and use the guidelines for communicating with the resident with ADRD. Be sure to thank residents for their participation.

Types of activities that may be useful include music, arts and crafts, games, exercise, gardening, pet therapy, spiritual activity, and remembering the past.

Stress Management for Residents Who Have ADRD

Stress increases confusion, agitation, and restlessness in residents with ADRD. Many of the stress management guidelines that are provided in Chapter 2 will be helpful to the resident. The guidelines and information included in the behavior management section of this chapter are appropriate stress interventions. Be sure that you are familiar with them and know how to use them.

SUPPORTING FAMILY AND FRIENDS

The impact of AD upon family members and friends can be devastating. They are suffering as they see the day-by-day progression toward death of a loved one. The resident with AD may not even recognize or respond to them. Visits can be so upsetting that visitors may stay away. As a result, family members are no longer available to support each other or the resident. They may feel guilt, anger, depression, and loneliness, which contribute to stress. Family conflict may occur as difficult decisions are made. It is frightening to realize that a loved one is suffering from AD, and it's easier to "look the other way." Financial resources may be quickly exhausted. Many community programs have long waiting lists and are unable to provide services to people needing a lot of care.

Most residents with AD have been cared for at home by a loved one. Safety issues and the demands of physical care eventually leave the caregiver exhausted. If the caregiver is an adult child, role reversal may be uncomfortable to both the parent and the child. If she is unable to continue providing care at home, the caregiver may have a sense of failure. When the resident with AD is admitted to the facility the caregiver may experience conflicting emotions, such as guilt and relief.

Family reactions to stress may result in emotional outbursts, complaints about their loved one's care, and hostility. Separate yourself from the hostility. The anger is not yours. They are angry about circumstances over which they have no control, and you may be the first person they encounter. Listen respectfully. Expressing emotions helps to relieve the anger. They also may be afraid to entrust the resident's care to the facility staff and exhaust themselves with constant visiting.

GUIDELINES

ASSISTING FAMILY AND FRIENDS

- Encourage family to communicate with each other.
- Seek suggestions from family members when possible; attending care plan meetings may be helpful.
- Respond calmly and respectfully regardless of the family's attitude.
- Help family members to be emotionally comfortable when visiting.
- Encourage the family to bring mementos of the past to share with the resident.
- Refer questions on ADRD to the nurse or the social worker.
- Be supportive, helping families to cope with changes as the disease progresses.
- Encourage the family to continue to share their grief with the resident.
- Suggest that they speak to the social worker about help from the community such as support groups.
- Encourage family participation in nursing home programs.
- Allow the family to participate in care of the resident as desired.

ENVIRONMENTAL ISSUES

Is important to maintain an environment that is safe and secure for residents, visitors, and staff. It should be supportive and restorative. The environment affects the behavior of residents with ADRD. Most facilities have a special unit that is small and homelike for residents with AD. It is a safe area, and is designed to allow wandering and independent movement. Colors are soothing and clutter is eliminated. Large social areas are provided, and a separate dining room is available for residents with AD. The best environment provides for sensory stimulation, orientation, and decision making. It allows for individual choices and changing abilities. Socialization is encouraged.

All staff members must have special training to work in an AD unit. Consistency in staffing and routine helps to provide predictability for the residents. Interaction between staff members and residents creates a homelike atmosphere. Teamwork is encouraged. A happy staff creates happy residents.

ETHICAL ISSUES AND ADRD

There are many ethical issues involved in caring for residents with AD. You may have strong feelings about some of these issues. However, most of the decisions about these issues are not under your control. It can be frustrating if your opinion differs from decisions that are made. It is important to provide the same quality care for all residents, regardless or your opinion about decisions that they or their families have made.

Autonomy is self-determination, or the freedom to make choices. Everyone has the right to autonomy. Questions and differences of opinion about autonomy include:

- Decision making—Should a confused person be allowed to make major decisions regarding health issues?
- Manipulation with lies—Is it acceptable to lie to a confused resident to get him to cooperate?
- Disclosure of the diagnosis—Should the resident be told he has AD?
- Safety versus autonomy—Should the resident be allowed freedom of choice if he is confused and could risk his safety?
- Competency—If mental incompetency is legally determined, should residents be allowed to continue making decisions for themselves?
- Informed consent—Should the confused resident be allowed to make a decision about something that he doesn't understand, for example, refusing medication?

As the justice system becomes involved, many of these ethical issues become legal issues. They also include nutrition and hydration, health care rationing, assisted suicide, mercy killing, mental competency, quality of life, and the continuation of treatment without the expectation of a positive outcome.

CHAPTER HIGHLIGHTS

1. Alzheimer's disease is the most common form of dementia in the United States.

2. Memory loss in ADRD is severe enough to interfere with normal life, while the loss in normal aging is mild.

3. Confusion, disorientation, wandering, and restlessness are characteristics of AD.

4. As residents with ADRD lose their ability to communicate, they may depend upon nonverbal communication.

5. Many chronic diseases cause symptoms that are similar to those of AD.

6. While there is no predictable progression of AD, it is usually divided into three stages: early, middle, and late.

7. Problems that may occur as AD progresses include agitation, aggression, and wandering.

8. The first guideline in managing problem behavior is to determine the cause.

9. Maintain a professional attitude when managing sexually aggressive behavior.

10. Understanding the reason for aggression will help you work with aggressive residents.

11. Encourage the depressed resident to talk about her feelings.

12. Maintaining the independence of the resident with ADRD should be the basis of all personal care.

13. As the brain deteriorates and chewing and swallowing decline, nutrition becomes a major problem for residents with ADRD.

14. Activities for residents with AD should be predictable and routine.

15. Be supportive, helping families to cope with change as AD progresses.

16. Maintain an environment that is safe and secure for residents, visitors, and staff.

17. Provide the same quality care for all residents, regardless of your opinion about decisions that they or their families have made.

VOCABULARY REVIEW

Fill in the blanks with the vocabulary term that best completes the sentence.

1. _____ means overly suspicious.

2. Seeing or hearing things that don't exist is _____.

3. _____ is an increase in wandering, restlessness, and confusion as evening occurs.

4. _____ is a progressive disorder of the brain that eventually destroys all mental function.

5. _____ is an impairment of mental function.

6. The loss of the ability to control urine or feces is called _____.

7. _____ is self-determination, or the freedom to make choices.

8. The inability to speak or express oneself is _____.

9. The _____ is all the conditions and influences around us.

10. _____ is a state of restlessness with no apparent cause.

CHECK YOUR UNDERSTANDING

The following questions cover the highlights of this chapter. Choose the best answer for each question.

1. The most common form of dementia in the United States is
   A. Parkinson's disease   C. Lewy disease
   B. Alzheimer's disease   D. Hallucination

2. Which of the following is a *true* statement about memory loss?
   A. Normal memory loss is more severe than the memory loss of AD.
   B. Normal memory loss in aging is severe enough to interfere with normal life.
   C. Memory loss in AD is severe enough to interfere with normal life.
   D. There are no other diseases that mimic AD.

3. Residents with later stages of ADRD continue to communicate primarily with

A. Nonverbal communication
B. Gestures
C. Normal verbal communication
D. Sign language

4. Which of the following is *not* a stage of AD?
   A. Early stage   C. Late stage
   B. Middle stage   D. Confusion stage

5. Which of the following is the first guideline in managing problem behavior?
   A. Observe for and determine the cause.
   B. Limit choices—avoid overwhelming the resident.
   C. Restrain the resident who has problem behavior.
   D. Islolate the resident who has problem behavior.

6. Which of the following is a *true* statement?
   A. The basis of personal care for the resident with AD should be to do everything for him.
   B. Activities for residents with AD should be predictable and routine.
   C. Residents with AD usually maintain adequate nutrition until the end of life.
   D. AD usually progresses through the stages in a predictable manner.

7. A confused resident keeps trying to go out the front door. Which of the following would be the best response to his behavior?
   A. Restrain him in his room.
   B. Tell him to please stay inside.
   C. Distract him with another activity.
   D. Call his family to stay with him.

8. What is the best response to an angry resident?
   A. Restrain her immediately.
   B. Ask the nurse to medicate her.
   C. Talk to her in a calm, soothing voice.
   D. Ignore her until she gets over it.

9. A depressed resident is crying. Which of the following responses would be most helpful?
   A. "Don't cry; that never helps."
   B. "I'd like to see a smile now."
   C. "It'll be alright tomorrow."
   D. "Would you like to talk about it?"

AGE-SPECIFIC TIP

Mild memory loss commonly occurs with normal aging. Since remembering and recalling may take more time, be patient and allow time for the elderly resident to process the information.

CULTURALLY SENSITIVE TIP

In many cultures, caring for a loved one at home is considered an honor and a duty. When they can no longer provide that care, family members may feel guilty and lash out in anger at health care workers. Respond calmly and respectfully, regardless of the family's attitude.

EFFECTIVE PROBLEM SOLVING

Mr. Archer has Alzheimer's disease and is very confused. While the nursing assistant is helping him go to the dining room, he suddenly stops and refuses to go any further. After trying unsuccessfully to convince him to move, the nursing assistant puts her hands on her hips and says, in an exasperated tone of voice, "Mr. Arthur, I don't care if you go to the dining room or back to your room, but you have to go somewhere."

Was the nursing assistant's communication appropriate? If not, what would have been more appropriate?

_____

_____

_____

_____

_____

INTERPERSONAL COMMUNICATION

Write a T or F to indicate if the statement is true or false.

_____ Communicate with confused residents in a calm, quiet manner.

_____ Expression of affection between residents should be discouraged.

_____ Scold a resident who becomes verbally aggressive.

_____ Your nonverbal communication is very important when communicating with confused residents.

_____ Touch the confused resident before you speak to him.

OBSERVING, REPORTING, AND RECORDING

Recognizing the signs of anger will help you to protect yourself and the resident. List five signs of aggressive behavior.

_____

_____

_____

_____

_____

_____

_____

_____

_____

*E*XPLORE *M*EDIA*L*INK

Check out www.prenhall.com/grubbs for additional chapter-specific interactive study and review activities.

$\mathcal{S}$UBACUTE CARE

$\mathcal{O}$BJECTIVES

1. List three reasons why a resident may be in a rehabilitation program in subacute care.

2. List ten guidelines for care of the resident on a mechanical ventilator.

3. Identify eight guidelines for care of the resident with a tracheostomy.

4. List ten guidelines for care of the resident with an IV.

5. Identify ten guidelines for care of the resident with a feeding tube.

6. List eight guidelines for care of the resident with a gastrointestinal suction pump.

$\mathcal{V}$OCABULARY

The following words or terms will help you to understand this chapter:

Mechanical ventilator

Tracheostomy

Intravenous (IV)

Nasogastric (NG) tube

Gastrostomy (G) tube

Nursing assistants have an important role in subacute care. Subacute care units provide care for residents with specific needs such as complicated respiratory care or rehabilitation. Combining resources, equipment, and trained personnel in one unit is efficient and cost-effective. Some subacute care unit residents already were in long-term care facilities, and others once were cared for in hospitals. These residents, who often require special equipment for survival, need assistance with personal care, moving, transferring between the bed and the chair, and other ADLs. Subacute care provides an opportunity for you to increase your knowledge and skills while caring for residents with many complicated needs (see Figure 25-1 ■).

REHABILITATION

Many subacute units specialize in rehabilitation. Physical therapy, occupational therapy, and speech therapy programs are provided to meet individual needs. Residents may be trying to overcome the effects of a stroke or disease such as diabetes or Parkinson's disease. Some are in rehabilitation because they have suffered a traumatic injury. They may be younger than the elderly residents you are used to caring for, and they may stay for a shorter period of time. Regardless of the reason they are in rehabilitation, nursing care should be provided in a restorative manner with an emphasis on indepen-

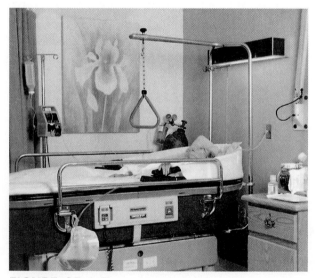

FIGURE 25-1 ■ Residents in subacute care can have complicated needs.

dence. Rehabilitation and restorative care are discussed in detail in Chapter 4. A review of that chapter would be helpful at this time.

CARE OF THE RESIDENT ON A MECHANICAL VENTILATOR

A **mechanical ventilator** is a machine that provides the resident with artificial respirations. It assists in the circulation and exchange of gases in the lungs. A person must move enough oxygen into and carbon dioxide out of the lungs to maintain body processes. When this does not occur naturally, mechanical ventilation is necessary. Ineffective respiration may result from a disease such as cancer or emphysema, drug reactions, or an injury. Mechanical ventilation does not cure the disease or injury, but it may prevent the resident's immediate death and prolong life. Although ventilators vary in design, most are equipped with controls and alarms that may be adjusted to meet individual needs (see Figure 25-2 ■). Ventilators are the responsibility of doctors, nurses, and respiratory therapists. Nursing assistants are *not* responsible for operating the equipment. Do not adjust the dials or controls on the ventilator or other equipment.

Meeting the Resident's Needs

Most residents on mechanical ventilation are completely dependent on others. Care must be taken to prevent the tubes attaching the resident to the ventilator from becoming twisted or disconnected while providing care. Residents on ventilators cannot speak while attached to the machine and must depend on nonverbal communication or writing notes. Communication can be stressful for both the caretakers and the residents. Some ventilator residents are comatose.

The resident on a ventilator has the same basic physical needs as any other resident. Turn and reposition the resident at least every 2 hours. Take care not to pull, twist, or disconnect the tubing. Good skin care and frequent oral care are important. Remember to touch and handle the resident gently, as this shows caring and compassion. A refreshing bath and clean bed linen will help the resident relax and feel less stressed.

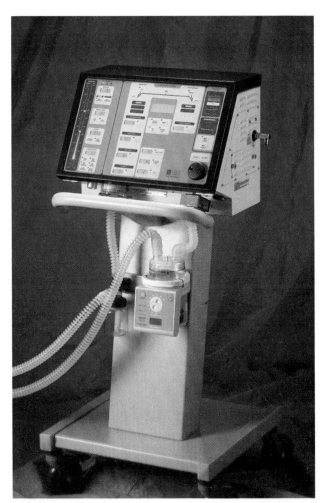

FIGURE 25-2 ■ The 740 Ventilator system. *Nellcor Puritain Bennett*

Conscious residents on ventilators often are anxious and frightened. Their breathing and their lives are totally dependent on a machine. Because they are extremely limited in activity, they can become bored and depressed. Complete dependency on others often creates feelings of hopelessness, despair, frustration, or anger. The difficulty in trying to communicate can be overwhelming. One of your most important responsibilities will be to provide emotional support and help ventilator-dependent residents meet psychological needs. Their families also may be anxious and need your reassurance and support.

The ventilator panel should be turned away from the resident, if possible. The alert resident will watch the dials and measurements and may become unnecessarily alarmed. Remember that even comatose residents may hear what is said.

Never make statements in front of the resident that might indicate something is wrong. A simple statement such as "I don't think the machine is working right" could cause the resident or the family to panic.

Place the call signal within reach and fasten it in place. Answer call signals immediately, no matter how often they are used. Residents who are afraid may use the call signal frequently. The more quickly you respond to the signal, the more comforted the residents will feel. Your prompt answer to their call for help is reassuring.

Most of the time, you will work with a nurse when providing physical care for residents on ventilators. The most basic tasks such as bathing or bedmaking become complicated when the resident is on a ventilator. Two people usually are needed for procedures that require moving the resident. One person moves the resident while the other person observes and assists with equipment, tubes, and wires. After you do a procedure—whether alone or with another nursing assistant—that involves moving or turning a resident, ask the nurse to check the resident and the equipment.

A nursing assistant *never* removes a resident from a ventilator. Being "weaned" off the ventilator may be difficult for a resident, and he or she will need support and reassurance. You may be asked to sit with a resident while he or she is off the machine. You also may be asked to measure the resident's vital signs during this period. Watch for cyanosis, confusion, and restlessness. Reassure the resident that he or she will be returned to the ventilator immediately if requested.

GUIDELINES

CARE OF THE RESIDENT ON A MECHANICAL VENTILATOR

- Remember that you are caring for a resident, not a machine.
- Offer your support and reassurance.
- Assist the resident to communicate.
- Place the call signal within the resident's reach and answer it promptly. (continued)

GUIDELINES (Continued)

- Get help before moving the resident.
- Allow the resident to have undisturbed periods of rest.
- Handle the resident gently.
- Turn and reposition the resident at least every 2 hours.
- Provide frequent oral care.
- Take care not to pull, twist, or disconnect tubing.
- Move the ventilator carefully and observe the gauge for changes.
- Measure, record, and report vital signs accurately.
- Notify the nurse immediately when an alarm sounds, the pressure gauge drops, or you observe anything unusual.
- Do not adjust the dials or controls on the ventilator or other equipment.
- Never remove a resident from the ventilator.

Care of the Resident with a Tracheostomy

A **tracheostomy** (a surgical opening into the trachea) is performed to create an artificial airway when a resident's natural airway is not functioning properly. A tube is inserted into the trachea through a surgical incision in the neck. The resident breathes through the tube rather than the nose or mouth (see Figure 25-3 ■). When used with a ventilator, the outer end of the tracheostomy tube is attached to the ventilator. The tracheostomy tube fits into the tracheostomy stoma (mouth of the surgical opening) and is secured by tapes, ties, or velcro fasteners.

In most areas, nursing assistants are not allowed to perform tracheostomy care. However, you may be providing personal care for tracheostomy residents. A new tracheostomy wound and the skin around it are cleaned and the dressing is changed several times a day, as needed.

If the tracheostomy tube has an inner cannula (an additional tube inside), it must be removed and cleaned once every shift or as needed. This procedure is done by a nurse or respiratory therapist because the resident must be disconnected from the ventilator. A spare tracheostomy tube is kept at the bedside in case immediate replacement is necessary.

Suctioning the Airway

A tracheostomy interferes with the resident's ability to cough and clear his or her airway of mucous. Mechanical suction may be necessary when secretions interfere with ventilation. On some occasions, the resident's nose and mouth may need to be suctioned. The nurse inserts a small catheter into the tracheostomy tube to suction a resident on a ventilator. The catheter is attached to a suction pump and collection bottle by a piece of tubing (see Figure 25-4 ■). It may be your responsibility to empty and record the contents of the collection

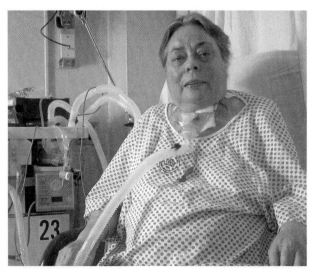

FIGURE 25-3 ■ A tracheostomy provides an artificial airway.

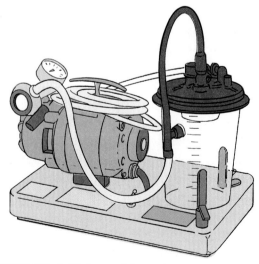

FIGURE 25-4 ■ A portable suction pump

bottle. Wear gloves and follow standard precautions when performing this procedure.

Nursing assistants generally are not allowed to suction residents. However, you are responsible for observing the resident, his or her breathing and the equipment, and for telling the nurse when a problem occurs.

Report to the nurse immediately if you observe any of the following:

- Bubbling, gurgling, rattling respirations
- Dyspnea (difficult breathing)
- Changes to pale, ashen or cyanotic color in skin, lips and/or nailbeds
- Complaints of shortness of breath or respiratory discomfort
- Sounding of the alarm on the ventilator

Always wear gloves and a mask when assisting the nurse with tracheostomy care or suctioning. Sometimes, a gown or goggles will be necessary. Dispose of contaminated materials according to facility policy. Follow standard precautions and wash your hands before and after the procedure.

GUIDELINES

CARE OF THE RESIDENT WITH A TRACHEOSTOMY

- Provide mouth care at least every 2 hours.
- Make sure that the tracheostomy tapes or ties are securely fastened.
- Avoid wetting the tracheostomy dressing while providing care.
- Check to see that a spare tracheostomy tube is available.
- Promptly report unusual observations such as bleeding from the tracheostomy site.
- Observe for signs that suctioning is needed and notify the nurse.
- Reassure the resident and family members.
- Follow standard precautions and wear gloves and a mask when assisting with tracheostomy care or suctioning.
- Never cover the opening of the tracheostomy or allow water to enter it.

ALTERNATIVE METHODS OF HYDRATION AND NUTRITION

Intravenous Therapy

Intravenous (IV) means "into the vein." The resident may receive fluid nutrients and/or medications through the IV. A needle or special catheter is inserted into the vein to give fluids by this method. A sterile dressing covers the insertion site. Tubing connects the needle or catheter to a container of fluid, which hangs from an IV pole. Usually, an IV control pump is attached to control the flow rate of the fluid. When a pump is used, the tubing from the container is threaded through the pump. The rate of flow is calculated and the pump preset by the nurse. The pump is equipped with an alarm that sounds when something is wrong. The control pump is plugged into an electrical outlet. Portable battery-operated pumps are available to allow for maximum mobility.

A nursing assistant may not start, stop, or adjust the flow rate of an IV. You are not allowed to change the sterile dressing. These tasks are the responsibility of the nurses. Observe the resident frequently and report any problems to the nurse immediately. The following guidelines will help you care for the resident with an IV.

GUIDELINES

CARE OF THE RESIDENT WITH AN IV

- Follow standard precautions and wear gloves if contact with body fluids is likely.
- Call the nurse whenever the pump alarm sounds.
- Observe for and report swelling, redness, bleeding, or leaking at the insertion site.
- Report complaints of pain or burning at the site of insertion.
- Report to the nurse if the flow rate changes or stops (see Figure 25-5 ■). Do not adjust the rate or turn off the pump.
- Report breathing problems or an elevated temperature.
- Call the nurse if the tubing disconnects. Do not attempt to reconnect it.   (continued)

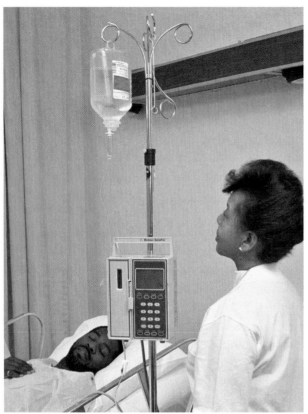

FIGURE 25-5 ■ Report to the nurse if the flow rate of the IV changes or stops.

GUIDELINES (Continued)

- Make sure the tubing is not kinked, tangled, or under the resident's body.
- Allow slack in the tubing to prevent tension on the needle or catheter.
- Give proper restraint care if the IV arm is restrained.
- Take blood pressures on the arm that does not have an IV.
- Assist the resident to turn and reposition, avoiding tension on the tubing.
- Keep the IV fluid container above the level of the insertion site.
- Use a portable IV stand to assist the resident in ambulation.
- Protect the IV site and keep the dressing dry.
- Handle the pump carefully, and avoid dropping or jarring it.

Keep the resident with an IV as comfortable as possible without disturbing the IV. Always ask the nurse to check the IV after you have completed the resident's care. The guidelines for changing the clothing of a resident with an IV are located in Chapter 13.

Feeding Tubes

Residents may need tube feeding to meet their nutritional needs. The two types of tubes most commonly used in a long-term care facility are nasogastric tubes and gastrostomy tubes.

A **nasogastric (NG) tube** is a tube placed through the nose into the stomach (see Figure 25-6 ■). ("Naso" is the medical term for nose and "gastric" means of the stomach.) An NG tube also may be attached to a wall suction outlet or to a suction machine to remove fluids from the stomach.

A **gastrostomy (G) tube** is a tube place directly into the stomach for feeding (see Figure 25-7 ■). A small surgical opening is made through the abdominal wall into the stomach. The tube may be held in place by an inflated balloon or it may be sutured. This type of tube often is used for residents who may need tube feedings for a long time.

Usually, the NG tube or the G tube will be attached to a container of commercially prepared formula ordered by the doctor. The tubing is

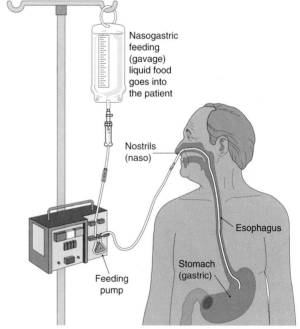

Nasogastric feeding (gavage) liquid food goes into the patient

Nostrils (naso)

Esophagus

Stomach (gastric)

Feeding pump

FIGURE 25-6 ■ An NG tube

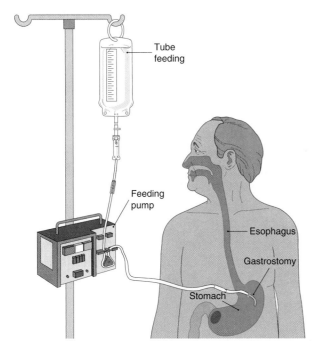

FIGURE 25-7 ■ A G tube

threaded through a pump that controls the amount and the rate of feeding. Some feeding pumps are turned off and the patient is disconnected from the pump when the feeding is complete. The pump has an alarm that sounds whenever the feeding tube becomes plugged. Notify the nurse immediately whenever the alarm sounds.

The resident who has a feeding tube should be observed frequently. If the pump is not working properly, the resident may receive the wrong amount of food. The fluid may enter too quickly and cause nausea, vomiting, and aspiration. Do not give a resident with a feeding tube anything to eat or drink without checking with the nurse. A resident with a feeding tube may be NPO (the abbreviation for "nothing by mouth"). The NG tube may cause pressure and sores inside or around the nose. Because the mouth and lips tend to dry out, frequent mouth care may be necessary.

The resident with a feeding tube should not lie flat. The head of the bed should be elevated at least 30°. Aspiration can result if the resident is not positioned properly. A major responsibility when caring for resident with a feeding tube is to report any unusual observations promptly. The following guidelines will help you carry out your responsibilities.

GASTROINTESTINAL SUCTIONING

Suctioning may be necessary to remove fluid, blood, or wastes from a resident's stomach. An NG tube is connected to a portable suction machine or a wall suction outlet (see Figure 25-8 ■). The machine may be set at a low level to suction continuously or intermittently (cycling on and off). This type of suctioning frequently follows surgery and is not

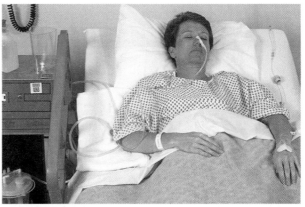

FIGURE 25-8 ■ Suctioning may be necessary to remove contents from the resident's stomach.

used often in subacute care. If you are caring for a patient with this type of pump, the following guidelines will be helpful.

GUIDELINES

CARE OF THE RESIDENT WITH A GASTROINTESTINAL SUCTION PUMP

- Wear gloves and follow standard precautions.
- Check for leaks in the tubing or the system.
- Keep collection containers below the level of the bed unless instructed otherwise.

GUIDELINES (Continued)

- Empty drainage containers only when instructed.
- Measure, describe, and record contents of the drainage container.
- Check to see that tubing does not become disconnected.
- Tell the nurse immediately if the amount of drainage in the container increases rapidly or if drainage stops or becomes bright red.
- Report complaints of nausea or abdominal discomfort.

CHAPTER HIGHLIGHTS

1. Subacute care units provide care for residents with specific needs such as rehabilitation or respiratory care.
2. Residents in subacute rehabilitation programs may be younger and stay for shorter periods of time.
3. Most residents on mechanical ventilators are completely dependent on others.
4. Nursing assistants are not allowed to adjust the dials or gauges on ventilators.
5. Never cover the opening of the tracheostomy or allow water to enter it.
6. Wear gloves and a mask when assisting with tracheostomy care or suctioning.
7. Nursing assistants may not start, stop, or adjust the flow rate of an IV.
8. Make sure the IV tubing is not kinked, tangled, or under the resident's body.
9. Keep the IV fluid container above the level of the insertion site.
10. The head of the bed must be elevated at least 30° for a resident with a feeding tube.
11. Notify the nurse immediately whenever the feeding pump alarm sounds.
12. Measure, describe, and record the contents of the gastrointestinal suction drainage container.

VOCABULARY REVIEW

Fill in the blanks with the vocabulary term that best completes the sentence.

1. A/An _____ is a machine that provides the resident with artificial respirations.

2. To choke when food or fluid enters the airway is to _____.

3. _____ is a gas, essential to life, that is found naturally in the air.

4. A surgical opening into the trachea is called a/an _____.

5. _____ means "into the vein."

6. Difficult breathing is called _____.

7. A/An _____ is a tube placed directly into the stomach through a surgical opening in the abdomen.

8. A/An _____ is a tube placed through the nose into the stomach.

9. A/An _____ is the mouth of a surgical opening.

10. The medical abbreviation NPO means _____.

CHECK YOUR UNDERSTANDING

The following questions cover the highlights of this chapter. Choose the best answer for each question.

1. You are assigned to bathe a 25-year-old rehabilitation resident who seems embarrassed about the situation. Which of the following statements is most appropriate?
   A. "I know you're used to bathing yourself, but you can't do that anymore."
   B. "I've never bathed anyone your age before."
   C. "Let me cover you with a bath blanket before we start your bath."
   D. "Maybe we should just skip your bath this morning."

2. A resident is in rehabilitation while recovering from injuries received in an auto accident. What is the best way to provide restorative care?
   A. Encourage him to do as much as possible for himself.
   B. Encourage him to rest while you provide all his care.
   C. Encourage his family to provide all his care.
   D. Encourage him to continue doing his own care, even if he becomes tired.

3. You observe that the resident on a ventilator has become extremely agitated. What is your *best* response?
   A. Tell him that everything will be all right.
   B. Sit by his bed and hold his hand.
   C. Tell him to calm down and he will feel better.
   D. Stay with him and notify the nurse immediately.

4. A resident who is being weaned from the ventilator looks nervous and anxious. Which statement is appropriate to make?
   A. "Don't worry. Everything looks okay."
   B. "You are really better off without the machine."
   C. "I can see you're upset. Can I help you?"
   D. "I don't know why you're upset. You ought to be happy."

5. Which statement about tracheostomy care is true?
   A. Cover the opening of the tracheostomy tube while providing care.
   B. Nursing assistants should remove and clean the inner cannula as necessary.
   C. Wear gloves and a mask when assisting with tracheostomy care.
   D. Make sure the tracheostomy ties are unfastened before you provide care.

6. How should you position the resident who has a feeding tube?
   A. on the abdomen
   B. with the head of the bed elevated
   C. flat on the back in the supine position
   D. with the head of the bed lowered

7. A resident is attached to a gastrointestinal suction pump. You observe that the amount of drainage has increased rapidly in the last hour. What should you do?
   A. Turn the suction pump off.
   B. Adjust the amount of suction on the pump.
   C. Move the collection device to a higher level.
   D. Notify the nurse immediately.

AGE-SPECIFIC TIP

The elderly resident on a respirator may find communicating to be stressful. Remain calm and supportive, and provide opportunities for writing notes or using nonverbal forms of communication.

CULTURALLY SENSITIVE TIP

Be aware that a resident may be able to speak and understand English but may not be able to read or write it. If that resident loses the ability to speak, you will need to pay close attention to nonverbal communication.

EFFECTIVE PROBLEM SOLVING

The nursing assistant is sitting with Mr. Loredo while he is being weaned from the ventilator. Mr. Loredo becomes anxious and requests to be returned to the ventilator. The nursing assistant says, "Just wait a few more minutes. You're doing very well."

Was the nursing assistant's communication appropriate? If not, what would have been more appropriate?

_____

_____

_____

_____

_____

_____

_____

_____

_____

INTERPERSONAL COMMUNICATION

Fill in the answer.

Be aware that residents with feeding tubes are usually NPO. Do not give the resident who has a feeding tube anything to eat or drink without _____ _____ _____ _____.

OBSERVING, REPORTING, AND RECORDING

Although nursing assistants do not generally suction a resident who has a tracheostomy, you are responsible for observing and reporting any problems. List five observations you would report that might indicate a need for suctioning.

_____

_____

_____

_____

_____

_____

_____

_____

_____

_____

_____

_____

_____

_____

EXPLORE MEDIALINK

Check out www.prenhall.com/grubbs for additional chapter-specific interactive study and review activities.

26

Coping with Death and Dying

Objectives

1. Explain how your attitude toward death affects your response to the dying resident.
2. Describe the five stages of grief.
3. Identify eight guidelines for meeting the dying resident's physical needs and six guidelines for meeting his or her psychosocial needs.
4. List six guidelines for helping the dying resident's family.
5. List six guidelines for assisting other residents to cope with their grief.
6. Identify four guidelines for coping with staff stress.
7. Describe hospice care.
8. Describe four signs and symptoms of approaching death.
9. List ten guidelines for providing postmortem care.

Vocabulary

The following words or terms will help you to understand this chapter:

Terminal illness
Denial stage
Anger stage
Bargaining stage

Depression stage
Acceptance stage
Psychosocial needs
Advance directives

Hospice
Cyanosis
Postmortem care

Death and dying is a subject that can be frightening and misunderstood. It involves a wide range of emotions such as fear, anger, guilt, empathy, and compassion. The more you learn about the dying process, the more you will be able to understand it. Understanding can help you to release fear and to accept death. This, in turn, will help you to become a more compassionate and effective caregiver. Keep that goal in mind as you study this chapter.

$\mathcal{A}$TTITUDES TOWARD DEATH AND DYING

It is important to remember that your attitude towards death directly affects your response to the dying resident. If you feel frightened or guilty, you will feel uncomfortable caring for residents who are dying. Because your attitudes about death and dying have a great influence on the care you give, it will help you to develop an attitude of acceptance of death. Your attitude is influenced by culture, religion, experience, and age.

Culture

You learned very early in life what your culture expected of you. You saw how your family and friends reacted to certain life events such as birth, marriage, and death. If they feared death, you may share the same feelings.

Religion

Religion has a great influence on attitudes toward death. Most religions hold beliefs about what happens after death. If you believe that death leads to a place of peace and beauty, it is not so frightening. However, for those who believe that death leads to eternal pain and suffering, fear is a normal reaction.

Personal Experience

Grieving is learned through experience. Your relationship with the dying person, your experience with grieving, and your expectations affect your attitude. For example, you may find it easier to accept a death that is peaceful and expected than one that is sudden or violent.

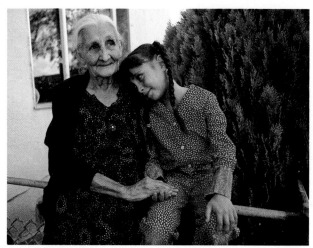

FIGURE 26-1 ■ There is often less fear of death in the very old and the very young.

Age

Age also affects your attitude toward death. Children do not fear death until they learn to do so from others. Young children often believe that death is only temporary and expect the dead person to return someday. The elderly usually have less fear of death. In fact, some see death as a release from suffering and loneliness. There seems to be less fear of death at both the beginning and the end of life (see Figure 26-1 ■).

$\mathcal{T}$ERMINAL ILLNESS

A **terminal illness** is an illness that is expected to end in death. There is little hope of recovery. Although many illnesses can be treated, controlled, or cured, there usually is no cure for a terminal illness.

$\mathcal{T}$HE STAGES OF GRIEF

The person who is dying feels intense grief. However, family members, friends, and caregivers also grieve.

Elizabeth Kubler-Ross, an expert on the care of terminally ill patients, divided grief into stages. The five stages of grief, according to Kubler-Ross, are denial, anger, bargaining, depression, and acceptance (see Figure 26-2 ■).

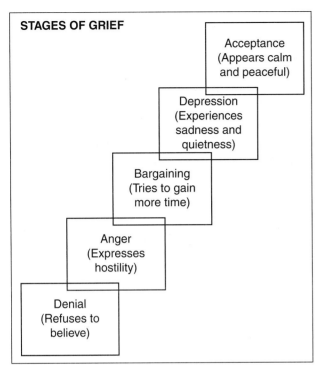

FIGURE 26-2 ■ The five stages of grief.

Denial Stage

In the **denial stage,** the grieving person refuses to believe what is happening. This first stage of grief is like a shock absorber, giving time to adjust. You cannot rush someone through denial. As much time as is needed should be allowed. A conflict also can arise when the resident is accepting while a family member is still in denial.

Anger Stage

During the second stage of grief, the **anger stage,** the grieving person expresses hostility. The most common target of this anger is the person with whom the grieving person spends the most time. At home, that usually is a family member. In the long-term care facility, it might be you. Remember that the anger is not about you; it is about dying.

Bargaining Stage

The **bargaining stage,** the third stage of grief, is an attempt to gain more time by promising something in return. Bargaining sometimes is expressed in the form of prayer. If the grieving person wants to talk to you, encourage hope, and respect his or her beliefs. Let the nurse know if the grieving resident indicates a need for spiritual assistance.

Depression Stage

The **depression stage** of grief is experienced with sadness and quiet. The grieving person may feel numb and unable to communicate. There is deep sadness with thoughts of loss of health, loss of independence, and eventually loss of life. Your help may be refused as the grieving person withdraws. Check on the resident frequently and continue to offer your assistance.

Acceptance Stage

In the **acceptance stage,** the fifth and last stage of grief, the dying person is calm and peaceful. You may hear the grieving resident say something like "I'm ready to die now." This doesn't always mean that death is really desired. It simply means that the resident has accepted that there is limited time left to live. You can help by trying to understand and accept the situation.

People do not always experience all the stages of grief in the same order. Some who never accept death die in denial or anger. Some people seem to get stuck in an earlier stage, while others move quickly to acceptance. There is no right or wrong way to grieve. It is important that you are aware of the stages and know what to expect when they occur. Your understanding that these are normal reactions will help you and the grieving person.

END-OF-LIFE CARE

It is easy to focus on the approaching death and lose sight of the needs of the whole person. Providing care for the dying involves responding to his or her psychosocial needs as well as physical needs. Be aware of end-of-life wishes of individual residents. Most residents will have advance directives (a document that provides instructions regarding a person's desires about health care). These directives, such as a living will or power of attorney for health care, must be honored.

Physical Needs

Physical needs are the most basic of all human needs and must be met first. It is difficult to provide emotional support to a resident who is physically uncomfortable. The dying resident may be in pain or discomfort. He may have dyspnea (difficult breathing). Dyspnea can be caused by disease or by anxiety and fear. The dying resident may lose interest in eating and drinking. The mouth, tongue, and lips may dry out from lack of fluids. Slowed circulation, decreased activity, and poor nutrition increase the risk of skin breakdown.

Meeting the Physical Needs of the Dying Resident

The nursing assistant plays an important role in providing comfort and prompt relief from pain. Keeping the dying resident comfortable should be your most important goal. Your observations and reporting help the health care team work together to meet the resident's needs. The following guidelines will help you meet the dying resident's physical needs.

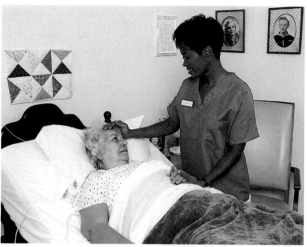

FIGURE 26-3 ■ The touch of your hand may be the dying resident's last memory.

GUIDELINES

MEETING THE DYING RESIDENT'S PHYSICAL NEEDS

- Report complaints of pain or discomfort promptly to the nurse.
- Watch for restlessness and facial expressions that may indicate pain.
- Turn and reposition the dying resident at least every 2 hours.
- Position the resident in correct body alignment.
- Stay with residents who are having difficulty breathing.
- Remain calm and reassuring.
- Encourage the resident with dyspnea to take slow, deep breaths.
- Offer small amounts of food frequently, if allowed.
- Provide mouth care for the dying resident at least every 2 hours.
- Lubricate the resident's lips to prevent cracking.
- Keep the resident's skin clean and dry.
- Massage with lotion each time you turn the resident.
- Handle the resident carefully and gently. The touch of your hand may be the resident's last memory (see Figure 26-3 ■).

Psychosocial Needs

The dying resident also has **psychosocial needs** (emotional, social, and spiritual needs). They include love and belonging, self-esteem, socialization, and spirituality. There is a need for communication and cultural acceptance. Residents who are dying often feel rejected and unloved. This is especially true if staff and family members avoid visiting the resident because they are uncomfortable being around people who are dying. It is important to remember that your presence is more comforting than anything you might say.

Communication with residents who are dying can be challenging. They may need to talk about subjects that are deep and troubling. They ask questions that have no answers, such as "Why did this happen to me?" Most of the time, rather than seeking answers, they just want to express their feelings and be heard.

It may be difficult for the dying resident to maintain self-esteem. Physical or mental changes such as incontinence or confusion may occur. Self-esteem is tied closely to independence. Maintaining some power and control increases self-esteem.

Religion is usually a source of comfort to the dying resident and family members. Spirituality needs can be met in many ways. Art, books, and music help raise spirits. The appreciation of natural beauty in the form of flowers, trees, and sunshine contributes to spirituality. Culture plays an important role in meeting the dying resident's psychosocial needs. Many cultures have beliefs and practices that relate to death and dying. Cultural experiences should be encouraged and respected at all times. The following guidelines will help you meet the psychosocial needs of the dying resident.

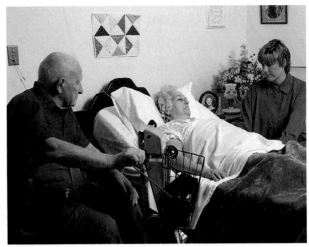

FIGURE 26-4 ■ The presence of family and friends comforts the dying resident.

GUIDELINES

MEETING THE DYING RESIDENT'S PSYCHOSOCIAL NEEDS

- Be caring, gentle, and empathetic.
- Listen carefully and answer appropriately.
- Allow the dying resident to make decisions whenever possible.
- Encourage and promote independence.
- Treat the dying resident with respect and dignity.
- Respect cultural beliefs and practices.
- Let the nurse know if the resident expresses a need for spiritual guidance.
- Ensure privacy for spiritual visits and rituals.
- Encourage the resident to express feelings.
- Allow the resident to talk about dying.

THE DYING RESIDENT'S FAMILY

One of the greatest needs of the dying resident is to be with family members. They need time to share memories and discuss the future. This provides an opportunity to make apologies and say goodbye. Visiting hours usually are extended to allow friends and family members to visit (see Figure 26-4 ■).

In many health care facilities, the family is encouraged to take an active role in caring for the dying resident. The person who is dying is comforted to know that a loved one is caring for him or her. Being as helpful as possible increases the family member's self-esteem and reduces some of the helpless feelings that death may bring. Participating in the dying resident's care helps to ease the feelings of

guilt that may be present now and/or come later. The family member is comforted by being available and useful.

Family participation does not relieve the staff of responsibility for the care of the dying person. The dying resident should receive as much of your time as your other residents. However, you will feel better knowing that the resident is not alone.

GUIDELINES

HELPING THE DYING RESIDENT'S FAMILY

- Check the care plan for family problems and interventions.
- Assist family members to meet their basic needs.
- Orient the family to the facility and be sure they know the location of rest rooms, water fountains, telephones, and vending machines.
- Check to see if guest trays are available.
- Offer pillows and blankets to family members who spend the night.
- Encourage family members to express their feelings.
- Be a respectful and supportive listener.
- Be accepting of cultural beliefs.
- Help family members and residents to have a comfortable, private visit (see Figure 26-4).

THE OTHER RESIDENTS

Residents of long-term care facilities often form close relationships. As they live together, they become a family. They share rooms, families, joys, and sorrows. Roommates frequently become close friends who depend on each other for companionship. Is it any wonder that they are saddened by the death of one of their own?

When a resident is dying, other residents may be upset. They may act out their emotions in irritability and anger. Some may withdraw and become depressed. Anxiety and fear affect their feelings and reactions. "I may be next" is a thought that may enter the minds of many residents.

GUIDELINES

ASSISTING OTHER RESIDENTS TO COPE WITH GRIEF

- Show concern for the resident's grief.
- Be aware that roommates have a relationship even if they do not seem to get along with each other.
- Take time to listen when they want to talk.
- Encourage expression of feelings.
- Be aware that talking about dying helps the resident work through his grief.
- Assure the grieving resident that feelings of anger, guilt, and fear are normal reactions.
- Watch for signs of depression.
- Share your observations with the nurse.

COPING WITH STAFF STRESS

When a resident dies in a long-term care facility, staff members also may grieve. Some residents have lived for years in the same facility. Because the staff knows and loves the residents, it is like a death in the family.

Working with dying residents can cause emotional conflict. Feelings of frustration, anger, and guilt are not uncommon. You may feel frustrated because you spend so much time with the resident, yet nothing you do seems to help. These are all normal feelings, so don't be too hard on yourself.

You may have to cope with the anger of a resident or family member. When you feel that you have done your best, you can't understand why they are angry. They are not angry at you, so don't take it personally.

GUIDELINES

COPING WITH STAFF STRESS

- Acknowledge the staff member's grief.
- Reassure the person that it is okay to grieve.
- Encourage expression of feelings.
- Remind staff members not to take outbursts of anger personally.
- Be empathetic and supportive.
- Encourage the staff member to take care of herself.
- Suggest stress relief techniques such as reading, exercise, or talking to a friend.
- If you are upset, discuss your feelings with a coworker and don't be ashamed to cry.

HOSPICE

Centuries ago in Europe, a hospice was a place of shelter for sick and weary travelers. Today, the old-fashioned idea of the hospice has been updated to meet the special needs of the dying and their families. **Hospice** is a program that provides care for the terminally ill and their families. Pain control, comfort measures, and continuity of care are provided by a team of health care workers and volunteers. Their goal is to improve quality of life by assisting the dying person to be as comfortable as possible and by providing supportive services to the family.

Care may be provided in a hospice facility or at home. Some hospice patients may be in a long-term care facility. The family or doctor may have requested hospice care. There may be no one avail-

TABLE 26-1 SIGNS AND SYMPTOMS THAT DEATH IS NEAR	
Circulatory System	*Cyanosis* (bluish color of the skin, lips, and nails due to lack of oxygen); weak, rapid, irregular pulse; decreased blood pressure; rise in body temperature with fever and perspiration.
Respiratory System	Dyspnea with shallow, noisy respirations; increased secretions and weak cough reflex causing a rattle in the throat; Cheyne-Stokes respirations (a repetitious pattern of ineffective breathing with periods of apnea).
Digestive System	Loss of appetite; difficulty swallowing; slow digestion and peristalsis (movement of food through the body); distended (swollen) abdomen; nausea and vomiting; bowel incontinence and irregularity.
Urinary System	Urinary incontinence; decreased urinary output; impaired kidney function that eventually fails.
Muscular System	Decreased body movement and muscle tone; muscles relax and become flaccid (limp); jaw drops and mouth remains partially open.
Nervous and Sensory Systems	Decreased awareness; decreased pain sensation; confusion; dilated pupils and eyes that seem to stare; decreased hearing ability; coma.

able to care for the person at home, or the family may have been providing the care but are unable to continue. It is very stressful to care for a loved one who is dying.

Hospice team members will visit the resident after admission to the facility. The hospice nurse will help the staff develop a plan that will provide continuity of care. The volunteer will make regular visits, and other hospice team members will be available as needed.

You may be assigned to care for hospice residents. Make sure you are familiar with each resident's care plan. Check for specific directives for end-of-life care. Treat the hospice worker with the same respect you show other staff members. Remember that they are part of the health care team and share your concern for the resident's quality of life.

SIGNS THAT DEATH IS NEAR

All the systems of the body gradually slow down as death approaches. The dying process varies from one person to another, and there is no set pattern. There are, however, some common signs that often are observed. Even when most of these signs are present, it is difficult to predict the time of death. Dying is as individualized as living. Remember that the last sense to fail is hearing. Assume that the dying resident can hear you, and continue talking even when there is no response.

Table 26-1 identifies signs and symptoms in each system that indicate that death is near.

Signs of Death

Death occurs when there is no pulse, no respirations, and no blood pressure.

POSTMORTEM CARE

Care of the body after death is called **postmortem care.** The purpose of postmortem care is to preserve the appearance of the body. Postmortem care includes positioning the body, straightening the room, and collecting the resident's personal belongings (see Figure 26-5 ■). The nurse will tell

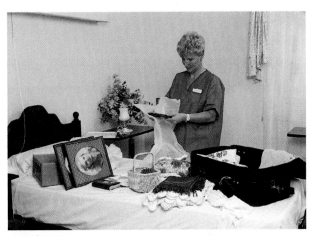

FIGURE 26-5 ■ Collecting the resident's belongings is part of postmortem care.

you when to begin this procedure. If you feel uneasy the first time you do postmortem care, talk about your feelings with the nurse.

The procedure for postmortem care is not the same in all facilities. In some facilities a shroud will be used. A shroud is a cover for wrapping the dead body. It is your responsibility to know the procedure where you work.

The Role of the Nursing Assistant

As a nursing assistant, your role in caring for the dying resident is very important. Because you provide so much of the hands-on care, the dying resident may turn to you in this time of need. Your comfort in working with the dying, as well as your knowledgeable and accepting attitude, can help the resident accept death more easily. Your presence at the bedside—your hand in the resident's hand—may help the resident take that final step on the journey through life (see Figure 26-6 ■).

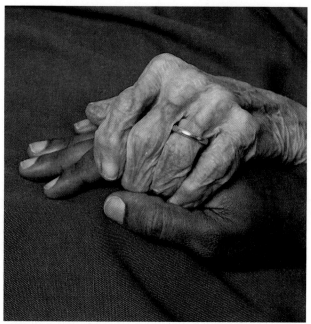

FIGURE 26-6 ■ Your hand in the resident's hand may help the resident take that final step on the journey through life.

GUIDELINES

PROVIDING POSTMORTEM CARE

- Wear gloves and follow standard precautions.
- Treat the body with respect, dignity, and privacy.
- Remove tubes and catheters according to facility policy.
- Bathe the body as needed.
- Place protective pads under the body to absorb urine and feces.
- Comb or brush the hair.
- Place the body in good body alignment, in a supine position, with the bed flat, if possible.
- Close the eyes gently.
- Elevate the head on a pillow, and place the arms at the side.
- Replace the dentures or put them in a labeled container.

GUIDELINES (Continued)

- Cover the body with a clean sheet, leaving the head and shoulders exposed.
- Remove supplies from the room. Leave the room neat and orderly.
- Provide privacy for the family if they wish to view the body.
- Handle jewelry according to facility policy.
- Leave identification on the body. You may need to apply additional identification according to facility policy.
- Wrap the body in a shroud or sheet if facility policy calls for it.
- Show respect for the resident's belongings by packing them carefully (see Figure 26-5).
- If belongings are not given to the family, they are cared for according to facility policy. A list of belongings may be required.
- Strip the unit after the body has been removed from the room.

CHAPTER HIGHLIGHTS

1. Your attitude toward death and dying affects your response to the dying resident.
2. People do not always experience all the stages of grief in the same order.
3. Be aware of the end-of-life wishes of individual residents.
4. Keeping the dying resident comfortable should be your most important goal.
5. It is important to meet the dying person's psychosocial needs as well as his or her physical needs.
6. You can help the family by being a supportive listener.
7. Discuss your feelings with a coworker, and don't be ashamed to cry.
8. Hospice provides care for people who are terminally ill.
9. All the systems of the body gradually slow as death nears.
10. The last sense to go is hearing, so talk to the dying resident.
11. The signs of death are no pulse, no respirations, and no blood pressure.
12. Follow your facility's policy when performing postmortem care.
13. The body must be treated with respect, dignity, and privacy at all times.
14. Pack the resident's belongings in a way that shows respect and caring.
15. Provide privacy for the family if they wish to view the body.

VOCABULARY REVIEW

Fill in the blanks with the vocabulary term that best completes the sentence.

1. The _____, the fourth stage of grief, is experienced with sadness and quiet.

2. A/An _____ is an illness that is expected to end in death.

3. A program that provides care for the terminally ill and their families is called _____.

4. In the _____ the grieving person refuses to believe what is happening.

5. During the second stage of grief, the _____, the grieving person expresses hostility.

6. _____ is a bluish color of the skin, lips, and nails due to lack of oxygen.

7. A document that provides instructions regarding a person's desires about health care is a/an _____.

8. Care of the body after death is called _____.

9. The _____ of grief is an attempt to gain more time by promising something in return.

10. The _____ are the dying person's emotional, social, and spiritual needs.

CHECK YOUR UNDERSTANDING

The following questions cover the highlights of this chapter. Choose the best answer for each question.

1. The *most* important factor affecting your response to dying residents is
   A. your age
   B. your religion
   C. your ability to perform postmortem care
   D. your attitude toward death

2. The dying resident starts talking to you about religion. What should you do?
   A. Tell him to wait and talk to his pastor.
   B. Encourage him to talk while you listen quietly.
   C. Change the topic immediately.
   D. Call the nurse immediately.

3. Which of the following statements about the dying resident's visitors is *false*?
   A. Visiting hours usually are extended when a resident is dying.
   B. Visitors promote the resident's well-being.
   C. You can help visitors meet their needs.
   D. Visitors usually are not allowed when a resident is dying.

4. Hospice specializes in care of residents who are
   A. acutely ill   C. chronically ill
   B. terminally ill   D. suddenly ill

5. Which of the following statements regarding postmortem care is *true*?
   A. The body always is wrapped in a shroud.
   B. Families should be prevented from seeing the dead body.
   C. All identification must be removed from the body.
   D. Handle the body with respect and dignity.

6. Which of these statements about caring for dying residents is *true*?
   A. Talk to dying residents and assume they can hear you.
   B. A dying resident cannot hear or understand you.
   C. Talk to the dying resident only if he responds.
   D. Ask the nurse if it is okay to talk to the dying resident.

7. Another staff member is crying because one of her residents died. What is the most appropriate response?
   A. "Stop crying or you'll upset everybody."
   B. "You're not acting in a very professional way."
   C. "I know you're upset about Mrs. Brady. Would you like to talk about it?"
   D. "Crying won't help. You need to get busy and care for your other residents."

AGE-SPECIFIC TIP

Elderly residents may become upset when another resident dies because they feel they will be next. Encouraging them to talk about it helps to relieve their fears.

CULTURALLY SENSITIVE TIP

Cultural reactions toward death and dying vary significantly. Avoid being judgmental toward individual behavior that makes you uncomfortable.

EFFECTIVE PROBLEM SOLVING

The nursing assistant is bathing Mrs. White, who is terminally ill. Mrs. White says, "I think I'm going to die pretty soon." The nursing assistant says, "I hope you'll feel better soon."

Was the nursing assistant's communication appropriate? If not, what would have been more appropriate?

_____

_____

_____

_____

_____

_____

_____

_____

_____

_____

_____

_____

INTERPERSONAL COMMUNICATION

Fill in the answer.

A coworker who is grieving over the death of a resident should be encouraged to _____

_____.

OBSERVING, REPORTING, AND RECORDING

Although it is difficult to predict the time of death, there are certain signs and symptoms that indicate that death is near. List six of these signs or symptoms that need to be reported and recorded.

_____

_____

_____

_____

_____

_____

_____

_____

_____

_____

_____

_____

_____

_____

_____

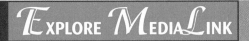

SURVEYS: ASSURING QUALITY CARE

QUALITY ASSURANCE

Quality assurance (QA) is a program conducted by facilities and corporations that consists of internal reviews and identification and resolution of problems. Through the QA process, resident care is evaluated on a continuous basis, and changes are made to improve the residents' quality of life. The QA committee is composed of various members of the health care team, and the nursing assistant may be a member of the committee. As conscientious nursing assistants provide continuous care, they not only help to ensure an optimum level of quality to the residents' lives, but also contribute significantly to the successful outcome of state and federal surveys.

HISTORY OF FEDERAL AND STATE REGULATIONS

The functions of long-term care facilities are directly regulated by federal and state governments. Many agencies set standards of care and conduct surveys for long-term care facilities. Each facility is licensed for business by the state. Additional certification is required for a facility to care for Medicare and Medicaid residents, whose care is paid for by these two federal programs. Legislation provides the basis for many facility policies and procedures that are designed to ensure a better quality of life for the elderly.

In the past, there were few regulations or controls, and care depended on the ethics of owners and operators of facilities. The federal government began focusing on long-term care facilities in the 1960s, and standards of care were developed. The first surveys concentrated on the physical environment and administrative policies of facilities. Later, when health and safety standards were implemented, infection control became a major issue. Finally, the government focused on patient/resident care standards. Laws were enacted, and standards of care became mandatory.

In 1987, the federal government passed the Omnibus Budget Reconciliation Act (OBRA), often called "The Nursing Home Reform Act." OBRA went into effect nationwide in 1990 and focuses on quality of life for residents in long-term care facilities. It specifically addresses residents' rights such as confidentiality and freedom of choice. It also mandates the training of nursing assistants in order to ensure the knowledge and skills of those who provide the residents' most basic care. Currently, both federal and state laws focus on the identification and prevention of elderly abuse. Long-term care facilities are required to do abuse and criminal checks for all employees before they begin to work.

UNDERSTANDING THE SURVEY PROCESS

State survey teams make annual visits to ensure that standards of care are being met, that residents' rights are being respected, and that the quality of life for residents is enhanced. Each facility is evaluated and given a rating according to the findings of the survey team. Regular inspections are also conducted by the federal government.

All areas of the facility are observed by a team of surveyors that includes representatives with experience in each of the individual areas or departments of the long-term care business. Surveyors tour the facility and observe the activities occurring during a usual day in the life of the residents. They interview residents, families, and staff members. Residents may be asked questions about their satisfaction with their care, and with the facility, the food, and the staff. Care will be taken to determine if the confused resident is satisfied with the quality of care provided. Some areas on which the surveyors focus include infection control, resident assessment, staff–resident interactions, and food service preparation and delivery. They also investigate staff credentials, the incidence of pressure sores, the use of restraints, hygiene and grooming, and residents' social activities. A surveyor may accompany you and observe the care that you give.

If problems (deficiencies) are found by the survey team, the inadequate care or substandard practices are addressed in writing. The facility is responsible for correcting existing problems that are cited by the team. Penalties such as fines, license revocation, and closure, as well as withdrawal of Medicare and Medicaid reimbursement, may be imposed upon facilities that are found to have severe problems. The survey team will return to follow up on deficiencies. Surveyors also respond to complaints about care within a facility that are reported by residents and visitors.

QUALITY CARE: THE REASON FOR IT ALL

A survey is a check-and-balance system to ensure that quality of care is provided on a continuous basis. The most important contributing factors that determine the quality of the care provided for residents include

- Infection control
- Safety
- Dignity
- Individuality
- Restorative approach to care
- Residents' rights

The purpose of a survey is to preserve the quality of the residents' lives.

There is no reason for staff anxiety during a survey if staff members are continuously conscientious in providing the best care possible. Greet surveyors as you would any visitor, and answer their questions briefly and truthfully. If you can't answer the question, tell the surveyor that you will get the information immediately. The responsibility lies with every staff member, and you, as a nursing assistant, play an integral role in maintaining the quality of each resident's life. This type of care will result in a successful survey. When a survey is approaching, it would be worthwhile to evaluate your resident care techniques and procedures. Evaluate the care you give as if you were a surveyor observing the use of your knowledge and skills. Be aware of the effect that you have upon the residents' well-being.

GUIDELINES

EVALUATING THE QUALITY OF RESIDENT CARE YOU PROVIDE

- Be continuously observant of residents' changing needs, and provide care accordingly. Report changes immediately to the nurse, and record information as care is provided.

- Prevent injury and disease by providing care in a safe manner. Review procedures to ensure that you are performing them correctly.

- Be aware of and follow the policies and procedures of the facility in which you work.

- Use each resident's care plan when providing care.

(continued)

GUIDELINES (Continued)

- Always encourage resident independence.

- Communicate respectfully with residents, visitors, and coworkers. Encourage resident communication. Listen attentively, and observe for nonverbal communication.

- Address residents according to their wishes. Do not use first names or nicknames without permission.

- Be a team member, and use the chain of command for problem solving.

- Take care of yourself, and work to maintain positive qualities and characteristics that will enhance your role as a nursing assistant.

- Maintain a professional appearance.

- Stay aware of your stress level, and use stress-reduction techniques as needed.

- Always perform your duties in an ethical and legal manner. Never threaten or force a resident.

- Follow the five basic steps before beginning each procedure: wash your hands, collect equipment, identify the resident, explain the procedure, and protect privacy.

- Use restraints only when ordered. Check restrained residents frequently. Remove restraints every 2 hours and provide fluids, toileting, exercise, and skin care.

- Use aseptic practices, and follow standard precautions. Wash your hands as needed.

- Wash your hands before putting on and removing gloves. Do not wear gloves in the hall. Discard them in the proper container.

- Remember that your first priority is to protect residents. Practice safety measures, and use correct body mechanics at all times.

- Always place the call signal within reach, and answer it promptly and politely.

- Treat each resident as an individual, and give praise frequently.

- Treat confused residents respectfully, and encourage communication. Respond professionally if the resident's behavior is inappropriate.

- Respect the cultural beliefs, practices, and choices of others.

- Keep residents' rooms neat by putting away supplies and equipment after use.

GUIDELINES (Continued)

- Change incontinent residents immediately. Wash, rinse, and dry the skin carefully.

- Return beds to the lowest level, fold gatch handles under the bed, lock wheels, and rinse side rails as appropriate.

- Maintain asepsis when handling clean and dirty linen by washing your hands, carrying linen away from your uniform, and following facility policy. Never put linen on the floor. Soiled linen must not be put on the overbed table.

- Keep linen containers covered. Position clean linen and food carts away from dirty linen and housekeeping carts.

- Maintain privacy and use aseptic techniques when providing personal care.

- Encourage residents to exercise and be as physically active as possible.

- Make sure that residents are properly clothed when being transported to and from the shower or tub room. This protects dignity.

- Be sure that residents are dressed tastefully in clean, wrinkle-free clothing that is in good repair.

- Prepare residents for mealtime. Comb the hair, and make sure clothing is neat and clean.

- Offer toileting and assist with handwashing as needed.

- Serve meals in a timely manner, check food trays carefully, and assist residents as needed.

- Position residents properly, and assist them to eat as independently as possible.

- Offer to replace any food item that the resident doesn't like.

- Do not hurry residents at mealtime.

- Offer fluids frequently, and assist as necessary.

- Maintain asepsis and safety in caring for residents with catheters.

- Check frequently to see that elastic support hose and bandages are not twisted or wrinkled.

- When working in subacute care, provide emotional support, answer call signals promptly, and notify the nurse immediately if an alarm sounds.

- Provide empathy for dying residents and their families.

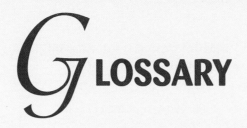GLOSSARY

Abbreviation: Shortened form of a word or phrase

Abduction: Moving away from the midline of the body

Acceptance stage: The fifth and last stage of the grieving process when the dying person is calm and peaceful

Activities of daily living (ADLs): Activities of personal care and hygiene that are performed daily

Acute illness: An illness that begins suddenly, is short-term, and is usually severe

Adapt: To change or to adjust

Adduction: Moving toward the mid-line of the body

Administrator: The person responsible for the operation of the entire facility

Adolescence: The teenage years between 13 and 18

Advance directive: A document that provides instructions regarding person's desires about health care

Agitation: State of restlessness and excitement with no apparent cause

AIDS (acquired immune deficiency syndrome): The term used to describe the final stage of HIV infection

Alzheimer's disease: A progressive nervous disorder that eventually destroys all mental function

Ambulate: Walk

Amputation: Removal of a body part, usually by surgery

Anatomy: The study of body structure

Anger stage: Stage two of the grieving process when the grieving person expresses hostility

Aphasia: The loss of the ability to talk or express oneself

Apical pulse: The pulse determined by listening to the heartbeat over the apex of the heart

Appendage: An extension of a body part; examples of appendages of the skin include fingernails, hair, and sweat glands

Asepsis: The absence of pathogens; the use of clear procedures

Aspirate: Choke

Aspiration: Choking

Aspiration pneumonia: Food or fluid entering the airway instead of the stomach

Assault: A threat to do bodily harm

Assess: Check or evaluate

Assistant Director of Nurses (A.D.O.N.): Assists the Director of Nurses, who has responsibility for the nursing department

Autonomy: Self-determination, or the freedom to make choices

Axillae: Underarms

Bargaining stage: Stage three of the grieving process is an attempt by the grieving person to gain more time by promising something in return

Battery: Touching another person's body without permission

Bedside commode: A portable chair with a toilet seat that fits over a container or regular toilet

Biohazardous medical waste: Waste material that has been contaminated with blood, body fluids, or body substances that may cause infection

Bioterrorism: An act intended to destroy large numbers of people by the release of biologically harmful agents

Blood pressure (BP): The force of blood against the artery walls as it is circulated by the heart

Bloodborne pathogen: A disease-causing microorganism found in blood, blood products, and body fluids that contain blood cells

Body alignment: A normal or correct anatomical position

Body mechanics: The use of the body to move

Body temperature: The amount of heat in the body

Bony prominence: Places where the bones are near the surface of the skin

Bruise: An injury that discolors but does not break the skin

Calorie: A unit of heat produced as the body burns food

Cardiopulmonary resuscitation (CPR): The procedure of emergency care to restore heart and lung function

Care plan: Plan of care for the resident

Cell: The basic building block of the body; the smallest unit of the body

Central processing unit (CPU): The controlling part of a computer or its "brain,"

which processes information and supervises the entire computer operation

Cerebrovascular accident (CVA): A stroke

Chain of command: The order of authority and problem solving within a facility

Chronic illness: An illness that usually begins slowly and lasts for a long time

Coccyx: The "tail bone" located at the base of the spine

Colon: The large intestine

Colostomy: A surgical opening into the colon where a section of the colon is brought to the surface of the abdomen for defecation

Comatose: Unconscious or unable to respond

Communicable disease: A disease or infection that spreads easily from one person to another

Communication: The sharing of information

Communication barriers: Problems that interfere with communication

Communication impairment: Difficulty in communication because of one or more disabilities, which may include problems with vision, speech, hearing, sense of touch, or movement

Complication: An additional problem that results from a disease or other condition

Confidentiality: The privacy of resident information

Constipation: The passage of hard, dry stool

Contaminate: To make dirty or expose to microbes

Contracture: A permanent shortening of a muscle due to lack of use or lack of exercise

Convalescence: The period of recovery after an illness or injury

Cross-training: Learning to perform additional skills that usually are performed by other members of the health care team

Cyanosis: A blue color of the lips, nails and skin that develops when the resident is not getting enough oxygen

Dangling: Sitting on the side of the bed

Defecation: Elimination of solid wastes from the body

Dehydration: The condition of having less than the normal amount of fluid in the body

Dementia: An impairment of mental function

Denial stage: Stage one of the grieving process when the grieving person refuses to believe what is happening

Dentures: False teeth

Depression stage: Stage four of the grieving process when the grieving person is sad and depressed

Developmentally disabled: A person who has not developed normally due to a birth defect, an injury, or an illness

Diarrhea: Loose, watery stool

Diastole: The stage of the cardiac cycle when the heart is resting and filling with blood

Diastolic pressure: The measure of the pressure of the flowing blood while the heart is resting

Director of Nurses (D.O.N.): Responsible for the entire nursing department

Discharge planning: The plans and arrangements for care of the resident after discharge

Disinfection: The use of chemicals to destroy many or all pathogens on objects

Disorientation: Confusion about the location, the time, and the identities of people (including the self)

Disoriented: Confused

Draw sheet: A small sheet, also known as a "pull sheet" or "turning sheet," that is placed across the middle of the bottom sheet. When tucked in, the draw sheet keeps the bottom sheet in place and free of wrinkles

Dyspnea: Difficult breathing

Edema: Accumulation of fluid that causes swelling of a body part

Emesis: Vomit

Emesis basin: A small kidney-shaped pan into which the resident spits or vomits

Empathy: Understanding how another person feels

Enema: The introduction of fluids into the rectum and colon to remove feces and cleanse the lower bowel

Environment: All the conditions and influences around us

Ethics: Guidelines for defining right or wrong behavior

Expectorate: Spit

Extremeties: The arms and legs

False imprisonment: Restraining or restricting a person's movements unnecessarily

Fecal impaction: A large amount of hard, dry stool

Feces: Solid waste eliminated by the body; stool; bowel movement

First aid: Immediate care for injuries or sudden illness given to prevent further injuries and save lives

Flatus: Gas or air expelled from the digestive system

Foley catheter: A urinary catheter that is left in place; an indwelling catheter

Fowler's position: A sitting or semisitting position

Fracture: Broken bone

Fracture pan: A bedpan with a flat end that is placed under the resident

Gastrostomy (G) tube: A tube that is placed through a surgical opening directly into the stomach

Geriatric resident: An elderly person who lives in a long-term care facility

Geriatrics: The branch of medicine that is concerned with the problems and diseases of the elderly

Geri-chair: A recliner on wheels often used for long-term care

Glossary: A small dictionary that includes words from this book and their definition

Graduate: A container that is used to measure fluids

Hallucinations: Seeing or hearing things that don't exist

Hazardous waste: Waste material that has been contaminated with blood, fluids, or body substances that may cause infection

Health: A state of complete physical, mental, and social well being

Health care team: The team that includes all the people who provide care and services for the residents

Heimlich maneuver: Immediate first aid for an airway obstruction

Hemiplegia: Paralysis of one side of the body

Hemorrhage: Severe bleeding

HIV (human immunodeficiency virus) infection: A disease that destroys the immune system and leaves the body unable to fight infection

Hormones: Chemicals in the endocrine system that regulate and control the activities of the body

Hospice: A program that provides care for the terminally ill and their families

Hydration: Supply of fluids

Hygiene: Activities that are performed for health and cleanliness

Hyperglycemia: High or above-normal level of blood sugar

Hypertension: Blood pressure that is abnormally high

Hypoglycemia: Low or below-normal level of blood sugar

Hypostatic pneumonia: A type of pneumonia that occurs because a person remains too long in one position

Hypotension: Blood pressure that is abnormally low

Incision: A clean, smooth cut of the skin

Incontinence: Lack of control urine or feces

Independence: The ability to care for yourself and to be in control of your life

Infection: A disease caused by germs (microorganisms)

Inflammation: A red, swollen, hot, and painful body part

Intake and output (I&O): Includes all fluids that are taken into the body and all fluids that are eliminated

Integument: Skin

Intravenous (IV): Into the vein

Intravenous (IV) fluids: Fluids administered through a needle into the vein

Invasion of privacy: Occurs when the privacy either of the resident's body or personal information is not protected

Laceration: A rough tear of the skin

Lateral position: Lying on the side

Libel: A written false statement that damages another person's reputation

Licensed practical nurse (L.P.N.): A person who is educated and licensed to assist the registered nurse in planning, providing, and evaluating nursing care. This position focuses on technical nursing skills and requires a 12- to 18-month training program and a state board examination.

Listening: Giving your attention to what you are hearing

Long-term care facility (LTCF): A facility that provides health care to people who are not able to care for themselves at home but are not sick enough to be in a hospital

Mechanical ventilator: A machine that provides the resident with artificial respirations

Menopause: The end of menstruation

Metabolism: The combination of all body processes

Microorganisms: Small living things that cannot be seen without the aid of a microscope; also called "microbes"

Mobility: The ability to move

Mouse: A hand-operated input device that also is used to control the computer

Muscle atrophy: Wasting or a decrease in the size of a muscle

Nasogastric (NG) tube: A tube placed through the nose into the stomach

Negligence: Failure to give proper care, which results in physical or emotional harm to the resident

Nonpathogens: Microorganisms that do not cause an infection

Nonverbal communication: The sharing of information without the use of words

Normal flora: Microorganisms that are necessary for good health and are harmless when found in certain locations

NPO: Nothing by mouth

Nursing assistant (N.A.): Assists nurses in providing care for residents

Nutrients: Food elements that are necessary for metabolism

Nutrition: The intake and use of food by the body

Obese: Overweight

Objective reporting: Reporting of factual information

Observation: A means of gathering information

Occupational Safety and Health Administration (OSHA): A government agency concerned with the safety and health of workers

Ombudsmen committee: A committee of concerned citizens appointed by the governor that investigates the complaints of resident abuse in health care facilities to protect the patient's rights

Omnibus Budget Reconciliation Act (OBRA): A federal law that protects all long-term care residents by assuring their safety, quality of care, and well-being

Oral hygiene: Mouth care

Organ: A group of tissues that work together to perform a certain function

Orient: Familiarize

Ostomy: A surgical opening into the body

Oxygen: A gas

Oxygen concentrator: A portable machine that pulls oxygen from the air and supplies it to the resident in a concentrated form

Paralysis: The inability to move a body part

Paranoid: Overly suspicious

Paraplegia: Paralysis of the lower half of the body

Pathogens: Microorganisms that are harmful and cause infection

Perineal care: Cleansing of the genital and rectal areas; peri-care

Peristalsis: The muscular contractions that move food through the digestive system

Petechiae: Patches of surface bleeding due to fragile blood vessels

Physical needs: The needs of the body

Physiology: The study of body function

PO: Oral feeding is allowed

Pollution: Environmental contamination

Postmortem care: Care of the body after death

Prefix: The element that is at the beginning of a word

Pressure sore: A breakdown of tissue that occurs when blood flow is interrupted; a bedsore

Prioritizing: Rating each task in its order of importance

Procedure: A list of steps to be taken in performing a task

Prone position: Lying on the abdomen

Prosthesis: An artificial body part

Psychosocial needs: Emotional, social, and spiritual needs

Puberty: The period of development when sex characteristics appear and the reproductive organs begin to function

Pulse: Heartbeat

Quadriplagia: Paralysis of both arms and legs

Radial pulse: The pulse located at the inner aspect of the wrist

Range-of-motion exercises: Exercises that are performed to take each joint through its normal area of movement

Rapport: A mutually trusting relationship

Reality orientation: Helps the resident to keep in touch with reality

Recording: Writing information about the resident is called "reporting" (charting), which creates a permanent communication of care given and other resident information

Registered nurse (R.N.): A person who is educated and licensed to plan, provide, and evaluate nursing care. Two-, 3-, or 4-year programs and a state board examination are required to become an R.N.

Rehabilitation: A method used to assist a person to achieve and maintain function at the highest possible level of independence

Report: The communication of resident information and assignments to those who are coming on duty

Resident: A person who lives in a long-term care facility

Residents' bill of rights: A list of the rights and freedoms of residents, guaranteed to all residents regardless of their illness or behavior

Respiration: Breathing; the intake of oxygen

Restorative care: Nursing care that assists each resident to function at the highest possible level of independence

Restorative environment: An environment that promotes independence and allows as much self-care as possible

Restraint: Any device used to restrict a person's freedom of movement

Root: The foundation of the word that contains the basic meaning

Sacrum: The bone directly above the coccyx

Seizure: A sudden spasm of muscles that is caused by abnormal brain activity

Self-actualization: "Proving oneself"; accepting challenges and meeting goals that one has set for oneself

Self-esteem: One's opinion of oneself

Shearing: A force upon the skin that stretches it between the bone inside and a surface outside the body

Slander: A false statement that damages another person's reputation

Software: The programs or sets of programs that cause the computer to perform a specific action

Specimen: A sample of material from the resident's body

Sphygmomanometer: The blood pressure cuff

Sputum: Thick, sticky mucus from the lungs or deep in the respiratory system

Standard precautions: Precautions used in the care of all residents; designed to protect the health care worker from infection through exposure to blood, fluids, and bodily substances

Sterile: Free from all microorganisms

Sternum: Breastbone

Stethoscope: An instrument used for listening to body sounds

Stoma: The mouth or opening of the ostomy

Stool: Solid waste material from the digestive system

Stress: Mental and physical tension or strain

Suffix: The element that is at the end of the word

Suffocation: The interruption of respiration

Sundowner's syndrome: An increase in wandering, restlessness, and confusion as evening occurs

Supine position: Lying on the back

Susceptible: Having an increased risk of developing an infection

Symptom: An evidence of a disease that cannot be observed

System: A group of organs that work together to perform a specific function

Systole: The stage of the cardiac cycle when the heart is contracting and pumping out blood

Systolic pressure: The measure of the pressure of the blood flowing while the heart is contracting

Terminal illness: An illness that is expected to end in death

Tissue: Group of cells that work together to perform a certain function

Toothettes: Sticks with small sponges to be used for oral care

Toxic: Poisonous

Tracheostomy: A surgical opening into the trachea to create an artificial airway when the resident's airway is not functioning

Transmission-based precautions: Include procedures that are used in the care of residents who are contagious or suspected of being infected with a communicable disease

Trauma: Physical or emotional injury or upset

Tympanic membrane: Eardrum

Urinal: A portable container that a male resident uses when urinating

Urinary meatus: The outer opening of the urinary system

Verbal communication: The use of words to share information; includes spoken and written words and sign language

Vital signs: Temperature, pulse, respirations, and blood pressure

Void: Urinate; to pass urine

ANATOMY AND PHYSIOLOGY

ILLUSTRATIONS

Musculoskeletal System

Skeleton

The skeleton is a living framework made by the joining of bones. It serves to provide support, body movement powered by muscular contractions, protection for the vital organs and other soft structures, blood cell production, and storage for essential minerals. There are 206 bones in the adult body, forming the two divisions of the skeletal system. The axial skeleton is comprised of the skull, vertebrae, rib cage, and sternum. The upper and lower extremeties and the shoulder and pelvic girdles form the appendicular skeleton.

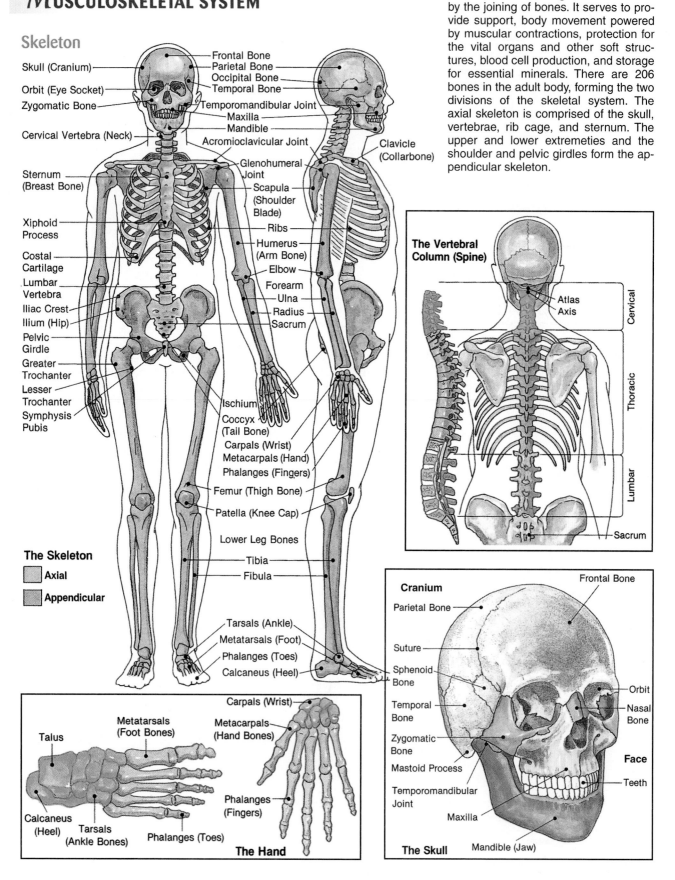

Skull (Cranium)
Orbit (Eye Socket)
Zygomatic Bone
Cervical Vertebra (Neck)
Sternum (Breast Bone)
Xiphoid Process
Costal Cartilage
Lumbar Vertebra
Iliac Crest
Ilium (Hip)
Pelvic Girdle
Greater Trochanter
Lesser Trochanter
Symphysis Pubis

Frontal Bone
Parietal Bone
Occipital Bone
Temporal Bone
Temporomandibular Joint
Maxilla
Mandible
Acromioclavicular Joint
Glenohumeral Joint
Scapula (Shoulder Blade)
Ribs
Humerus (Arm Bone)
Elbow
Forearm
Ulna
Radius
Sacrum

Clavicle (Collarbone)

Ischium
Coccyx (Tail Bone)
Carpals (Wrist)
Metacarpals (Hand)
Phalanges (Fingers)
Femur (Thigh Bone)
Patella (Knee Cap)
Lower Leg Bones
Tibia
Fibula

Tarsals (Ankle)
Metatarsals (Foot)
Phalanges (Toes)
Calcaneus (Heel)

The Skeleton

Axial
Appendicular

The Vertebral Column (Spine)

Atlas
Axis
Cervical
Thoracic
Lumbar
Sacrum

Talus
Metatarsals (Foot Bones)
Calcaneus (Heel)
Tarsals (Ankle Bones)
Phalanges (Toes)

Carpals (Wrist)
Metacarpals (Hand Bones)
Phalanges (Fingers)

The Hand

Cranium
Parietal Bone
Suture
Sphenoid Bone
Temporal Bone
Zygomatic Bone
Mastoid Process
Temporomandibular Joint
Maxilla

Frontal Bone
Orbit
Nasal Bone
Face
Teeth
Mandible (Jaw)

The Skull

MUSCULOSKELETAL SYSTEM

Muscles

The tissues of the muscular system comprise 40 to 50 percent of the body's weight. The skeletal muscles of the body are voluntary muscles, subject to conscious control. They exhibit the properties of excitability; that is, they will react to nerve stimulus. Once stimulated, skeletal muscles are quick to contract, and can relax and very quickly be ready for another contraction. There are 501 separate skeletal muscles that provide contractions for movement, coordinated support for posture, and heat production. Muscles connect to bones by way of tendons.

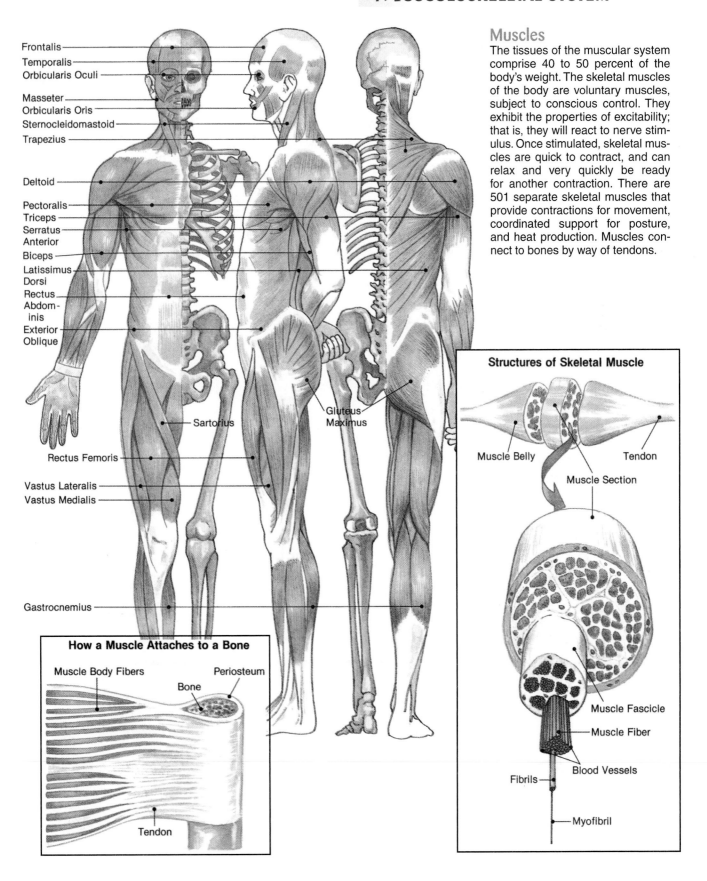

Frontalis
Temporalis
Orbicularis Oculi

Masseter
Orbicularis Oris
Sternocleidomastoid
Trapezius

Deltoid

Pectoralis
Triceps
Serratus Anterior
Biceps
Latissimus Dorsi
Rectus Abdominis
Exterior Oblique

Sartorius

Gluteus Maximus

Rectus Femoris

Vastus Lateralis
Vastus Medialis

Gastrocnemius

Structures of Skeletal Muscle

Muscle Belly
Tendon
Muscle Section
Muscle Fascicle
Muscle Fiber
Blood Vessels
Fibrils
Myofibril

How a Muscle Attaches to a Bone

Muscle Body Fibers
Periosteum
Bone
Tendon

NERVOUS SYSTEM

Brain and Spine

The Brain

The nervous system includes the brain, spinal cord, and nerves. Structures within the system may be classified according to divisions: central, peripheral, and autonomic divisions of the nervous system. The central nervous system includes the brain and spinal cord. The sensory (incoming) and motor (outgoing) nerves make up the peripheral nervous system. The autonomic nervous system has structures that parallel those of the spinal cord and then share the same pathways as the peripheral nerves. This division is involved with motor impulses (outgoing commands) that travel from the central nervous system to the heart muscle, blood vessels, secreting cells of glands, and the smooth muscles of organs. The impulses will stimulate or inhibit certain activities.

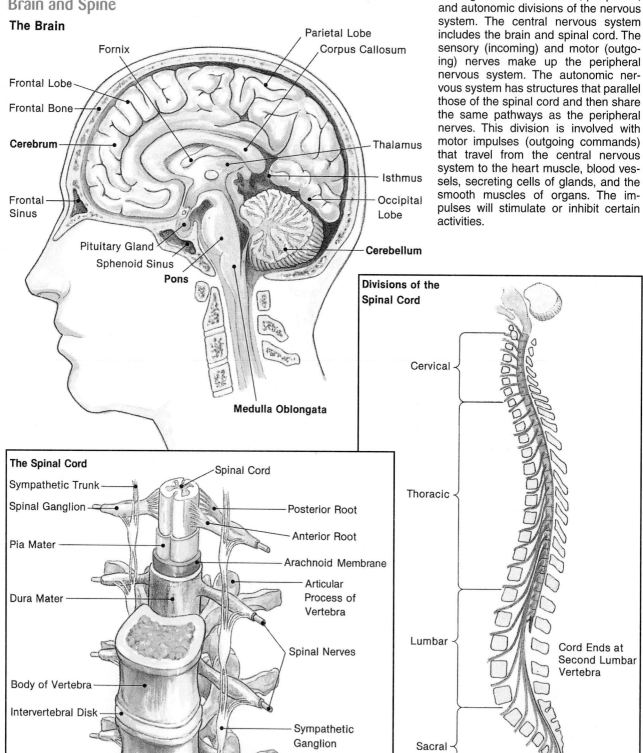

The Brain labels:
Fornix
Frontal Lobe
Frontal Bone
Cerebrum
Frontal Sinus
Pituitary Gland
Sphenoid Sinus
Pons
Parietal Lobe
Corpus Callosum
Thalamus
Isthmus
Occipital Lobe
Cerebellum
Medulla Oblongata

Divisions of the Spinal Cord
Cervical
Thoracic
Lumbar
Sacral
Cord Ends at Second Lumbar Vertebra
Coccyx Bone

The Spinal Cord
Sympathetic Trunk
Spinal Ganglion
Pia Mater
Dura Mater
Body of Vertebra
Intervertebral Disk
Spinal Cord
Posterior Root
Anterior Root
Arachnoid Membrane
Articular Process of Vertebra
Spinal Nerves
Sympathetic Ganglion
Transverse Process of Vertebra

NERVOUS SYSTEM

Nerves

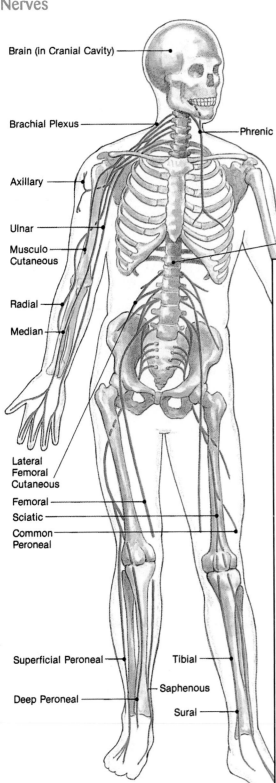

- Brain (in Cranial Cavity)
- Brachial Plexus
- Phrenic
- Axillary
- Ulnar
- Musculo Cutaneous
- Radial
- Median
- Spinal Cord (in Spinal Cavity)
- Lateral Femoral Cutaneous
- Femoral
- Sciatic
- Common Peroneal
- Superficial Peroneal
- Tibial
- Deep Peroneal
- Saphenous
- Sural

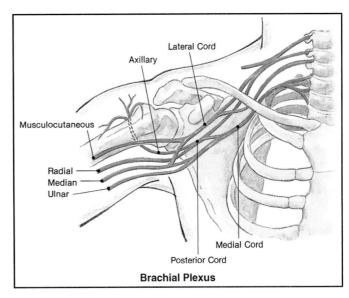

- Lateral Cord
- Axillary
- Musculocutaneous
- Radial
- Median
- Ulnar
- Medial Cord
- Posterior Cord

Brachial Plexus

Autonomic Nervous System

The autonomic nervous system affects the heart, blood vessels, digestive tract, salivary and digestive glands, pancreas, liver, spleen, anal sphincter, kidneys, urinary bladder, urinary sphincter, adrenal glands, thyroid gland, gonads, genitalia, nasal lining, larynx, bronchi, lungs, iris and ciliary muscles of the eyes, tear glands, and hair muscles. Impulses can increase or slow heart rate, stimulate dilation or constriction of blood vessels, cause glands to secrete or decrease secretion, initiate or inhibit contractions in the bladder, stimulate or decrease a wave of muscle contraction along the digestive tract, and many other essential body activities.

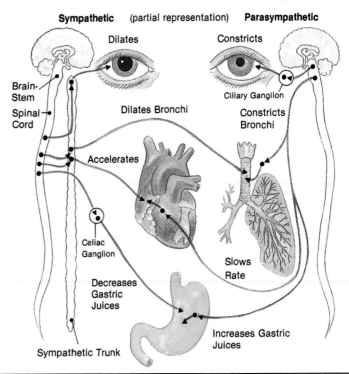

Sympathetic (partial representation) **Parasympathetic**

- Dilates
- Constricts
- Brain-Stem
- Spinal Cord
- Ciliary Ganglion
- Dilates Bronchi
- Constricts Bronchi
- Accelerates
- Celiac Ganglion
- Slows Rate
- Decreases Gastric Juices
- Increases Gastric Juices
- Sympathetic Trunk

CARDIOVASCULAR SYSTEM

Heart

The heart is a hollow, muscular organ that pumps 450 million pints of blood in the average lifetime. Its superior chambers, the atria, receive blood. Both atria fill and then contract at the same time. The inferior chambers are the ventricles. They pump blood out of the heart. Both ventricles fill and then contract at the same time. When the atria are relaxing, the ventricles are contracting.

The right side of the heart receives blood from the body and sends it to the lungs (pulmonic circulation). The heart's left side receives oxygenated blood from the lungs and sends it out to the body (systemic circulation).

The heartbeat originates at the sinoatrial node (pacemaker) and spreads across the atria to stimulate contraction. After a slight delay, the impulse is sent from the atrioventricular node, down the bundles of His, and out across the ventricles. This stimulates the ventricles to contract while the atria are relaxing.

The heart muscle (myocardium) receives its blood supply by way of the right and left coronary arteries. These vessels are in the first branches of the aorta.

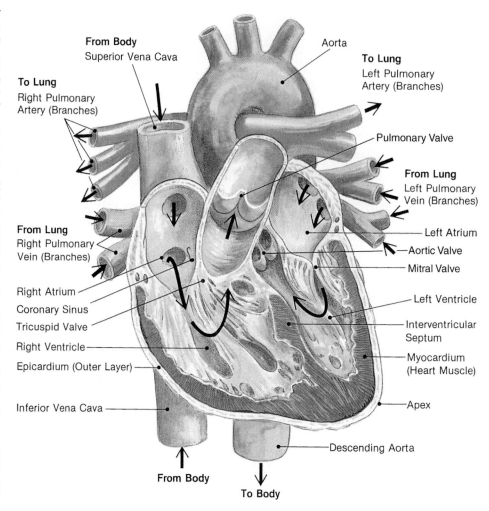

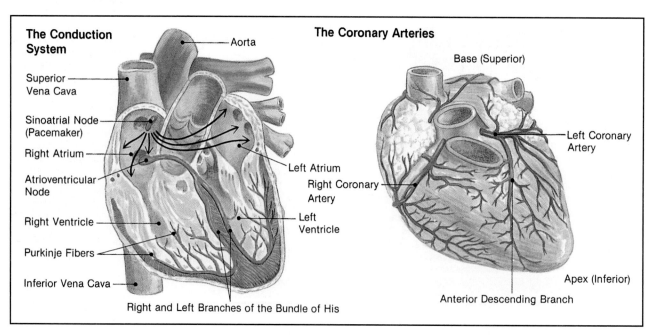

CIRCULATORY SYSTEM

Blood Vessels

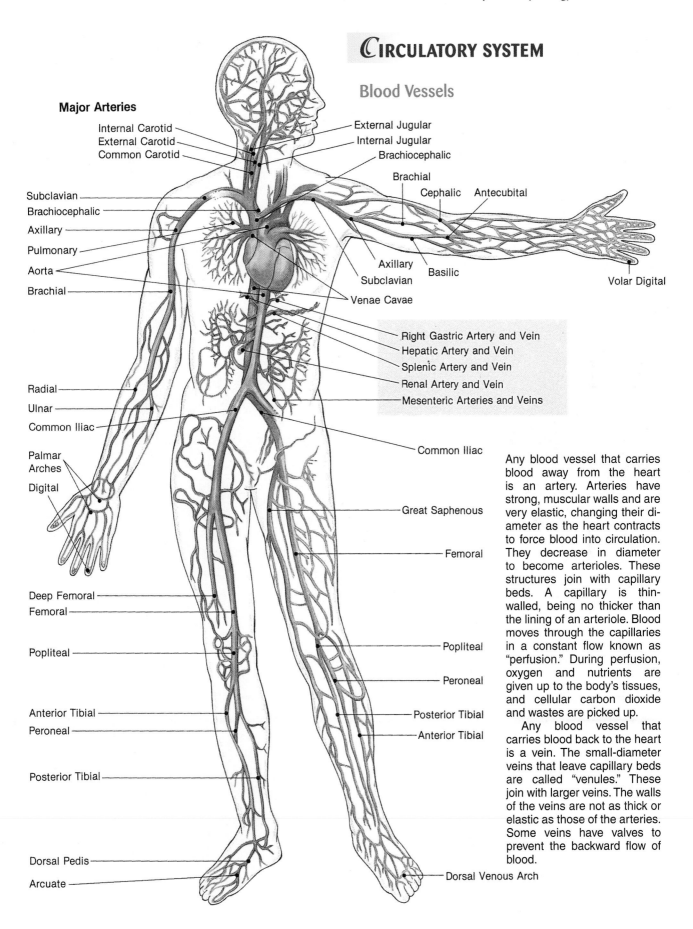

Major Arteries

Internal Carotid
External Carotid
Common Carotid

External Jugular
Internal Jugular
Brachiocephalic

Brachial
Cephalic   Antecubital

Subclavian
Brachiocephalic
Axillary
Pulmonary
Aorta
Brachial

Axillary
Basilic
Subclavian

Venae Cavae

Volar Digital

Right Gastric Artery and Vein
Hepatic Artery and Vein
Splenic Artery and Vein
Renal Artery and Vein
Mesenteric Arteries and Veins

Radial
Ulnar
Common Iliac

Common Iliac

Palmar
Arches
Digital

Great Saphenous

Femoral

Deep Femoral
Femoral

Popliteal

Popliteal

Peroneal

Anterior Tibial
Peroneal

Posterior Tibial
Anterior Tibial

Posterior Tibial

Dorsal Pedis
Arcuate

Dorsal Venous Arch

Any blood vessel that carries blood away from the heart is an artery. Arteries have strong, muscular walls and are very elastic, changing their diameter as the heart contracts to force blood into circulation. They decrease in diameter to become arterioles. These structures join with capillary beds. A capillary is thin-walled, being no thicker than the lining of an arteriole. Blood moves through the capillaries in a constant flow known as "perfusion." During perfusion, oxygen and nutrients are given up to the body's tissues, and cellular carbon dioxide and wastes are picked up.

Any blood vessel that carries blood back to the heart is a vein. The small-diameter veins that leave capillary beds are called "venules." These join with larger veins. The walls of the veins are not as thick or elastic as those of the arteries. Some veins have valves to prevent the backward flow of blood.

RESPIRATORY SYSTEM

The airway consists of structures involved with the conduction and exchange of air. Conduction is the movement of air to and from the exchange levels of the lungs. Air enters through the nose (primary) and mouth (secondary) and travels down the pharynx to enter the larynx. After passing through the larynx, air enters the trachea. At its distal end, the trachea branches into the left and right primary bronchi. These bronchi branch into secondary bronchi, which then branch into the bronchioles. Some of the bronchioles end as closed tubes. Air movement in them helps the lungs expand. The rest of the bronchioles carry the air to the exchange levels of the lungs.

Pharynx

Trachea

Bronchiole

Pleura

Right Main Bronchus

Left Main Bronchus

Diaphragm

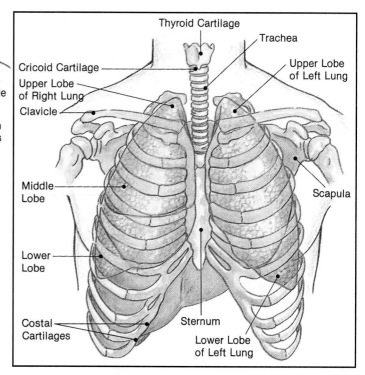

Thyroid Cartilage

Trachea

Cricoid Cartilage

Upper Lobe of Left Lung

Upper Lobe of Right Lung

Clavicle

Middle Lobe

Scapula

Lower Lobe

Costal Cartilages

Sternum

Lower Lobe of Left Lung

Bronchiole

Respiratory Bronchiole

Alveolar Duct

Alveolus

Alveolar Sac

Alveolar Sacs

The respiratory bronchioles turn into alveolar ducts. These form alveolar sacs that are made up of the alveoli. Gas exchange takes place between the alveoli and the capillaries in the lungs.

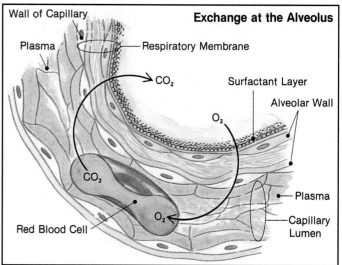

Wall of Capillary

Exchange at the Alveolus

Plasma

Respiratory Membrane

Surfactant Layer

CO_2

Alveolar Wall

O_2

CO_2

Plasma

O_2

Capillary Lumen

Red Blood Cell

DIGESTIVE SYSTEM

The digestive system includes the digestive tract and various supportive structures and accessory glands. The tract begins at the oral cavity with the teeth and tongue. This salivary glands release saliva into the mouth to moisten food for swallowing. The tract continues down the throat to the esophagus, through the cardiac sphincter, and into the stomach. Acid and digestive enzymes are added to the food to produce chyme. The chyme passes through the pyloric sphincter to enter the small intestine. Digestive enzymes from the pancreas and bile from the liver are added to the chyme. The processes of digestion and absorption are completed in the small intestine. Wastes are carried through the ileoceccal valve into the large intestine. The wastes are moved to the rectum, from where they can be expelled through the anus.

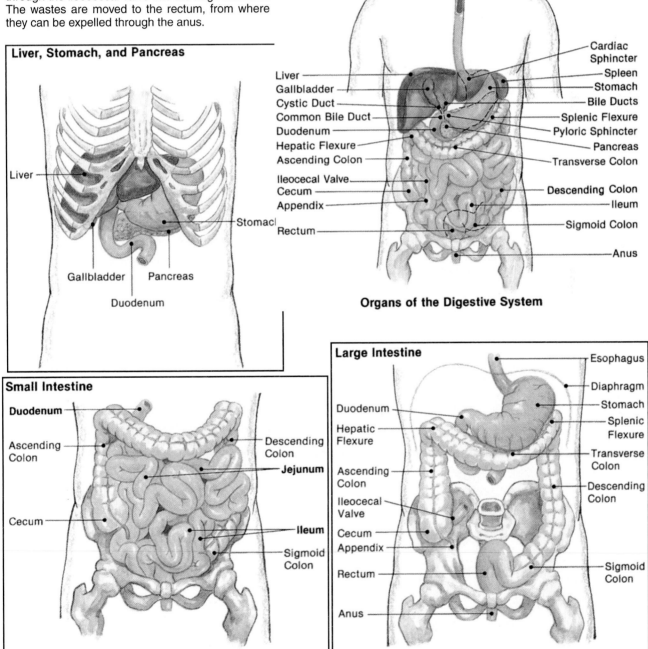

Liver, Stomach, and Pancreas

Organs of the Digestive System

Small Intestine

Large Intestine

URINARY SYSTEM

Organs of the Urinary System

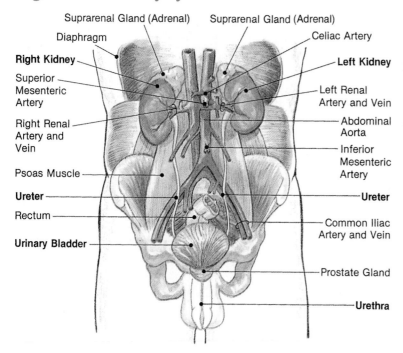

Suprarenal Gland (Adrenal)
Diaphragm
Right Kidney
Superior Mesenteric Artery
Right Renal Artery and Vein
Psoas Muscle
Ureter
Rectum
Urinary Bladder

Suprarenal Gland (Adrenal)
Celiac Artery
Left Kidney
Left Renal Artery and Vein
Abdominal Aorta
Inferior Mesenteric Artery
Ureter
Common Iliac Artery and Vein
Prostate Gland
Urethra

The urinary system is part of the body's excretory structures (urinary system, lungs, sweat glands, and intestine). The kidneys remove the wastes of chemical activities (metabolism) in the body. These wastes are removed from the blood to produce urine. At the same time, the kidneys remove certain excess compounds, regulate the blood pH (acid–base balance), and the concentration of sodium, potassium, chlorine, glucose, and other important chemicals.

The Nephron

Each kidney is made up of microscopic nephrons. Both wastes and needed chemicals are filtered from the blood. As these materials are passed through the nephron, the needed compounds (including water) are sent back into the blood. Wastes are collected as urine.

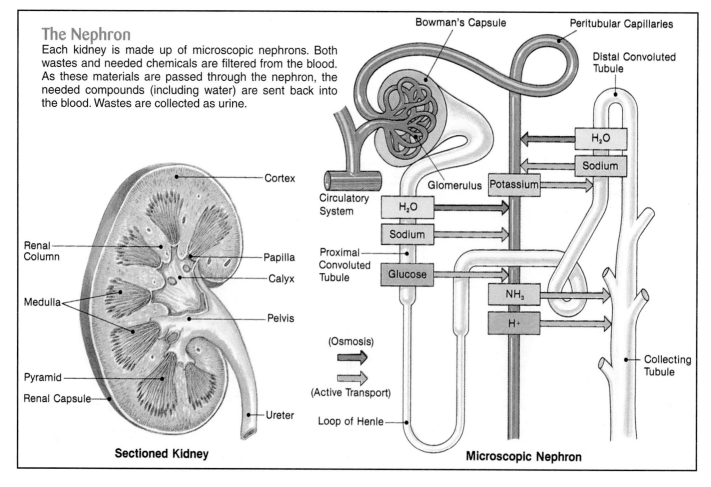

Renal Column
Medulla
Pyramid
Renal Capsule

Cortex
Papilla
Calyx
Pelvis
Ureter

(Osmosis)
(Active Transport)

Sectioned Kidney

Bowman's Capsule
Peritubular Capillaries
Distal Convoluted Tubule
H_2O
Sodium
Glomerulus
Potassium
Circulatory System
H_2O
Sodium
Proximal Convoluted Tubule
Glucose
NH_3
H^+
Loop of Henle
Collecting Tubule

Microscopic Nephron

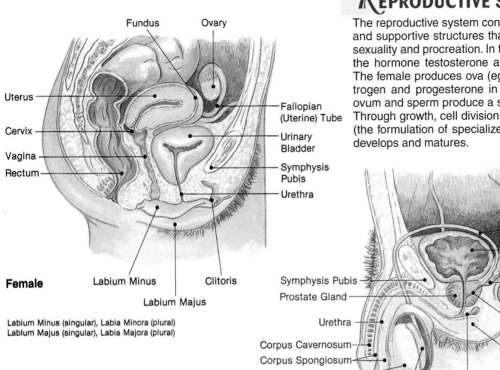

Female

Labium Minus (singular), Labia Minora (plural)
Lablum Majus (singular), Labia Majora (plural)

REPRODUCTIVE SYSTEM

The reproductive system consists of the organs, glands, and supportive structures that are involved with human sexuality and procreation. In the male, spermatozoa and the hormone testosterone are produced in the testes. The female produces ova (eggs) and the hormones estrogen and progesterone in her ovaries. The union of ovum and sperm produce a single cell called a "zygote." Through growth, cell division, and cellular differentiation (the formulation of specialized cells) the new individual develops and matures.

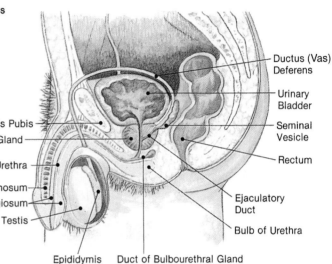

Male

The Ovary

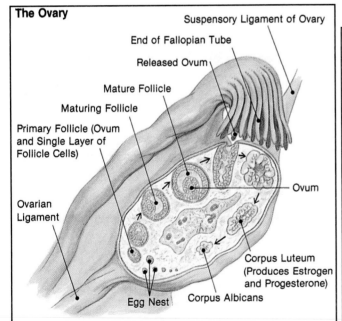

The developing ovum and its supportive cells are called a follicle. Each month, follicle-stimulating hormone (FSH) from the pituitary gland starts the growth of several follicles. Usually, only one will mature and release an ovum (ovulation). During its growth, the follicle produces estrogen. After ovulation, the remaining cells of the follicle form a specialized structure that produces both estrogen and progesterone.

The Breast

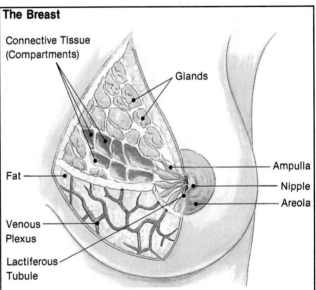

The breasts contain the mammary glands that produce milk (lactation). A mammary gland is a highly modified form of sweat gland. Estrogen stimulates the growth of the ducts, while progesterone stimulates the development of the secreting (milk-producing) cells. Lactic hormone from the pituitary stimulates milk production. Another pituitary hormone, oxytocin, stimulates the milk-producing cells to eject their milk into the ducts.

*I*NTEGUMENTARY SYSTEM

The Skin

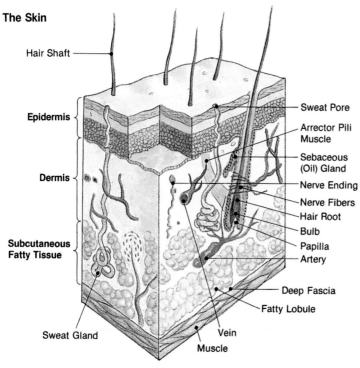

Skin

The skin is the largest organ of the body. In the adult the skin covers about 3000 square inches (1.75 square meters) and weighs about 6 pounds. It is involved with protection, insulation, thermal regulation, excretion, and the production of vitamin D.

The Peritoneum

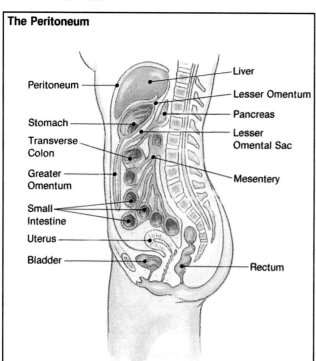

Membranes

Membranes cover or line body structures to provide protection from injury and infection. There are four major classes of membranes. Mucous membranes line those structures that open to the outside world (for example, the mouth, the airway, digestive tract, urinary tract, and vagina). Serous membranes line the closed body cavities and cover the outsides of organs. The cutaneous membrane is the skin. Synovial membranes line joints to reduce friction during movement.

A serous membrane that covers an organ is called a "visceral layer." The term "parietal layer" is used for the part of the serous membrane that lines a cavity. The serous membrane in the thoracic cavity is called "pleura" (for example, the parietal pleura lines the chest cavity). In the abdominal cavity, it is called "peritoneum" (for example, the parietal peritoneum). A double layer of peritoneum is called "mesentery." The membrane that lines the sac surrounding the heart is called "pericardium."

Synovial Joint

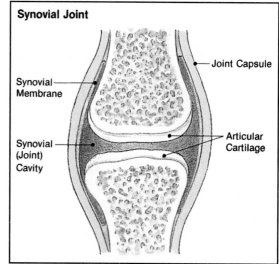

The Pleura

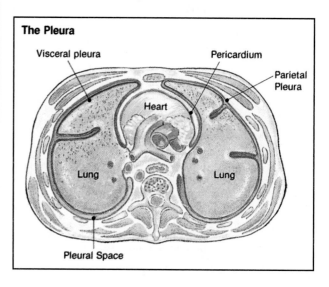

SENSES

Eye and Ear

The Eye

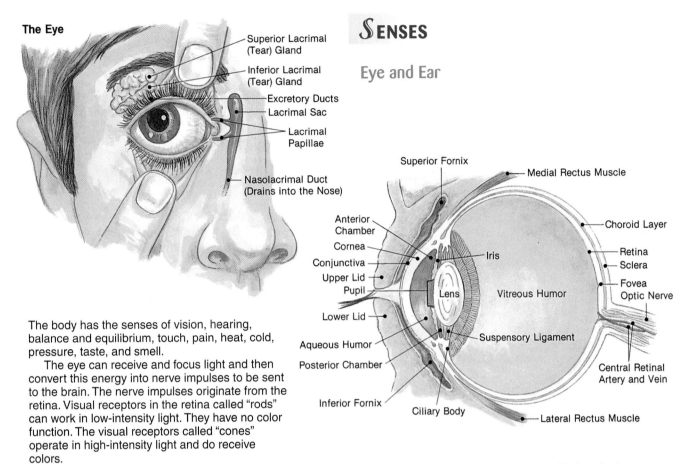

- Superior Lacrimal (Tear) Gland
- Inferior Lacrimal (Tear) Gland
- Excretory Ducts
- Lacrimal Sac
- Lacrimal Papillae
- Nasolacrimal Duct (Drains into the Nose)

- Superior Fornix
- Medial Rectus Muscle
- Anterior Chamber
- Cornea
- Conjunctiva
- Upper Lid
- Pupil
- Lower Lid
- Aqueous Humor
- Posterior Chamber
- Inferior Fornix
- Iris
- Lens
- Vitreous Humor
- Suspensory Ligament
- Ciliary Body
- Choroid Layer
- Retina
- Sclera
- Fovea
- Optic Nerve
- Central Retinal Artery and Vein
- Lateral Rectus Muscle

The body has the senses of vision, hearing, balance and equilibrium, touch, pain, heat, cold, pressure, taste, and smell.

The eye can receive and focus light and then convert this energy into nerve impulses to be sent to the brain. The nerve impulses originate from the retina. Visual receptors in the retina called "rods" can work in low-intensity light. They have no color function. The visual receptors called "cones" operate in high-intensity light and do receive colors.

The ear's functions include hearing, static equilibrium (balance while standing still), and dynamic equilibrium (balance when moving). The outer and middle ear are responsible for sound gathering and its transmission. The inner ear has the nerve endings for hearing and equilibrium.

The Ear

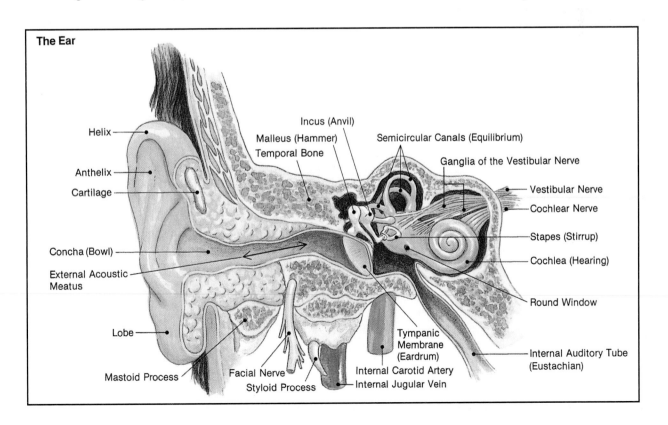

- Helix
- Anthelix
- Cartilage
- Concha (Bowl)
- External Acoustic Meatus
- Lobe
- Mastoid Process
- Facial Nerve
- Styloid Process
- Incus (Anvil)
- Malleus (Hammer)
- Temporal Bone
- Semicircular Canals (Equilibrium)
- Ganglia of the Vestibular Nerve
- Vestibular Nerve
- Cochlear Nerve
- Stapes (Stirrup)
- Cochlea (Hearing)
- Round Window
- Tympanic Membrane (Eardrum)
- Internal Carotid Artery
- Internal Jugular Vein
- Internal Auditory Tube (Eustachian)

*I*NDEX